Current Diagnostic Pediatrics

Series Editor: Alan R. Chrispin

John L. Gwinn   Philip Stanley

Diagnostic Imaging in Pediatric Trauma

With Contributions by
G.F. Gates   F.A. Lee   J.G. McComb   J.H. Miller
C.J. Schatz   H.D. Segall   F.Y. Tsai

With 275 Figures in 468 Separate Illustrations

Springer International 1980

Series Editor
Dr. Alan R. Chrispin
The Hospital for Sick Children, X-Ray Department, Great Ormond Street, London WC1N 3JH, England

John L. Gwinn, MD
Philip Stanley, MD
University of Southern California, Childrens Hospital of Los Angeles, 4650 Sunset Boulevard, P. O. Box 54700, Los Angeles, CA 90054, USA

ISBN-13: 978-1-4471-3102-1 e-ISBN-13: 978-1-4471-3100-7
DOI: 10.1007/978-1-4471-3100-7

Library of Congress Cataloging in Publication Data. Gwinn, John 1922-. Diagnostic imaging in pediatric trauma. (Current diagnostic pediatrics; v. 3) Bibliography: p. Includes index. 1. Children-Wounds and injuries. 2. Wounds-Radiography. 3. Diagnosis, Radioscopic. 4. Pediatric, radiology. I. Stanley, Philip, 1941- joint author. II. Title. III. Series. RD93.5.C4G88 617.1'07'572 79-24971

Softcover reprint of the hardcover 1st edition 1980

Preface

Trauma to various organ systems is a common medical problem in the pediatric age group. With the increase in vehicular traffic and active participation in contact sports, as well as a change in the social atmosphere, the incidence of injury to children is increasing. There is considerable morbidity associated with these injuries and accidents are the most common cause of death in this population group.

The radiologist, using the various diagnostic radiological modalities available, becomes involved in practically all cases of trauma of any degree of seriousness. The radiological methods lend themselves not only to determining the specific diagnosis but also to assessing the extent of the injury. This is important in determining the management of the patient as in recent years a more conservative type of therapy is advocated in several types of injury.

As has been said, "Children are not like adults," hence injuries are of different types from those seen in adults. The ligaments and tendons of children are stronger than the bone structure, thus sprains and strains are not as common as fractures. Certain organs are in a less protected position in a child and may readily be injured from relatively minor trauma. Injury due to violent action of others such as gunshot and stab wounds are not as common as in the adult population but they are increasing in the teenage group. Blunt trauma or that due to rapid deceleration is the usual type of trauma seen in childhood.

Many textbooks, as well as articles published in various journals, deal with trauma in general, but only a few specifically pertain to children, and the majority of these are mainly related to management of the injury. In this volume, the emphasis is on the radiological approach and diagnosis of childhood injury. Special attention is given to the way in which pediatric trauma differs from that in the adult.

The material included in this volume is, for the most part, taken from cases seen at the Childrens Hospital of Los Angeles. The authors are on the radiological staff at Childrens Hospital and they have drawn heavily on their own personal experiences in handling pediatric patients who have been injured.

The chapters are broken down into the various organ systems for easy reference, and pertinent articles from the literature are included in each chapter bibliography. A section on ultrasound and nuclear medicine is included which covers the use of these modalities, when indicated, in all trauma.

We would like to express our gratitude and thanks to Florence Stubbins and Carolyn Eya for the hours of time and frustration spent in transcribing the manuscripts. We also wish to express our appreciation to Deryl Davis for the production of the photographic prints used in the text. Finally, our thanks to Springer-Verlag and the many people involved for their tolerance and help in the preparation of this book.

John L. Gwinn
Philip Stanley

Contents

Contributors

Gates, Gary F., MD
Director of Nuclear Medicine, Good Samaritan Hospital, Portland, Oregon

Gwinn, John L., MD, MS in Pediatrics
Professor of Radiology and Pediatrics, University of Southern California; Radiologist-in-Chief, Childrens Hospital of Los Angeles

Lee, Fred A., MD
Clinical Professor of Radiology, University of Southern California; Attending Radiologist, Childrens Hospital of Los Angeles

McComb, J. Gordon, MD
Assistant Professor of Surgery (Neurological), University of Southern California School of Medicine; Head, Neurosurgery, Childrens Hospital of Los Angeles

Miller, John H., MD
Clinical Assistant Professor of Radiology, University of Southern California School of Medicine; Chief, Nuclear Radiology and Diagnostic Ultrasound Division, Childrens Hospital of Los Angeles

Schatz, Charles J., MD
Assistant Clinical Professor of Radiology and Otolaryngology, University of Southern California School of Medicine, Director of ENT Radiology, Hollywood Presbyterian Hospital, Los Angeles

Segall, Hervey D., MD
Professor of Radiology (Neuroradiology), Director of Neuroradiology, University of Southern California School of Medicine; Head, Neuroradiology, Childrens Hospital of Los Angeles and Los Angeles County – University of Southern California, Medical Center

Stanley, Philip, MD
Clinical Associate Professor of Radiology, University of Southern California: Associate Attending Radiologist, Childrens Hospital of Los Angeles

Tsai, Fong Y., MD
Associate Professor of Radiology (Neuroradiology), University of Southern California School of Medicine: Neuroradiologist, Los Angeles County – University of Southern California, Medical Center

1 Introduction

John L. Gwinn and Philip Stanley

Childhood trauma is a common problem in pediatrics and requires rapid, complete, and accurate diagnosis. In some instances the diagnosis can be made from the history and physical examination and no further diagnostic studies are needed. However, it is frequently necessary to have additional information, and imaging studies provide the best way to gain this knowledge. This book is intended to cover, in one volume, the use of the various imaging modalities available to the radiologist for the proper assessment of childhood trauma and to present the radiological findings which allow the proper diagnosis to be made. The plan of management is often developed from these procedures.

An attempt has been made to present concepts and material which have been utilized over a period of time by experienced pediatric radiologists in their daily encounters with childhood trauma. For the most part, a pragmatic method has been taken to indicate how to approach the problem and how best to utilize the imaging modalities in order to obtain the most desirable information for correct diagnosis. Children should, at least, have the same diagnostic expertise and equipment available for their benefit as does the adult.

In children, there are particular differences which make them more susceptible to certain types of injuries and because of the developing tissues the response to trauma may be different from that in adults. These variances are cited throughout the book.

The book is arranged so that each chapter deals with a specific organ system, with the exception of the chapter on nuclear medicine and ultrasound. In this chapter the use and the findings of these two modalities in injuries to all organ systems are dealt with.

Admittedly, there is often more than one way of arriving at a solution to a diagnostic problem. In this book the approach used is that favored by the individual author or, in some circumstances, that developed as a policy of the Department of Radiology at the Childrens Hospital of Los Angeles. This is not to say that deviations are not made, at times, and particularly in the child with multiple injuries in whom one specific factor may supersede all others. There are pertinent references so that the reader can review other literature on the subject.

We hope this book will be of value to all those physicians who are involved in the care of children.

2 Urinary Tract Trauma

John L. Gwinn and Philip Stanley

In the child and teenager, urinary tract trauma is not uncommon, but fortunately severe injury does not occur with the frequency one might expect [10, 20, 21]. There is an increasing incidence due to the greater vehicular mobility and active participation in sports [23].

Blunt, nonpenetrating trauma to the urinary tract is much more common than penetrating trauma in children [6, 20, 24, 38, 41]. In the urinary tract, renal injury is the most frequent, followed by bladder and urethral injury. Ureteral trauma is rare and occurs mainly with instrumentation and penetrating forces [5, 10, 24].

Radiological studies make a major contribution in the investigation of a child suffering from urinary tract trauma, enabling both the identification of the lesion and determination of the extent of the injury. This is a great aid for planning therapy [17, 38]. In addition, radiological studies can be used to help assess prognosis.

There are several diagnostic modalities available, and a combination of studies may be required. Even though McDonald et al. [33] concluded, from their study of 209 clinically stable patients with renal trauma, that an emergency intravenous urogram was not necessary, it is the belief of many that an emergency bolus/infusion intravenous urogram, often with nephrotomography, should be performed in cases of renal trauma [24, 29, 30, 38, 39, 47, 55, 57, 60]. The bolus/infusion injection method presents a higher concentration of contrast medium to the glomerulus. As the contrast material is filtered in the kidney by the glomerulus without tubular absorption or excretion, a much better urogram is obtained [56]. This may be the only study that need be done.

In recent years, radionuclide studies have gained greater acceptance in evaluating renal trauma [25]. These can be done easily and rapidly and are noninvasive. Freeman et al. [15] state that in case of a negative scan, the angiogram has never been positive. Scans can show both the location and extent of a defect in renal cortical tissue and there have not been any known false positives or false negatives [53].

Ultrasonography is another noninvasive technique now being used in renal trauma. This technique may show interruption of the normal kidney outline or demonstrate collections of fluid about the kidney.

Arteriography is extremely important in evaluating the extent of injury in certain instances and should be available for children [4, 9, 12, 17, 19, 22, 28, 29, 32, 37, 45, 47, 48, 50, 51, 54, 58, 59, 61, 62]. Angiography is of particular value in patients with multiple organ injury as the extent of injury to all these structures can be evaluated [13, 22, 26, 28, 44].

Up to the present time, computerized tomography (CT) of the body has not been used enough in children with renal trauma to enable its effectiveness to be accurately assessed. It is, however, a promising type of study which only needs more data to prove its usefulness.

Retrograde pyelography is not now of much value in relation to renal trauma, but it is useful ureteral injuries [5].

Voiding cystourethrography and retrograde urethrography are important in investigating bladder and urethral trauma [3, 16].

A scheme of approach to diagnosis can be worked out for each involved area of the urinary tract that is suspected of being traumatized.

2.1 Renal Trauma

Renal trauma is not as common as injury to other abdominal organs such as the spleen and, as a rule, it does not cause death [14]. Nevertheless, any child with a history of trauma to the abdomen and/or kidney area, and particularly with any degree of hematuria, must be investigated radiologically [20, 30, 40, 60]. Injury to multiple sites, often severe, is relatively common in association with renal injury [9, 22, 29, 34, 38, 41, 52, 58, 63].

In children, it must be kept in mind that up to 22% of renal injuries occur in patients with abnormal kidneys [1]. These may include previously unrecognized Wilms' tumor, hydronephrosis, ectopic kidneys, and other renal anomalies [1, 10, 14, 20].

Some anatomical features peculiar to children tend to make them more susceptible to renal trauma than adults. Perirenal fat, which serves as a protection in adults, is poorly developed in children.

The lower portions of the kidneys extend below the rib cage and the peritoneal covering of the anterior surface of the kidney is thin. In addition, the kidney is mobile, to a certain degree, and fixed only at the vascular origin with the aorta and vena cava [1, 10, 14, 20, 57]. All these factors contribute to an increased susceptibility to trauma of the kidney in children.

The increasing use of diagnostic studies, such as renal biopsy, add the iatrogenic type of trauma, which also requires radiological investigation.

In a series of 64 consecutive patients, seen at Childrens Hospital of Los Angeles who had renal trauma, the injury was associated with vehicular accidents, or auto versus pedestrian or motorcycles in 29. Sixteen were due to falls, 5 to sports activity (including skateboards) 2 were in battered children, 2 followed direct, an accidental blows, and in 10 the cause not stated in the record. This is similar to other reports [31, 38].

Twenty-four (37.5%) had other significant injuries and some of these were severe. Other workers have reported similar findings [9, 22, 29, 38, 41, 44]. All trauma in this group was due to blunt non-penetrating type injury.

As in other reported series [6, 7, 15, 20, 31, 43, 57] among those injured were 52 boys (81%) and 12 girls (19%). There was a rather equal distribution across the age span from 1 year to 17 years. The largest grouping (28 cases, 43.7% of the total) was between ages 5 and 9 years. This has been noted by others [31]. Surgery was performed on 13 (20%), including five nephrectomies (7.8%). There was one death due to multiple severe injuries and not primarily due to the renal trauma. Most of the nephrectomies were performed early in the series, with more conservative

Table 2.1. Radiological evaluation of renal trauma in children

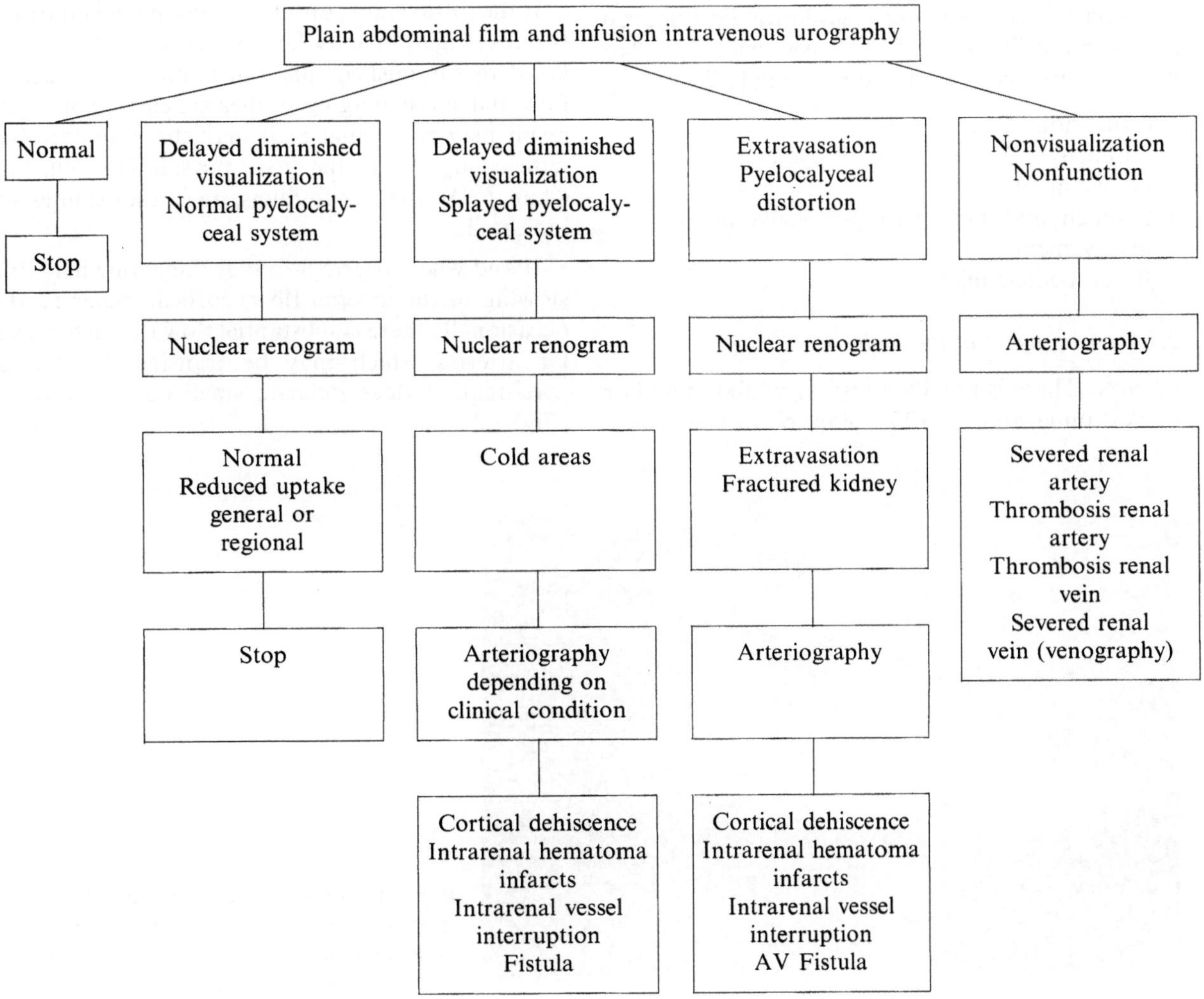

management being practised later, because the radiological evaluation of renal trauma improved dramatically.

Most renal trauma in children is not life-threatening and is due to blunt injury, so there is time to evaluate the patient adequately and to determine the extent of the injury [10, 37, 48, 61]. In penetrating trauma, there is other abdominal organ injury in up to 80% of the cases, and these injuries may take precedence over the kidney injury [18, 20].

The therapy of renal trauma should be directed to conserving the maximum amount of renal tissue [1, 17, 22, 27, 60]. An aggressive and thorough radiological evaluation leads to a more rational approach to management [1, 27, 28, 29, 50, 58]; see Table 2.1.

2.1.1 Classification of Injury

Numerous classifications have been proposed, combining clinical and radiological findings [4, 6, 12, 13, 17, 20, 21, 31, 38, 45, 49, 50, 55, 59, 60, 62, 63]. In recent years the emphasis has been on the radiological aspects because the clinical findings can be misleading [20, 48, 60, 61]. Here we have elected to use the classification offered by Lang [27]:

1. Contusion of the kidney
2. Parenchymal injury without pyelocalyceal involvement
3. Parenchymal injury with pyelocalyceal involvement
4. Renal pedicle injury

2.1.1.1 Contusion of the Kidney

Clinical: There is usually a history of abdominal or flank trauma, and up to 95% of the patients will have either microscopic or gross hematuria [14, 37, 41, 44]. However, the degree of hematuria does not reflect the severity of the injury [20, 37, 38, 39, 63]. Flank pain or tenderness may be present [14, 20, 37, 38, 41]. Other more serious injury may obscure the fact that renal injury is present (Table 2.2).

Radiology: Plain films of the abdomen and high dose intravenous urography, with or without nephrotomography, are obtained as soon as possible following the injury [2, 14, 20, 41]. If there is shock, it must, of course, be dealt with in order to obtain satisfactory studies.

The plain films are not often diagnostic, but sometimes a soft tissue mass density may be seen [1]. The bony structures can be assessed for fractures [63]. Obliteration of the psoas shadow is not a reliable sign in children. The intravenous urogram is often normal but may show delayed or diminished function, the pyelocalyceal system being intact [13, 38] (Fig. 2.1). It is important to evaluate the contralateral kidney on the urogram [1, 52].

If the intravenous urogram is completely normal, the investigation may be discontinued. When delayed or diminished function is observed, nuclear flow and static imaging studies are carried out. The result may be normal or it may show an even but reduced uptake in the involved side [15, 39], (see Chap. 6). With these findings, no further studies are indicated.

If and when arteriography is done, one may find slowing of the arterial flow, cortical ischemia and occasionally there is substantial flow through capsular arteries which may be transient. If this is persistent, it does indicate small cortical infarcts (Fig. 2.2).

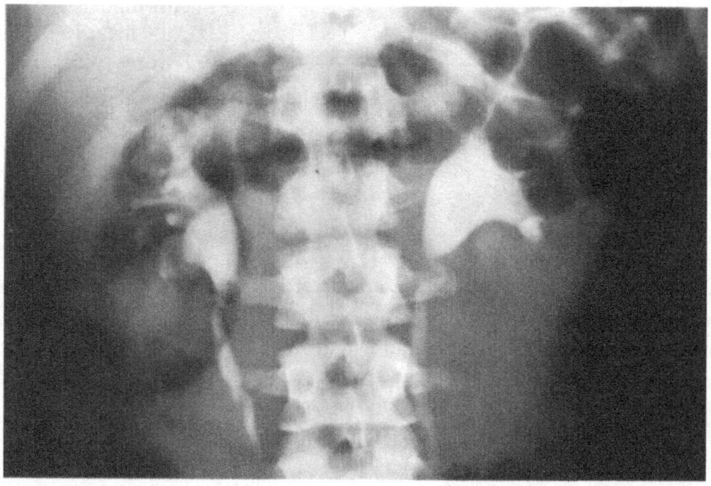

Fig. 2.1. Trauma of the left flank. Excretory urogram with good visualization of both renal collecting structures. The lucent area in the left renal pelvis represents a blood clot

Table 2.2. Renal contusion

Clinical	Intravenous urography	Radionuclide	Arteriography
History of trauma Hematuria (often microscopic) Pain/tenderness	Delayed/diminished function Normal pyelocalyceal system Contralateral kidney normal	Normal Even but reduced uptake	Slow arterial flow Cortical ischemia AV shunting Increased capsular flow

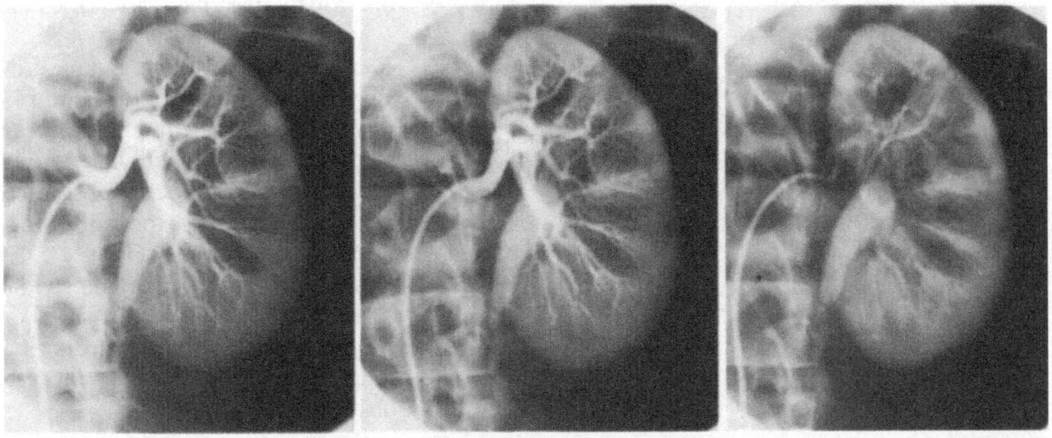

Fig. 2.2. Contusion of the left kidney (three views). Selective left renal arteriogram. There is slight slowing of the arterial blood flow but with early filling of a vein in the upper pole. There is good parenchymal perfusion

2.1.1.2 Parenchymal Injury Without Pyelocalyceal Involvement

Clinical: Hematuria is the hallmark of all degrees of renal trauma and most patients with this type of injury do have hematuria. Flank pain is present, and occasionally a flank mass is palpable due to blood and fluid within Gerota's fascia (Table 2.3).

Radiology: The plain films may show fractures of the ribs or of the transverse spinal processes and a soft tissue mass density in the region of the kidney. Intravenous urography, done as soon as possible after the injury, will show delayed and/or diminished function and frequently splaying or displacement of the pyelocalyceal structures. Occasionally, the irregularity of the renal outline is noted and nonvisualization of some of the calyces [38, 39] (Figs. 2.3, 2.4).

Radionuclide renography should be introduced in these cases. There will be generalized or regionally diminished renal tubular function [15, 39]. With ^{99m}Tc-DTPA scintigraphy, a halo of diminished radioactivity around the kidney, or a portion there of, is often demonstrated, indicating rupture of the capsule and perirenal hematoma (see Chap. 6). Ultrasonography will confirm these findings with a sonolucent region found adjacent to the kidney.

The arteriogram may show cortical dehiscence, intrarenal hematoma, disruption of the intrarenal arterial or venous circulation, an AV fistula, or an infarct. However, the vast majority of patients in

Table 2.3. Parenchymal injury without pyelocalyceal involvement

Clinical	Intravenous urography	Radionuclide	Arteriography
History of trauma Hematuria Pain/tenderness/mass	Delayed/diminished function (general or local) Splaying of pyelocalyceal struct. Occasional cortical fracture Mass	Diminished tubular function (generalized or regional) Halo of diminished radioactivity around kidney	Cortical dehiscence Intrarenal hematuria Perirenal hematoma AV fistula Infarct

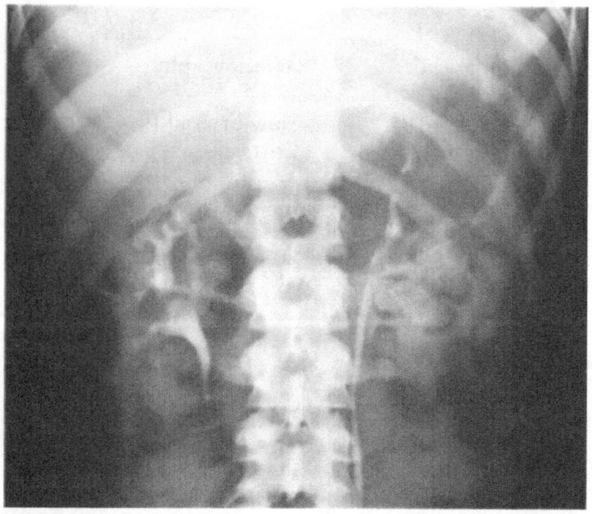

Fig. 2.3. Excretory urogram – 3 min film. There is delayed and diminished function of the left kidney. The right is normal

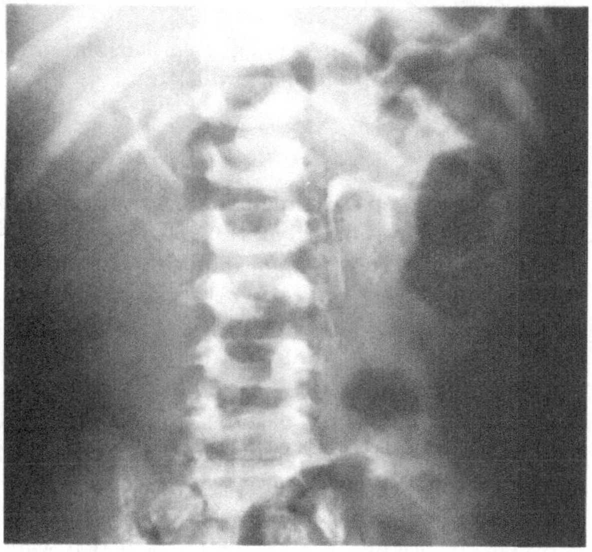

this classification are treated conservatively so the invasive arteriogram should be used sparingly (Fig. 2.5).

2.1.1.3 Parenchymal Injury with Pyelocalyceal Involvement

Clinical: This is a more severe injury to the kidney, but the clinical presentation is the same as in the previously described categories (Table 2.4).

Radiology: Plain films, again, are not very helpful. The intravenous urogram shows distortion of the pyelocalyceal system, extravasation of the contrast media into the parenchyma, perirenal or periureteric areas, and on rare occasions, into other organs [20, 38]. Disruption of the collecting structures must occur to produce such (Figs. 2.6, 2.7). Multiple knife wounds in the parenchyma, without involving the calyceal structure, do not show extravasation [39]. Blood clots, as filling defects, may be seen in the renal pelvis or ureter and these may cause obstruction.

Renography and scintigraphy are valuable in studying these patients since an assessment of renal tubular function can be made. The fracture of the kidney and hematomas can usually be seen. The extravasation is demonstrated by an increased uptake outside the confines of the kidney [15, 39, 53].

The arteriogram may show the same findings as in patients with parenchymal injury without pyelocalyceal involvement. In addition this study may demonstrate severe or multiple fracture sites, wide separation of the fragments, loss of perfusion of the

◁
Fig. 2.4. Excretory urogram – 8-min film. The middle and inferior calyceal group the on right are not visualized. The nephrogram is absent in the lower half of the right kidney. The left kidney is normal

Table 2.4. Parenchymal injury with pyelocalyceal involvement

Clinical	Intravenous urography	Radionuclide	Arteriography
History of trauma Hematuria (clots) Pain/tenderness/mass	Distortion of pyelocalyceal struct. Extravasation of contrast Fistulization Blood clots in pelvis/ureter	Diminished tubular function Kidney fracture demonstrated Extravasation	Intrarenal hematoma Perirenal hematoma Parenchymal tear Infarct AV fistula Severe fractures of kidney Loss of perfusion Number of renal arteries

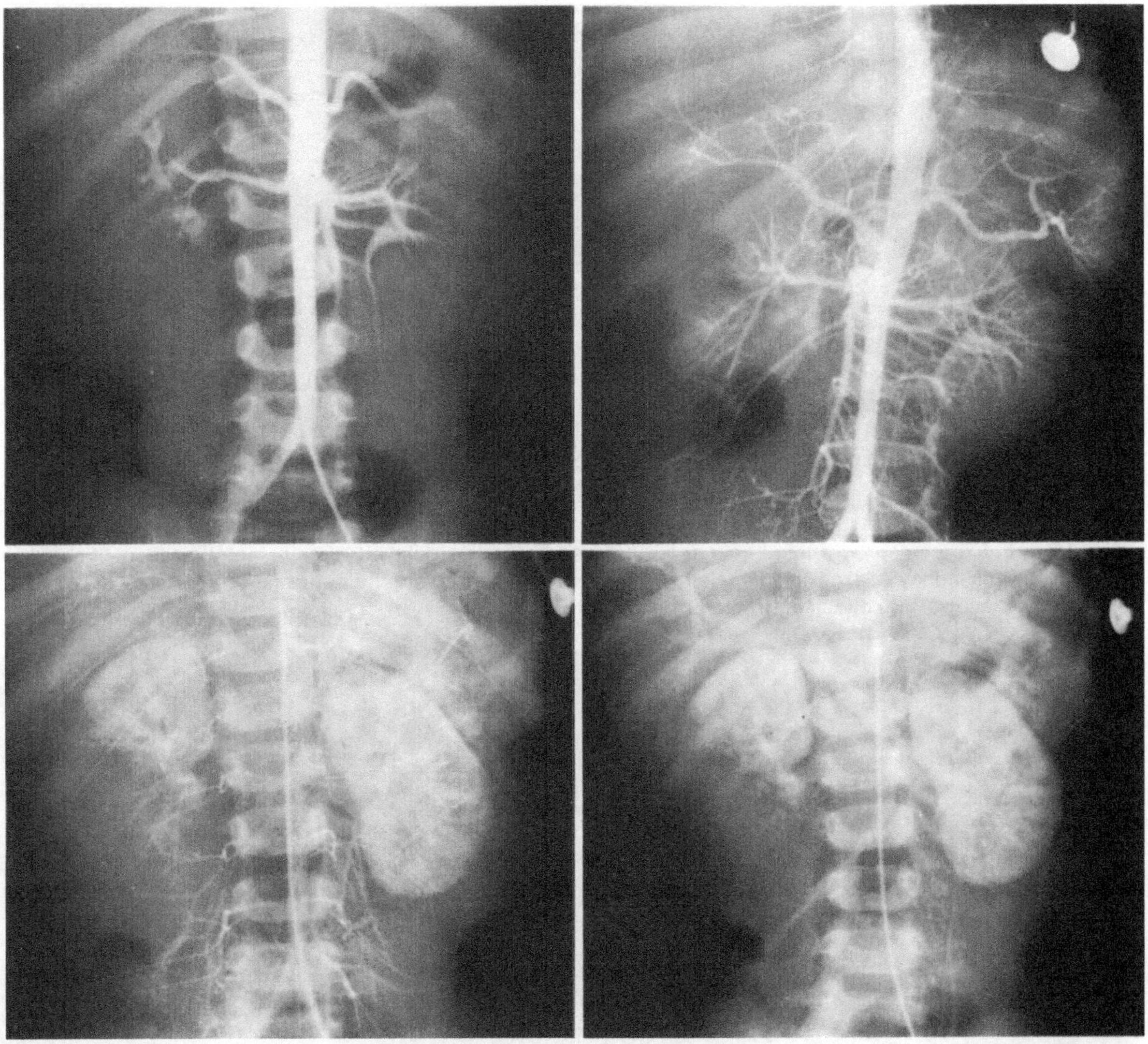

Fig. 2.5. Flush aortogram (four views) – same patient as in Fig. 2.4. Vessels are stretched over the lower half to the right kidney. There is no extravasation. There is poor perfusion of the lower portion of the right kidney

edges or to regional areas of the kidney, and large interposed hematomas [12] (Figs. 2.8, 2.9).

Even though the majority of these patients will now be treated conservatively, when surgery is contemplated as much tissue as possible must be saved. The arterial study is the most realistic way of determining the extent of the injury [12].

2.1.1.4 Renal Pedicle Injury

Clinical: This is the most severe form of renal injury, and if there is to be any success in preserving renal function, rapid and accurate diagnosis is mandatory [32]. Fortunately, this type of injury is rare.

These children often present with severe clinical symptoms of pain and gross hematuria. However, hematuria of any degree is absent in one-third of the cases. Frequently there is injury to other organs, however.

This type of renal trauma is seen with both blunt and penetrating injury. Penetrating trauma is almost always surgically explored [19]. When blunt forces are responsible they are usually those of sudden deceleration which causes a whiplike action on the renal pedicle [44]. The kidney in a child is mobile and fixed primarily at the vascular attachments. Thus, sudden deceleration can cause a rapid and marked shearing force on renal vessels. Such force may cause complete severance of either artery or vein. However, more often these forces tear the intima, resulting in thrombus formation and occlusion of the vessel (Table 2.5).

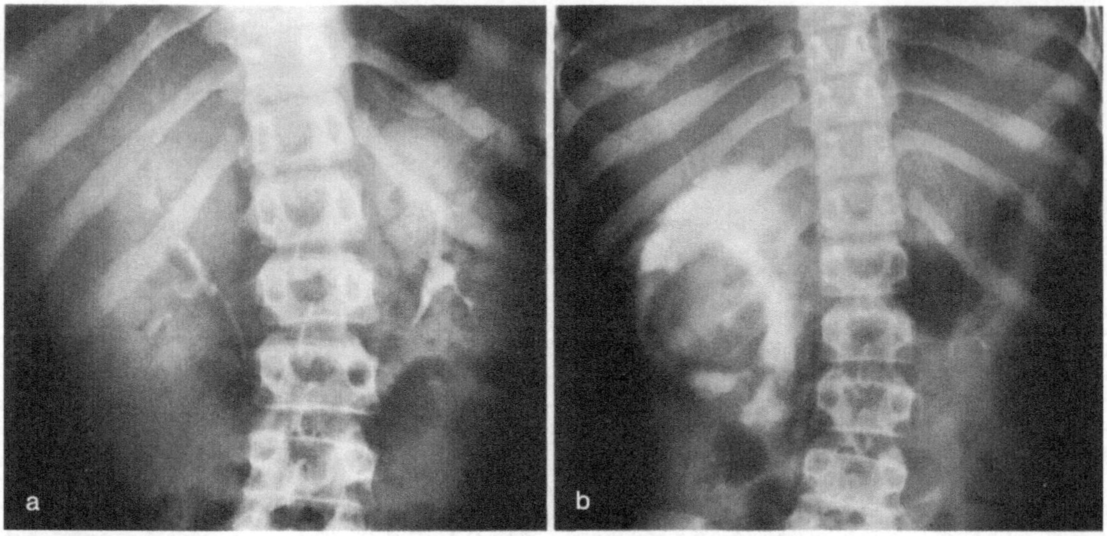

Fig. 2.6 a, b. Excretory urogram. **a** 8-min and **b** delayed films. The right kidney is larger than the left and there is poor visualization of the collecting structures on the right. On the delayed film (**b**) extravasation of the contrast medium into the perirenal area is shown

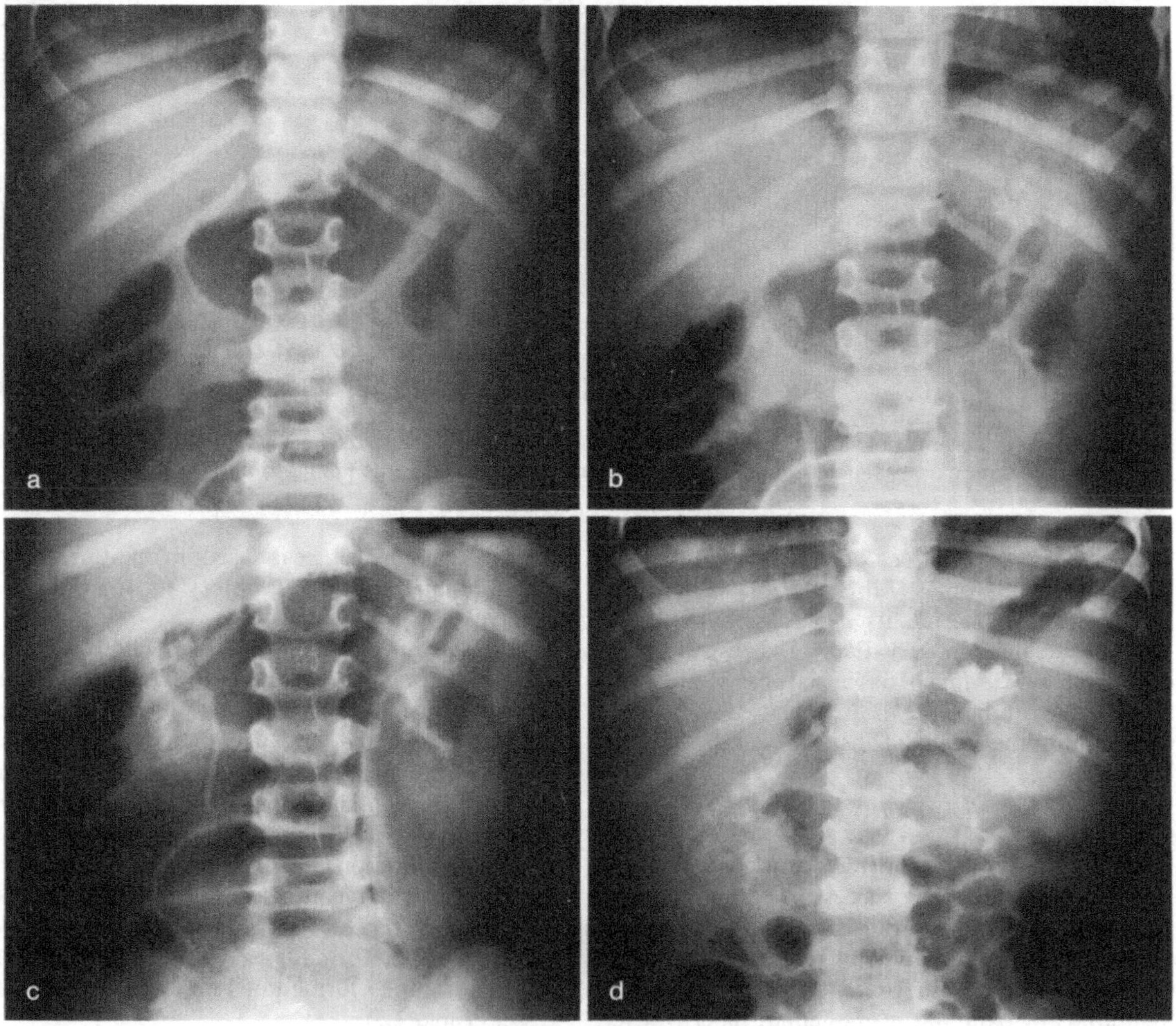

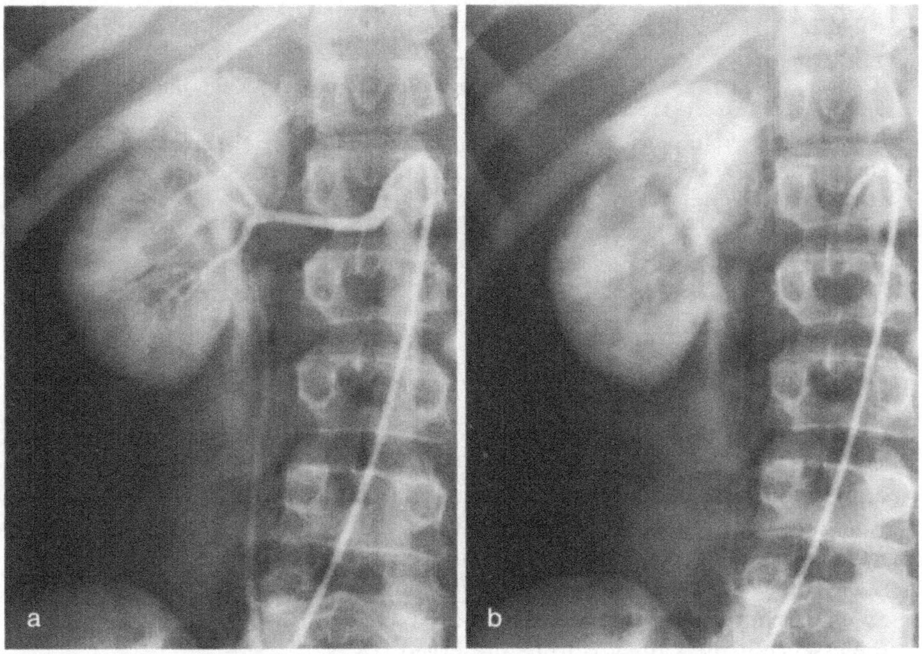

Fig. 2.8 a, b. Selective right renal arteriogram – same patient as in Fig. 2.6. **a** The arterial vessels are spread and a fracture of the kidney is well demonstrated. **b** Nephrogram phase illustrating the fracture through the upper pole of the right kidney

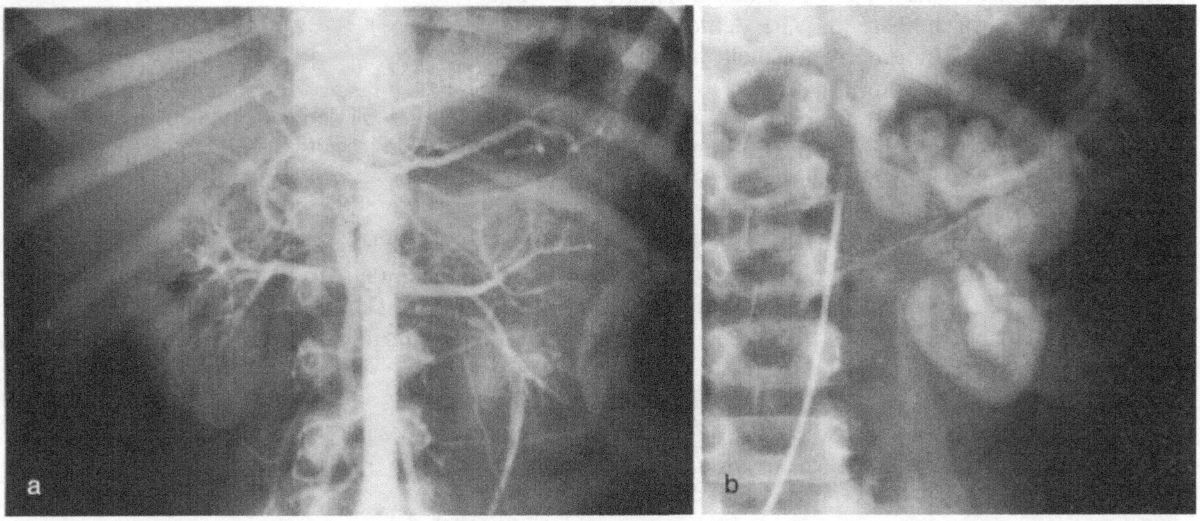

Fig. 2.9 a, b. Flush aortogram – same patient as in Fig. 2.7. **a** Early arterial phase with splaying and stretching of the vessels; **b** nephrogram with the fracture of the kidney demonstrated. The edges are poorly perfused

◁ **Fig. 2.7 a–d.** Plain film of the abdomen and excretory urogram. **a** Obliteration of the left psoas shadow; **b** splaying and distortion of the left collecting structures; **c** extravasation of contrast material along the left ureter; **d** intrarenal extravasation of contrast material

Table 2.5. Renal pedicle injury

Clinical	Intravenous urography	Radionuclide	Arteriography
History of severe trauma Hematuria (66%–75%) Often associated injury	Nonvisualization Normal contralateral	No activity renal bed	Severance renal artery Thrombosis renal artery Thrombosis renal vein Severance renal vein (venography) Number of vessels

Radiology: The intravenous urogram in these cases has the value of demonstrating the contralateral kidney [6]. On the involved side, there will be nonvisualization and nonfunction, shown by intravenous urogram and radionuclide studies [23, 26, 39]. At the Childrens Hospital of Los Angeles the nuclear study is usually not done, but in preference an emergency arteriogram is performed. Time is of the essence if the kidney is to be preserved [18, 32, 37].

The arteriogram may show one of several features. There may be complete severance of the renal artery, or thrombosis of the renal artery. When the renal vein is thrombosed there is a dense nephrogram, and the thrombosis may be demonstrated (Figs. 2.10, 2.11). Venography is usually necessary to show renal vein severance.

In venous obstruction, it has been shown experimentally that the roentgenographic findings depend upon the level of venous obstruction in relation to the ovarian or spermatic vein. When the renal vein was ligated on the caval side of this collateral circulation the urogram and arteriograms were normal. If the vein was ligated at the hilum, then the urogram and arteriogram showed a persistent dense nephrogram. The nuclear scan showed significant increase in tubular uptake regardless of the ligated area [54]. Free floating fragments of the kidney can be shown. This information is critical for the proper

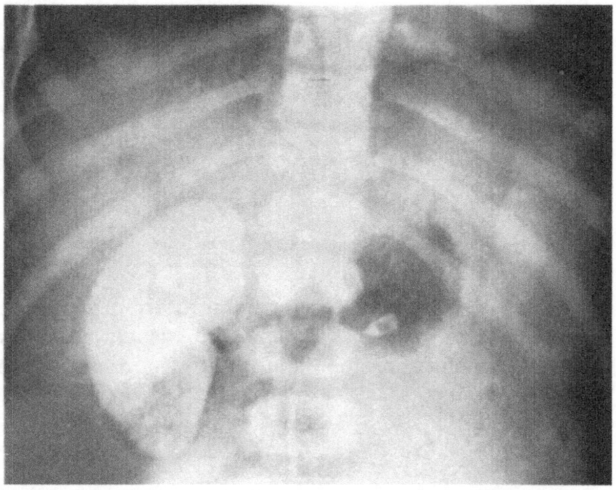

Fig. 2.11. Late phase of aortogram with a normal nephrogram on the right and complete obstruction of the left renal artery due to intimal tear and clot

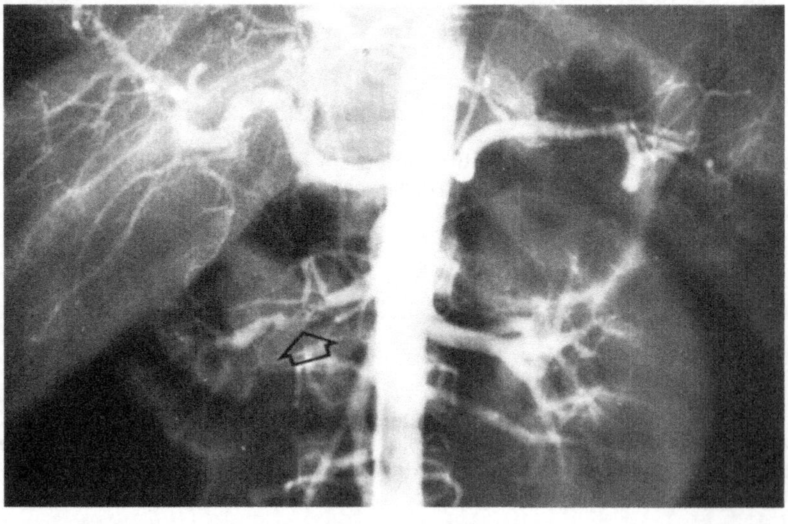

Fig. 2.10. Flush aortogram with partial obstruction of the right renal artery due to intimal tear and clot (*arrow*)

surgical approach. If surgery is to be done immediately and prior to the usual arteriogram, an intraoperative angiogram is very helpful. This study is more sensitive and specifically diagnostic than the direct examination of the kidney during operation [32].

2.1.2 Iatrogenic Trauma

Percutaneous renal biopsy for diagnosis and management of various renal disorders in children, including renal transplantation, is being done more frequently. These patients can have postbiopsy bleeding and arteriovenous fistulas.

The nuclear scan 1 Fig. 2.12 shows an even uptake in a transplanted kidney. A percutaneous renal biopsy was done as rejection was being clinically considered. Following this, the clinical condition deteriorated and another scan was performed (Fig. 2.13). This shows an area of decreased uptake, interpreted as being blood. About one-half unit of blood was removed and the scan repeated 1 week later when an even distribution of uptake was demonstrated. The noninvasive techniques of nuclear scanning and ultrasonography are of great help in evaluating these patients.

2.1.3 Management and Complications

There is considerable discussion in the literature concerning the management of renal trauma, but the trend seems to be in the direction of a more conservative approach. There is still a wide range of opinion regarding the exact indication for surgery and the timing of the procedure [40].

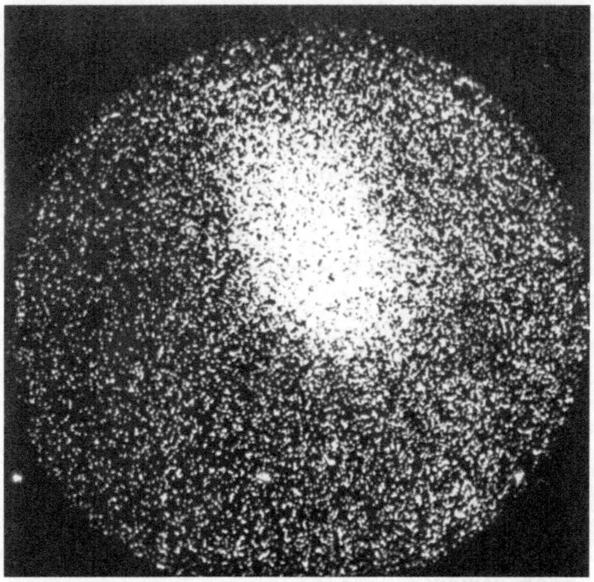

Fig. 2.12. Renal scan in a transplanted kidney showing an even, normal distribution and uptake of the radionuclide

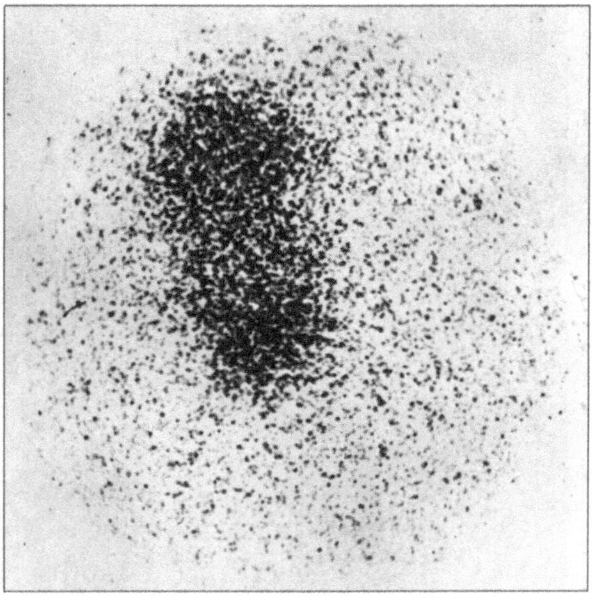

Fig. 2.13. Renal scan in a transplanted kidney following percutaneous biopsy of the kidney with an area of decreased uptake due to hematoma. One-half unit of blood was removed from this area

There is concern about the complications of kidney trauma and their later sequelae. Early complications consist of pararenal abscess, hematoma, and gradual loss of function [14, 20]. Hypertension may be a later complication and has been reported in up to 6% of patients [14]. Hypertension, as a complication, in children is rare [17, 20, 57]. Palavatana et al. followed 14 cases of childhood renal trauma from 10 months to almost 14 years [42]. There were no adverse clinical manifestations. There was slight shrinkage and some distortion in the intravenous urogram in one case, and calcification in another. These changes are uncommon.

2.2 Ureteral Trauma

Ureteral injury in children is rare, and mostly of due to surgical procedures and instrumentation [24]. When injured in other circumstances the cause is usually penetrating injury and not blunt trauma [5, 10, 46]. In children, in particular, there may be disruption of the ureteropelvic junction due to sudden hyperextension associated with abrupt deceleration [50].

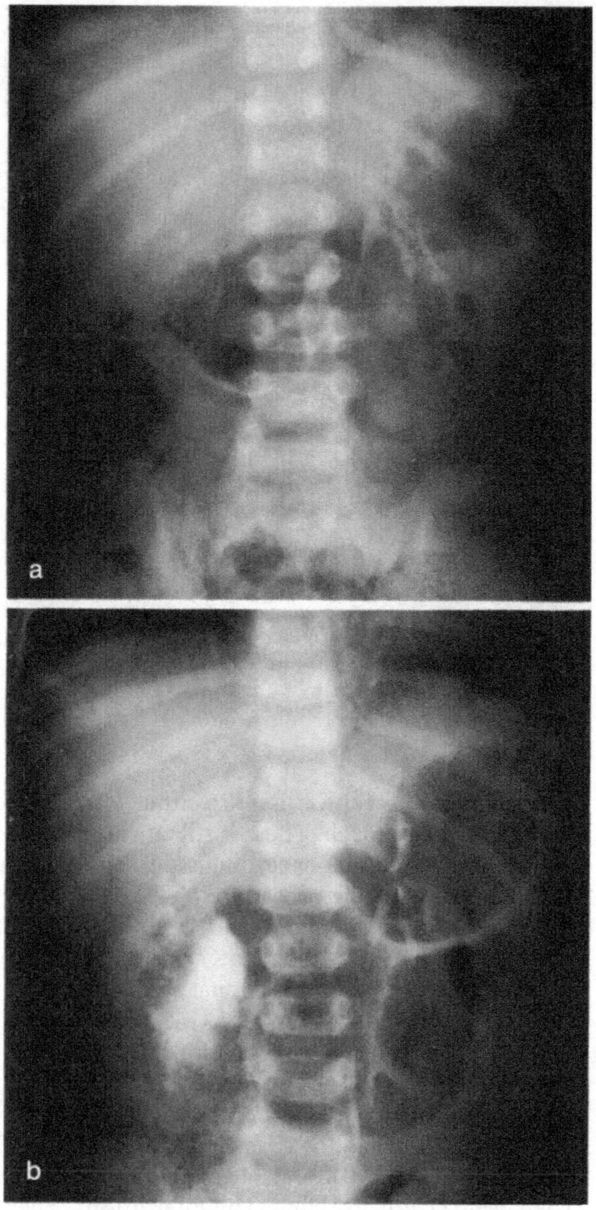

Fig. 2.14 a, b. Excretory urogram. **a** The right renal collecting structures are not as well visualized as on the left; **b** delayed film. There is extravasation of contrast medium at the ureteropelvic junction on the right, indicating a tear at this point

Clinical: The history is often that of a surgical procedure, including instrumentation prior to the symptoms, or penetrating abdominal injury such as gunshot wounds [46]. The patient complains of pain. There may be flank enlargement and/or signs of peritoneal irritation.

Radiology: These patients should have intravenous urography and retrograde pyelography performed. In one series, 42% of the patients with ureteral injury demonstrated extravasation from the ureter on intravenous urography (Fig. 2.14). The remainder showed varying degrees of obstruction [5]. The intravenous urogram also provides the opportunity to evaluate the kidneys. Retrograde pyelography is the definitive study for ureteric injury [5] (Fig. 2.15). The point of extravasation is easily shown as are the area and degree of ureteral obstruction.

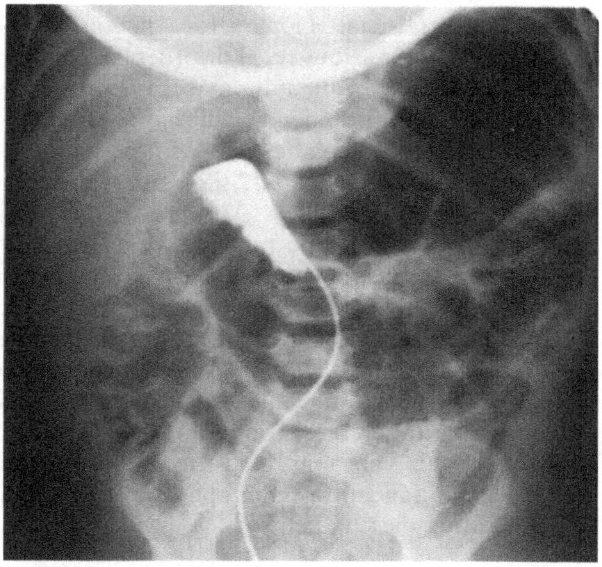

Fig. 2.15. Retrograde pyelogram with perforation of the ureter by the ureteral catheter and extravasation of the contrast material

2.3 Bladder Trauma

Probably the most common cause of bladder injury in children is an endoscopic procedure [35]. However, both blunt and penetrating trauma are factors, with 10%–25% being due to penetrating trauma [35]. Fractures of the pelvis are commonly associated with bladder injury [11, 24, 50]. Montie states that 75% of blunt bladder injuries have an associated fracture [35].

The degree of bladder trauma can be classified in four groups [3]:

1. Contusion
2. Extraperitoneal rupture
3. Intraperitoneal rupture
4. Combined extra- and intraperitoneal rupture

The differentiation can be made with radiological studies and this is important in dictating the management.

Contusion is the most common type of bladder injury. In one series, the cystogram demonstrated 31

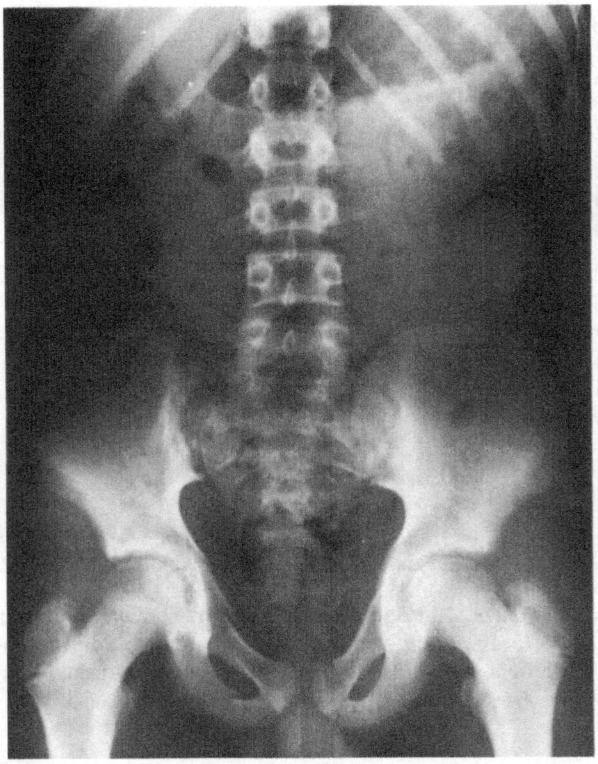

Fig. 2.16. Supine film of the abdomen demonstrating the fractures of the ischium and pubis

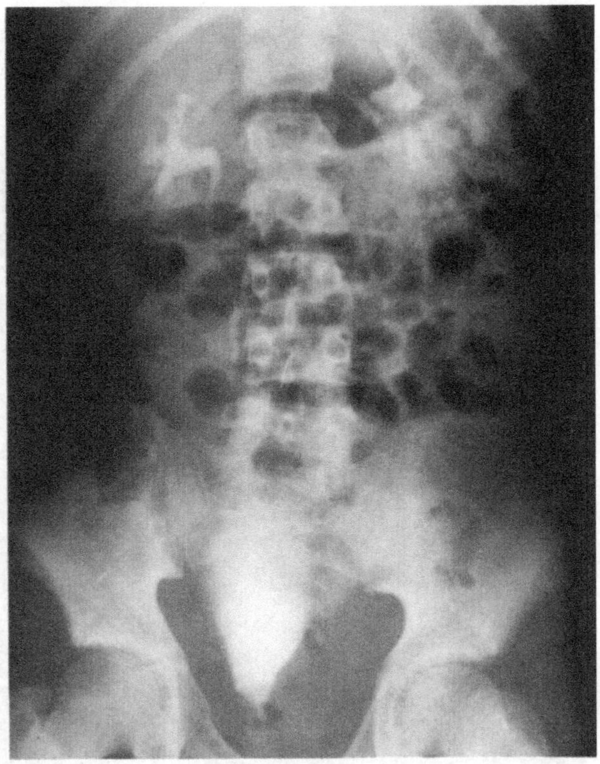

Fig. 2.17. Excretory urogram – same patient as in Fig. 2.16, showing normal upper urinary tracts. The bladder is elevated and has a "teardrop" deformity secondary to bladder trauma and pelvic hematoma

with contusion, 17 with intraperitoneal rupture, and 13 with extraperitoneal rupture [8].

Clinical: The child with bladder trauma complains of lower abdominal pain and dysuria. There may be an inability to void [10]. Hematuria of varying degrees is present, and shock may occur.

Radiology: Plain films of the abdomen with particular reference to the pelvic area will show the fractures so frequently seen in patients with bladder trauma (Fig. 2.16). Such radiographs may also demonstrate fluid in the peritoneal cavity.

Cystograms and retrograde cystourethrography are the studies of choice. Excretory urography should be done to evaluate the kidneys and to exclude renal involvement [50] (Fig. 2.17). The retrograde cystourethrogram permits evaluation of the urethra, as well as the bladder, and the bladder can be completely avulsed [10] (Fig. 2.18). For the cystogram, the volume of contrast used must be sufficient for the purpose and roentgenograms in multiple projections must be obtained; these include postvoiding studies.

The cystographic findings in the various classifications of bladder trauma, according to Brosman [3], are listed in Table 2.6.

The classification of bladder trauma should not be difficult. Care must be taken to do a complete study.

Table 2.6. Cystographic findings in bladder trauma

Contusion	Extraperitoneal	Intraperitoneal
Elevated bladder	Base of bladder obscured	Contrast around bowel
Deviation of bladder	by contrast	Contrast outlined
"Teardrop" bladder	Small lines of contrast to	Hourglass bladder
Obliteration soft tissue	extensive lines in fascial planes	Opaque bands in reflections
No extravasation		Contrast around liver and spleen

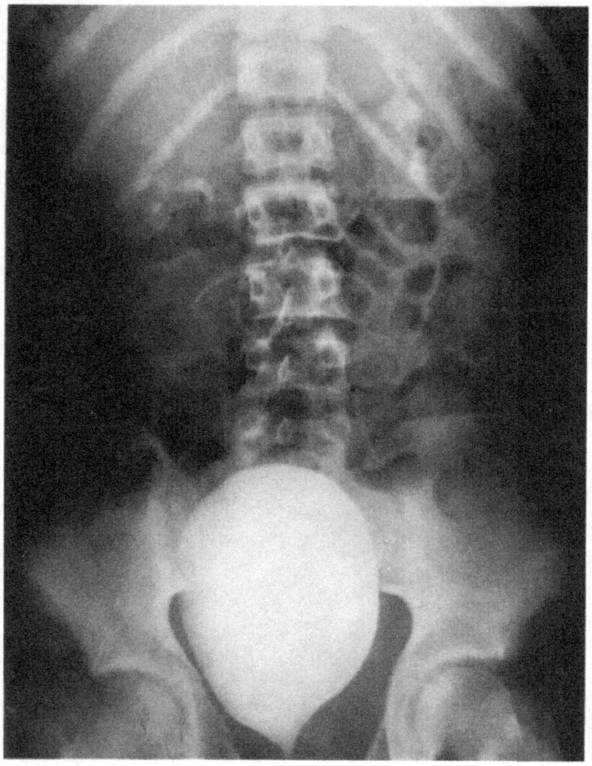

Fig. 2.18. Cystogram – same patient as in Figs. 2.16 and 2.17 with elevation and deformity of the bladder

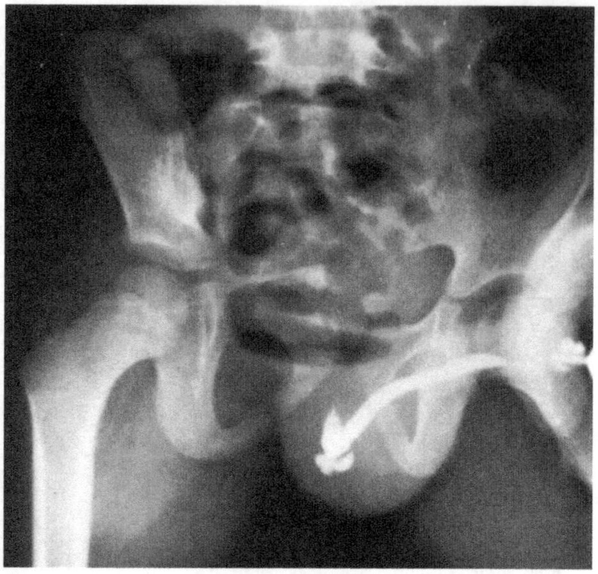

Fig. 2.19. Retrograde urethrogram showing traumatic perforation and severance of the urethra. Contrast medium is seen outside the confines of the urethra, and no contrast medium entires the bladder

But a relatively minor injury must not be converted into a major one by the procedure.

2.4 Urethral Trauma

Urethral trauma is rare in children [16] but may be caused by instrumentation or by blunt or penetrating trauma. Tears are more common than total severance of the urethra [16]. The most significant injury is prostamembranous disruption (often associated with pelvic fracture) with the urethra lacerated close to the apex of the prostate. The puboprostatic ligament is ruptured and the bladder is displaced upward and posteriorly [36]. In rupture below the urogenital diaphragm, the extravasation is often contained in Buck's fascia [46]. The pendulous urethra lends itself to trauma due to sharp instrumentation or projectiles [16].

Clinical. Urethral injury should be suspected in a child with a pelvic fracture. There will be an inability to void and frequently a drop of blood may be seen at the urethral meatus.

Radiology. A retrograde urethrogram should be performed (Fig. 2.19). This will easily demonstrate the area of tear or severance with extravasation of the contrast (Fig. 2.20). Multiple projections and positions are required. An incomplete tear is present when extravasation of contrast from the urethra occurs in conjunction with contrast medium in the bladder.

Intravenous urography is also required as this will demonstrate the configuration and position of the bladder. An upward deviation and a "teardrop" deformity of the bladder are usually associated with complete severance of the urethra [36] (Fig. 2.21).

Complications do occur following urethral tear or severance. Urethral stricture is the major complication [10, 16, 50]. There may be impotence or incontinence following some injuries to the urethra, hence it is important to establish the correct diagnosis as soon as possible so that adequate treatment may be instituted.

References

1. Banowski LH, Wolfel DA, Lackner LH (1970) Considerations in diagnosis and management of renal trauma. J Trauma 10:589–597
2. Bogash M, Pollack H, Cates JL (1974) Renal injuries caused by external blunt trauma. Urology 4:509–513
3. Brosman SA, Fay R (1973) Diagnosis and management of bladder trauma. J Trauma 13:687–694
4. Capek V, Fostik F (1963) The significance of selective renal angiography in injuries of the kidneys in childhood. AJR 90:75–80

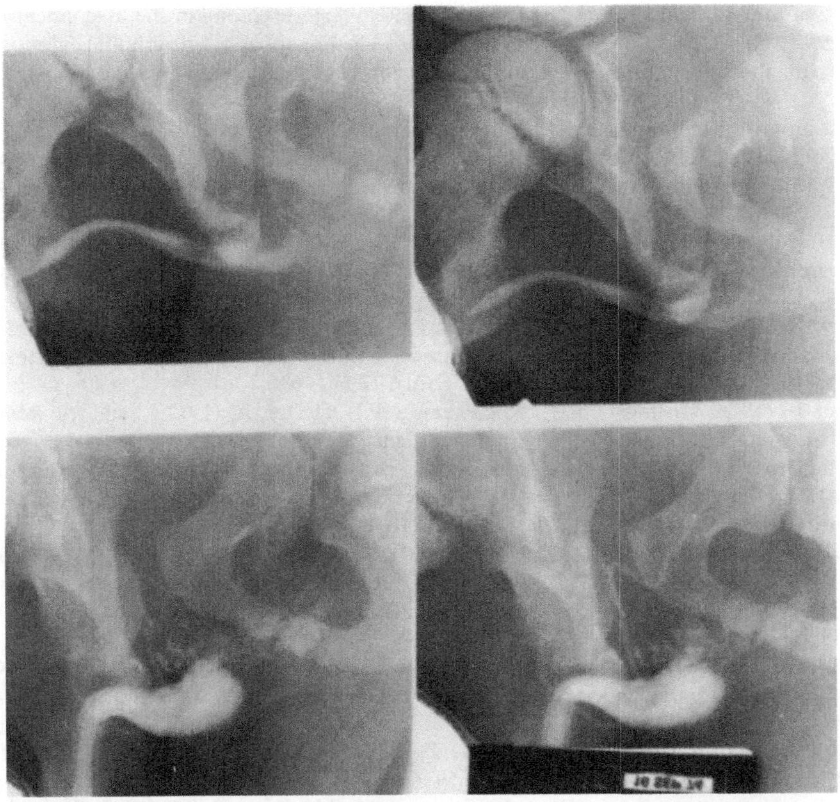

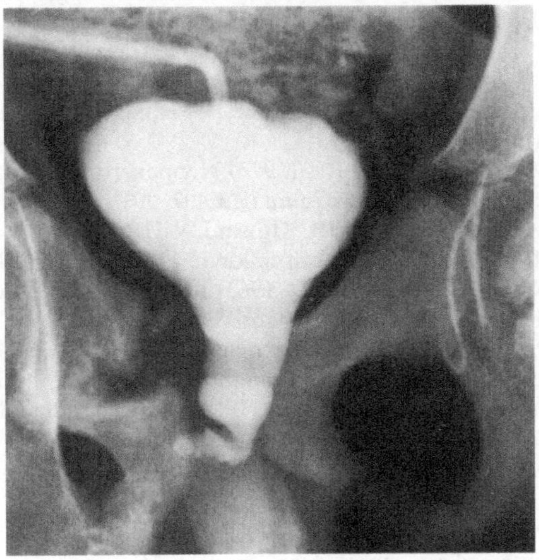

Fig. 2.20. Retrograde urethrogram with complete obstruction of the urethra due to trauma. Contrast material is seen in the ductal system and none in the bladder (*above*). Antregrade cystogram through a cystostomy catheter with complete disruption of the urethra. Fracture of the pubis noted on the right (*below*)

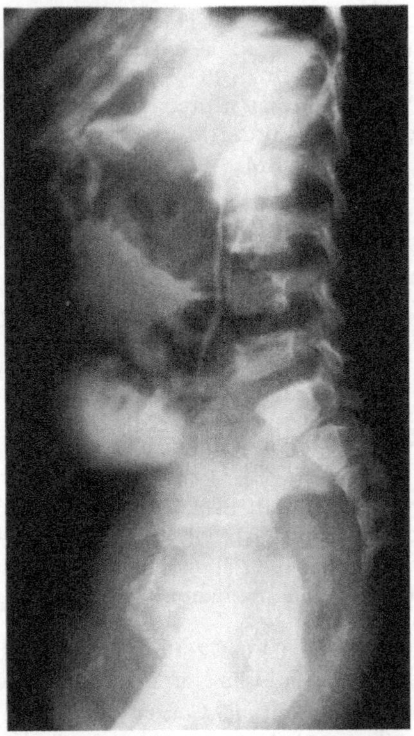

Fig. 2. 21. Excretory urogram – lateral projection – same patient as in Figs. 2.19 and 2.20 with normal upper urinary tract. The bladder is elevated and displaced anteriorly, and the base of the bladder is deformed

5. Carlton CE, (1977) Injuries to the ureter. Urol Clin North Am 4:33–44
6. Cass AS, (1975) Renal trauma in the multiple injured patient. J Urol 114:495–497
7. Cass AS, Ireland GW (1973) Comparison of conservative and surgical management of more severe degrees of renal trauma in multiple injured patients. J Urol 109:8–10
8. Cass AS, Ireland GW (1973) Bladder trauma associated with pelvic fracture in severely injured patients. J Trauma 13:205–212
9. Cockett ATK, Frank IN, Davis RS, Linke CA (1975) Recent advances in the diagnosis and management of blunt renal trauma. J Urol 113:750–754
10. Cook FT, Barkin M, Schillinger JF (1975) Urologic injuries – part II. Upper and lower genitourinary tract. In: Surgical Staff of the Hospital for Sick Children, Toronto, Canada (ed) Care for the injured child. Williams & Wilkins, Baltimore, pp 166–169
11. Donohue JP, (1975) Ureteral and bladder injuries in children. Pediatr Clin North Am 22:393–399
12. Elkin M, Meng CH, de Paredes RG (1966) Roentgenologic evaluation of renal trauma with emphasis on renal angiography. AJR 98:1–26
13. Emanuel B, Weiss H, Gollin P (1977) Renal trauma in children. J Trauma 17:275–278
14. Engle RME (1977) Trauma of the genitourinary system. In: Ballinger WF II, Rutherford RB, Zuedema GD (eds) Management of trauma. Saunders, Philadelphia, pp 456–478
15. Freeman LM, Kay CJ, Meng CH (1966) The contribution of renal scanning in the evaluation of renal trauma. Radiology 86:1021–1029
16. Garret RA (1975) Pediatric urethral and perineal injuries. Pediatr Clin North Am 22:401–406
17. Glenn JR, Harward BM (1960) Injured kidney. JAMA 173:1189–1195
18. Guerriero WG (1977) Penetrating renal injuries and the management of renal pedicle injury. Urol Clin North Am 4:3–12
19. Guerriero WG, Carlton CE Jr, Scott R Jr, Beall AC (1971) Renal pedicle injuries. J Trauma 11:53–62
20. Hessel SJ, Smith EG (1974) Renal trauma: comprehensive review and radiological assessment. CRC Crit Rev Clin Radiol Nucl Med 5:251–293
21. Hodges CV, Gilbert DR, Scott WW (1951) Renal trauma: a study of 71 cases. J Urol 66:627–637
22. Javadpour N, Guinan P, Bush LM (1973) Renal trauma in children. Surg Gynecol Obstet 136:237–240
23. Jevtich MJ, Montero GG (1969) Injuries to renal vessels by blunt trauma in children. J Urol 102:493–496
24. Kaufman JJ, Brosman SA (1972) Blunt injuries of the genitourinary tract. Surg Clin North Am 52:747–760
25. Kazmin MH, Swanson LE, Cockett ATK (1967) Renal scan: the test of choice in renal trauma. J Urol 97:189–195
26. Koenigsberg M, Blaufox MD, Freeman LM (1974) Traumatic injuries of the renal vascularity and parenchyma. Semin Nucl Med 4:117–132
27. Lang EK (1975) Arteriography in the assessment of renal trauma. The impact of arteriographic diagnosis on preservation of renal function and parenchyma. J Trauma 15:553–566
28. Lang EK, Trichel BE, Turner RW, Fontenotra RA, Johnson B, St Martin EC (1971) Renal angiography in the assessment of renal trauma. Radiology 98:103–112
29. Linke CA, Frank IN, Young LW, Cockett ATK (1972) Renal trauma in children: diagnostic workup and management. NY State J Med 72:2414–2420
30. Lucey DT, Smith MJV, Koontz WW, Jr (1972) Modern trends in the management of urologic trauma. J. Urol 107:641–646
31. MacPherson RI, Decter A (1971) Pediatric renal trauma. J Can Assoc Radiol22:10–21
32. Marks LS, Brosman SA, Lindstrom RR, Fay R (1974) Arteriography in penetrating renal trauma. Urology 3:18–22
33. McDonald EJ Jr, Korobkin M, Jacobs RP, Minagi H (1976) The role of emergency excretory urography in evaluation of blunt abdominal trauma. AJR 126:739–742
34. Mertz JHO, Wishard WN Jr, Nourse MH Mertz HO (1963) Injury of the kidney in children. JAMA 183:730–733
35. Montie J (1977) Bladder injuries. Urol Clin North Am 4:59–67
36. Morehouse DD, MacKinnon KJ (1977) Posterior urethral injury: etiology, diagnosis and management. Urol Clin North Am 4:69–73
37. Morrow JW, Mendez R (1970) Renal trauma. J. Urol 104:649–653
38. Morse TS (1975) Renal injuries. Pediatr Clin North Am 22:379–391
39. Morse TS, Harris BH (1973) Nonpenetrating renal vascular injuries. J Trauma 13:497–501
40. Morse TS, Smith JP, Howard WHR, Rowe ML (1967) Kidney injuries in children. J Urol 98:539–547
41. Nation EF, Massey BD (1963) Renal trauma: experience with 258 cases. J Urol 89:775–778
42. Palavatana CG Sr, Silverman FN (1964) Delayed sequels to renal injury in childhood. AJR 91:659–665
43. Persky L, Forsythe WE (1962) Renal trauma in childhood. JAMA 182:709–712
44. Peters PC Bright TC, III (1977) Blunt renal injuries. Urol Clin North Am 4:17–28
45. Peterson NE, Stables D (1977) Blunt renal injuries of intermediate degree. Urology 9:11–16
46. Pontes JE (1977) Urologic injuries. Surg Clin North Am 57:77–96
47. Pryor JP, Williams JP (1975) A study of 137 cases of renal trauma. Br J Urol 47:45–49
48. Radwin HM, Fitch WP, Robinson JR (1976) A unified concept of renal trauma. J Urol 116:20–22
49. Reid LS (1973) Renal trauma in children: a ten year review. Aust NZ J Surg 42:260–266
50. Richter MW, Lytton B, Myerson D, Grnja V (1973) Radiology of genitourinary trauma. Radiol Clin North Am 11:593–631

51. Rothfeld SH, Stein H (1972) Renal trauma in children: angiography as an aid to treatment. Angiology 23:426–450
52. Salvatierra O (1975) Management of urologic injuries – trauma rounds. West J Med 122:257–261
53. Samuels LD, Smith JP (1968) Kidney scanning in pediatric renal trauma. J Trauma 8:583–592
54. Schiller M, Harris BH, Samuels LD, Clatworthy HW, Morse TS (1972) Diagnosis of experimental renal trauma. J Pediatr Surg 7:187–193
55. Scott R Jr, Carlton CE, Ashmore AJ, Duke HH (1963) Initial management of nonpenetrating renal injuries: clinical review of 111 cases. J Urol 90:535–539
56. Smalley RH, Banowsky LHW (1971) Evaluation of renal trauma by infusion urography. J Urol 105:620–622
57. Smith MJV, Seidel RF, Bonacarti AF (1966) Accidental trauma to the kidneys in children. J Urol 96:845–847
58. Solheim K, Resch F, Kordt KF (1972) Closed renal injuries. Injury 3:185–195
59. Thompson LM (1977) Expectant management of blunt renal trauma. Urol Clin North Am 4:29–32
60. Vermillion CD, McLaughlin AP, Pfister RC (1971) Management of blunt renal trauma. J Urol 106:478–484
61. Williams JE (1976) Radiology now – renal trauma: the place of arteriography. Br J Radiol 49:743–744
62. Wein AJ, Arger PH, Murphy JJ (1977) Controversial aspect of blunt renal trauma. J Trauma 17:662–666
63. Young LW, Wood BP, Linke CA (1975) Renal injury from blunt trauma in childhood: radiological evaluation and review. Ann Radiol (Paris) 18:359–376

3 Neuroradiology in Head Trauma[1]

Hervey D. Segall, J. Gordon McComb, Fong Y. Tsai, and John H. Miller

3.1 Introduction

3.1.1 General Comments

Radiological studies available for assessment of children with head trauma include plain skull X-rays, arteriography, computerized tomography (CT), air studies, echoencephalography, and radionuclide brain scanning. The radiological approach will vary, depending on whether the investigation is being carried out under the emergent circumstance of acute head trauma or whether the delayed consequences of trauma are being evaluated. Obviously, it is best to admit a child with an acute head injury to a hospital where CT, as well as facilities for emergency surgery are available.

In the acute situation, the rapidity with which radiological studies must be accomplished depends on the severity of head injury and the patient's neurological status [38]. Thus, if a patient is showing rapid neurological decline, routine skull X-rays are frequently omitted and a CT scan is the diagnostic study of choice. If the child's condition is deteriorating very rapidly, it may even be necessary to eliminate a CT scan and proceed to the operating room without any X-ray studies whatsoever, relying solely on clinical findings for the localization of a suspected mass lesion. Treatment, surgical or medical, is obviously of little value once extensive and irreversible central nervous system (CNS) changes have taken place [14].

The child with a serious head injury should be transported in a semiprone position so that nasopharyngeal secretions may drain. Once the child has arrived in the X-ray department and is undergoing radiological studies, it is always important to make certain that he is observed carefully for changes in cardiopulmonary status. Respiratory insufficiency and hypovolemia must always be treated before proceeding with various diagnostic X-ray studies. In dealing with small infants it should be remembered that there may be enough blood loss into the scalp to produce a significant hypovolemia which can lead to circulatory collapse. Other injuries may occur and priority for these injuries must be established.

With *all* severe head injuries it is necessary to obtain a lateral X-ray of the cervical spine. Once cervical spine injury has been excluded, manipulation of the head and neck for various radiological studies can be undertaken with a reasonable degree of confidence.

There is no role for lumbar puncture in acute head trauma; it will add no new information and, on occasion, it may worsen a patient's neurological status by producing serious shifts within the cerebrospinal fluid (CSF) spaces resulting from the removal of fluid from the lumbar subarachnoid space. Loss of CSF from the lumbar subarachnoid space may provoke herniation of the cerebellar tonsils, resulting in serious neurological deficit, and even death.

The presence or absence of a skull fracture and its location may influence whether or not the patient need be admitted for observation. However, various other parameters are of equal or greater importance. These parameters include the presence or absence of loss of consciousness (the duration of the episode of unconsciousness is also to be considered) in addition to other aspects of the patient's neuological status, and whether it is improving or deteriorating. Vomiting, headache, focal neurological findings, and seizures are also significant. The reliability of the parents and their ability to bring the child back to the hospital without undue delay are important considerations as well.

Fractures of the skull may also raise the question of whether or not a child has been battered. In the case of battered children, the history on admission is frequently vague and inconclusive and may not fit the clinical findings. Early suspicion of child abuse is of obvious importance since early detection of battering is beneficial not only to the child [85] but to his siblings as well. If there is any suspicion of battering, a skeletal survey is indicated to determine if other fractures exist [50]. It is important to note, however, that one should not rely solely on the

[1] *Note on illustrations:* All CT scans are oriented as if the reader were looking at the head from *above*. Thus, a patient's right side is on the reader's right. The front of the head is at the top and the occiput is at the bottom. EMI CT 1005 and CT 1010 scanners were used.

All X-rays (skull films, air studies, angiograms) are conventionally presented, with the patient's right on the reader's left.

radiological finding of multiple skeletal fractures to ascertain the diagnosis of child abuse. An abused child may not have skeletal fractures [44].

3.1.2 Skull X-rays

Routine skull X-rays have become more limited in value with the advent of CT scanning. In an acute situation, it is always necessary to weigh the value of skull X-rays against the time incurred in obtaining them. The routine ordering of skull X-rays after a child has sustained a very minor head trauma should be discouraged as the yield is very low.

Skull films will usually reveal the presence and site of skull fracture. Furthermore, skull films will show the relationship of the fracture line to meningeal grooves and dural sinuses in children who might have extradural hematoma. In severe acute head trauma, skull films utilizing appropriate projections, and occasionally tomography, may be beneficial in ascertaining the presence and extent of a depressed skull fracture. Follow-up skull examinations in certain fracture cases will show widening of the defect at the fracture site which leads to consideration of lesions producing a "growing skull fracture" (see later). Plain skull films in older children following trauma may show shift of the pineal when it contains sufficient calcium to be identified roentgenographically. Such a finding may indicate the presence of intracerebral or extracerebral hematoma or posttraumatic cerebral swelling. Of course, it should be remembered that the pineal may be shifted *to* the side of an atrophic hemisphere. Other radiological data and historical data will usually alert the physician to the likelihood of an atrophic lesion. Furthermore, shift of the pineal toward an atrophic hemisphere may be secondary to earlier trauma. Additional findings resulting from trauma that can be identified on skull films include pneumocephalus, air-fluid levels within the paranasal sinuses and intracranial or extracranial foreign bodies.

Chronic changes resulting from posttraumatic lesions may also be evident on skull films; for example, skull thinning and bulging in chronic subdural hematoma may be evident. Calcification within chronic subdural hematoma or extradural hematoma may be appreciated on skull films. Changes secondary to atrophy, including a Dyke-Davidoff-Masson syndrome, may become apparent on skull films obtained in posttraumatic instances.

Despite the spectrum of posttraumatic abnormalities that can be detected on skull films [6], this examination usually does not adequately portray the pathological changes resulting from trauma on which to base treatment. Frequently, it is not possible to establish the presence of a mass or localize it following trauma. In addition, skull films usually do not permit the diagnosis of the nature of an intracranial traumatic lesion when one is present. Generalized sutural diastasis following trauma indicates the presence of increased intracranial pressure only and is of no localizing value. Physiological calcification under the age of 10 years is extremely rare so that one cannot usually lateralize a posttraumatic lesion by examining skull roentgenograms in this age group.

Finally, although the skull film is usually the best method for demonstrating a skull fracture, such a lesion may be missed with this technique even when tomography is utilized.

Obviously, therefore, the plain skull film is inadequate to give all information needed about the intracranial compartment. If there is clinical evidence of an intracranial mass lesion, further diagnostic radiological evaluation is warranted.

3.1.3 Angiography

Before the development of CT scanning, angiography was frequently used to ascertain whether or not a surgically treatable intracranial mass was present. Even today, in places where CT scanning is not available or on those occasions when the CT scanner is not functioning, angiography is still necessary. Angiography is able to define the size and location of a mass lesion and whether it is intra- or extra-axial in the majority of cases. Specific vascular abnormalities associated with head trauma are rarely found in the pediatric age group, and angiography to rule out their presence is infrequently warranted; angiography is indicated in the unusual circumstance when a lesion that may benefit by treatment (usually surgery) is suspected on clinical grounds. Such vascular abnormalities include displacement of the middle meningeal artery or dural sinuses, vascular spasm, traumatic aneurysm, vessel occlusion, meningeal pseudoaneurysms, and arteriovenous fistulas. Angiography may be useful in ascertaining cerebral death, as with cerebral death there is no evidence of contrast material extending beyond the intracranial portion of the carotid arteries [75]. A fuller discussion of these entities will follow under the heading "Traumatic Vascular Lesions."

3.1.4 Computerized Tomography

Since its clinical introduction in 1973, CT scanning has been the primary diagnostic X-ray procedure of choice in both acute and chronic head trauma. The size, location and, frequently, age of the hematoma are much better delineated with CT scanning than with angiography. The nature of an acute mass lesion can frequently be much better delineated by CT scanning. As an example, cerebral edema can be separated from a hematoma, which generally is not the case with angiography. This is particularly helpful from a clinical standpoint since edema does not warrant surgical intervention while the presence of a hematoma may.

CT scanning done from the foramen magnum to the vertex will diminish the chance of missing a lesion, or make certain that multiple lesions are not present (Figs. 3.1, 3.2). In addition to the size of the ventricles, visualization or nonvisualization of the subarachnoid spaces, as well as shifts of midline structures, may give an indication as to the degree of cerebral swelling. The CT findings, when correlated with the patient's neurological status, may suggest a need for intracranial pressure monitoring. CT scans are very helpful in ascertaining whether or not delayed hemorrhage, subdural hematomas, or post-traumatic hydrocephalus is developing. Delayed posttraumatic residues involving the brain such as atrophy and porencephaly (Fig. 3.3) may be shown. CT findings will be discussed further in subsequent sections, including the use of intravenous contrast material in head trauma.

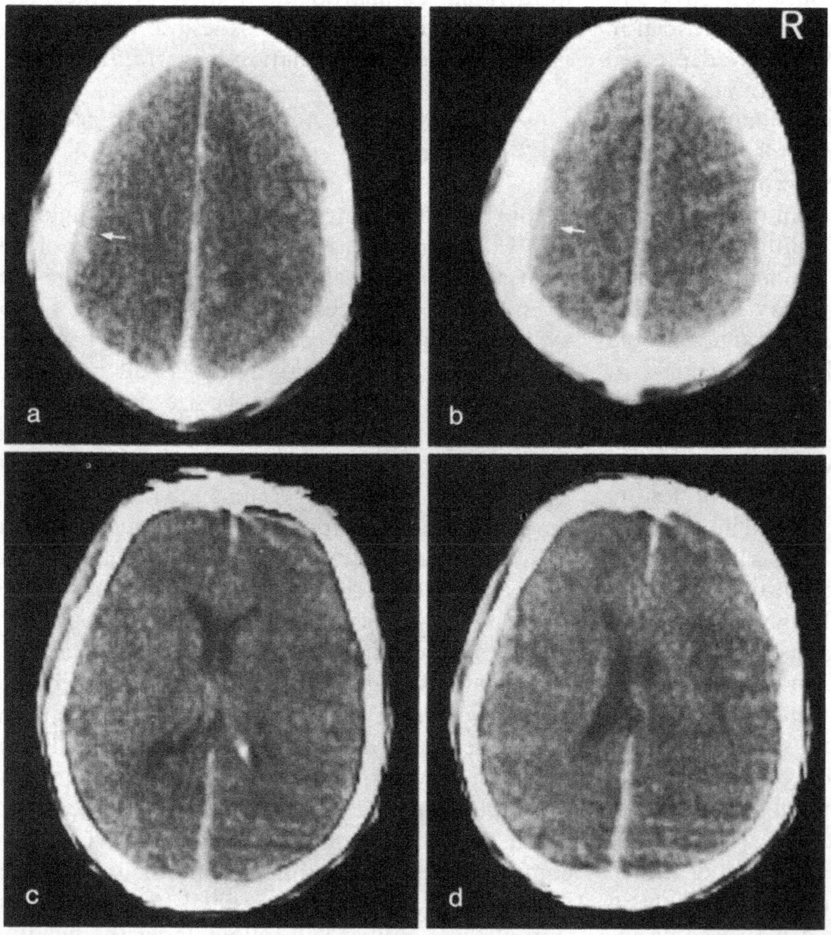

Fig. 3.1 a–d. Four slices from a CT study in an older child with head trauma. The upper two slices are above the level of the lateral ventricles and show a small left-sided epidural hematoma (*small white arrow*) which was barely seen on a lower slice at the level of the top of the left lateral ventricle (**d**). The lowest slice of the four (**c**) was below the hematoma. This series shows the importance of obtaining higher slices in children with head trauma if all abnormalities are to be seen

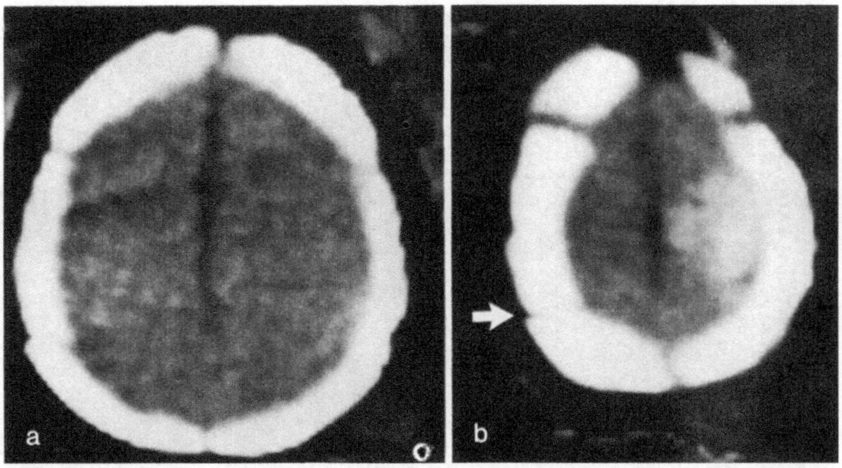

Fig. 3.2 a, b. CT scans in an infant. These scans show the importance of imaging the head all the way to the vertex in head trauma. The second highest scan (**a**) shows a fracture involving the left parietal bone. However, the highest slice (**b**) shows, in addition to the left parietal fracture (*arrow*), a superfical right-sided high density blood collection. Note the anterior fontanel, coronal sutures, and sagittal suture on the same slice

3.1.5 Echoencephalography

Echoencephalography is used primarily to determine whether or not there is a shift of the third ventricle. Echoencephalography is also able to ascertain, in many cases, the size of the lateral ventricles. Although some clinicians like to use echoencephalography in the emergency room to determine the presence of midline shift, CT scans are better at defining the intracranial anatomy and, as a result, echoencephalography has diminished considerably in use.

3.1.6 Air Studies

The use of air introduced either into the ventricles (Fig. 3.4) or into the lumbar subarachnoid space has had limited use in the management of patients with head injuries and has become much less indicated with the advent of CT scanning.

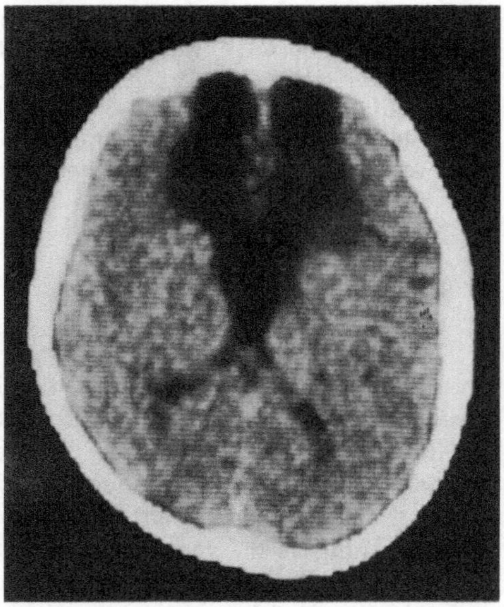

Fig. 3.3. Bilateral frontal porencephaly. CT scan in a 6-year-old child, the victim of child abuse. Bilateral low density areas (note that their density is similar to that of ventricular fluid) are noted to extend anteriorly into the frontal lobes from the frontal horns. These porencephalies are secondary to earlier trauma which resulted in bilateral frontal intracerebral hemorrhages and contusions

3.1.7 Radionuclide Brain Scanning

The use of radiopharmaceuticals in head trauma has had a very limited role [103] but radionuclide scanning has been helpful in the subacute or chronic stage of head trauma and has been useful in defining the presence or absence of subdural hematomas[13]. It was not useful at all, however, in acute head trauma as acute subdural hematomas would not be shown; in fact, the development of membrane surrounding the hematomas takes 7–10 days before there is evidence of increased radionuclide delineation. Radionuclide brain scanning can sometimes demonstrate a subdural hematoma that is isodense on the CT scan but, as a rule, certain precontrast CT findings are strongly suggestive of an extracerebral

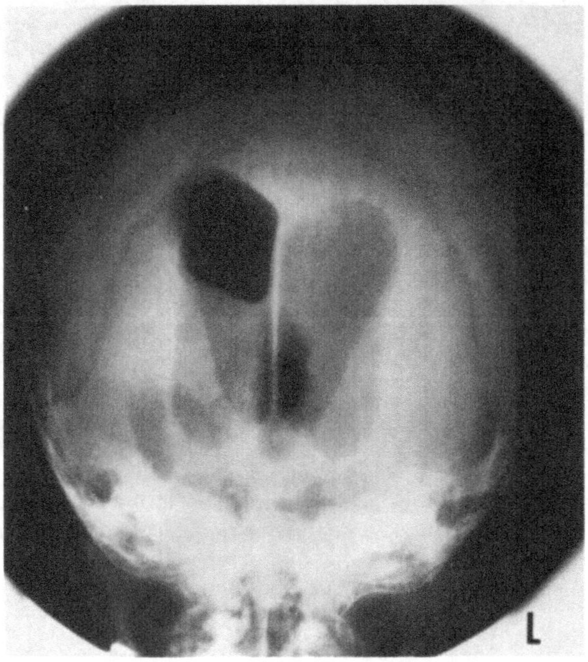

Fig. 3.4. Posttraumatic hydrocephalus. Ventriculogram, brow-up position, AP Towne projection. The air study shows the moderate to marked dilatation of the frontal horns and third ventricle. The communicating hydrocephalus resulted from previous trauma with extensive intraventricular and subarachnoid hemorrhage

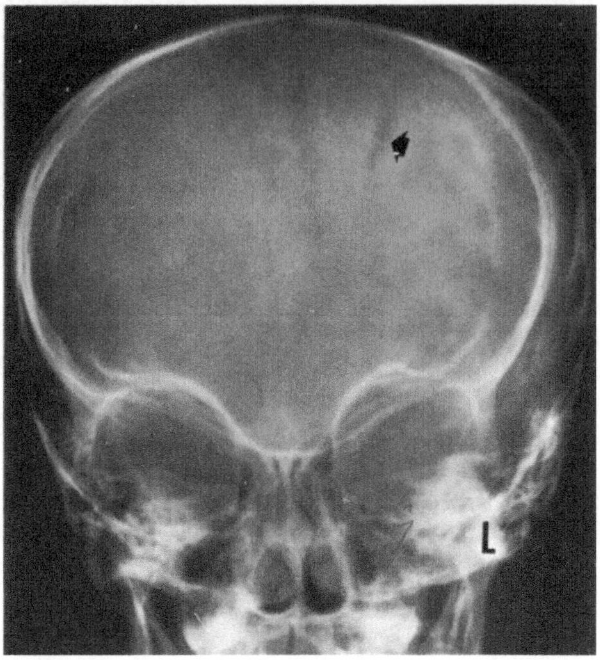

Fig. 3.5. Laceration simulating fracture. An AP skull film in a child following head trauma shows a linear area(*arrow*) which could be confused with a fracture but there was a laceration on the left side. When the laceration was sutured, repeat skull films showed no lucent line in that area. The findings seen on the above skull film represent air within the laceration

collection and good postcontrast CT scans are generally diagnostic [66, 97].

Intrathecal radiopharmaceuticals still continue to be of great help in roughly locating the site of a CSF leak occurring as a result of head trauma. Posttraumatic hydrocephalus, which was once evaluated mainly with the use of intrathecal radionuclides [7] or by the introduction of air, is now best defined by CT scanning as the ventricular size can be easily evaluated and monitored. Radionuclide brain scanning is still helpful in determining the presence and direction of CSF flow, which may become abnormal following head trauma.

As with angiography, it is also possible to define the absence of cerebral blood flow and thus confirm the presence of brain death after radionuclide injection.

3.2 Trauma Involving the Pediatric Skull

3.2.1 Skull Fractures – General Comments

The radiologist should become familiar with the appearance of normal vascular grooves involving the calvarium in childhood so as to avoid misinterpreting them as fractures. In childhood, vascular grooves in the frontal region tend often to be more prominent than in adults. Many variants and artifacts must be appreciated to avoid an erroneous diagnosis of fracture. Various linear shadows may simulate a fracture; for example, air between the edges of a laceration can result in a lucent line that suggests a fracture (Fig. 3.5). Linear fissures extending laterally from the posterior portions of the sagittal sutures in newborns may simulate fracture. Independent interparietal bones occur in over 10% of newborns and should not be confused with fractures. The appearance of other normal structures such as the mendosal suture and innominate synchondrosis may also be mistakenly interpreted as fractures in the newborn [12]. The curvilinear configuration of "ripple lines" (which represent simple folds in the soft tissues of the scalp) should be readily appreciated as such on newborn skull films [12]. In addition, there are numerous other normal childhood variants that can easily be confused with fracture lines [9].

The most common finding on skull X-rays following trauma is that of skull fracture [26]. The majority of such fractures have little clinical significance as they are infrequently associated with other pathological processes. The finding of a skull fracture does, however, indicate that a significant force has been applied to the skull [46]. The majority of fractures are linear and nondisplaced and thus require no surgical intervention. If the fracture crosses the middle meningeal artery or major dural sinus, there is an increased likelihood of an extra-axial hematoma. The vast majority of such fractures, however, are not associated with hematomas requiring surgical intervention. On the contrary, the absence of a fracture crossing a major vascular channel does not exclude the possibility of a hematoma developing.

One series showed that the commonest causes of skull fracture in childhood were falls and automobile accidents [40]. Of children with skull fractures 80% had external evidence of trauma to the head. Fractures were ipsilateral to the external scalp lesion in 84% and contralateral in 16% [40].

The finding of skull fracture by no means indicates the presence of a significant intracranial injury. It only confirms that a force has been applied to the skull [45]. It is well appreciated that it is not uncommon to find a fracture in patients who have never had impairment of consciousness; nor is it unusual to have serious brain damage without a fracture [45]. Thus, the presence of a skull fracture may be relatively insignificant and may not affect treatment or prognosis in the individual case. Depressed fractures and those associated with CSF rhinorrhea, however, command greater attention [40].

Roberts and Shopfner evaluated 570 children with head injuries referred to the X-ray department for skull examinations. They concluded that the presence of a fracture did not affect treatment except in one case where a depressed fracture was found, and in an additional case where there was a foreign body [80].

Both lateral views of the skull, anteroposterior or posteroanterior views and Towne projections, are obtained routinely in the evaluation of head trauma. The value of obtaining cervical spine views prior to manipulation of the head and neck should also be remembered. *Every* child with significant head trauma should at least have a lateral view of the cervical spine. In addition to the standard views, a base view of the skull may also be useful, but basal skull fractures frequently require tomography for their demonstration. Tomography may also be useful in other areas where the bony anatomy is complex [90]. When it is desired to assess the presence and extent of a depressed skull fracture, tangential views may be indicated (Fig. 3.11) (see later).

New fractures have sharp margins (Fig. 3.7). The margins become less distinct as healing occurs. This, however, is a slow process since skull fractures tend to heal more slowly than other types of fractures. In small children, the fracture line tends to disappear faster radiographically than in older children. A fracture may not be visible within 3–6 months in a small child, whereas in older children radiographic disappearance of a fracture may take up to a year [93].

Diastatic fractures are fractures which involve the cranial sutures, causing them to spread. Diastasis

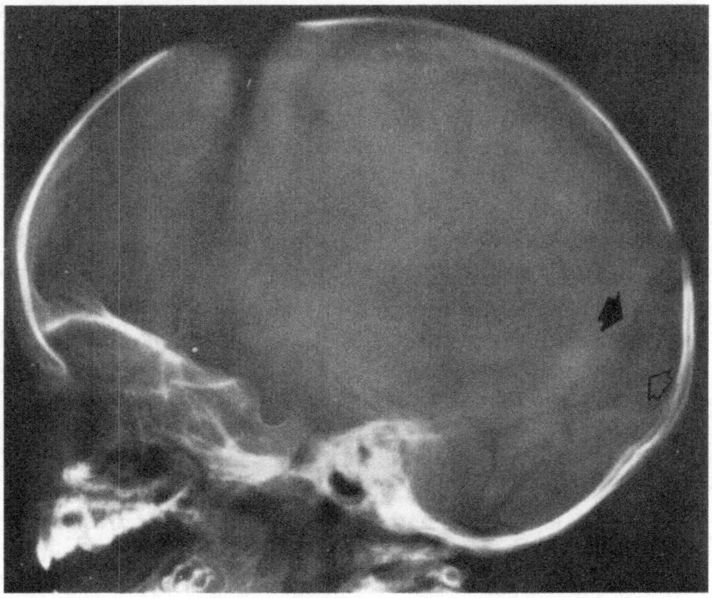

Fig. 3.6. Diastatic skull fracture. Lateral view of the skull shows diastasis of the right lambdoidal suture (*closed black arrow*), secondary to local trauma. The opposite lambdoidal suture (*open black arrow*) served as a comparison and was not widened. There was bilateral coronal diastasis due to increased intracranial pressure

may be readily appreciated by comparing a diastatic suture with a normal suture on the opposite side (Fig. 3.6). We have also found the following simple rule of help in the evaluation of sutural width in childhood: (1) no suture should measure more than 3.0 mm after the 3rd month of life, and (2) the sagittal suture, or the coronal suture, measured at its top, should not measure more than 2.0 mm after the first birthday.

A fracture may be present but not demonstrable roentgenographically [99]. It may be found only subsequently at operation or at postmortem examination. For example, in one series concerning 40 children with extradural hematoma, only 40% had fractures (16 cases). The fracture was demonstrated roentgenographically in only ten of those. Operation (in four) and postmortem examination (in two) yielded the six additional fractures [40].

Most children who develop subdural hematomas do not have skull fractures. Overall, only 15% of children with subdural hematomas had fractures in one series [40]; however, fractures associated with subdural hematoma were commoner in older children than in babies [40]. Furthermore, the site of the fracture is not a reliable index for the location of a subdural hematoma when both fracture and subdural hematoma are present. When there was a fracture, the subdural hematoma was commonly located contralateral to the fracture [40].

Fractures may also be associated with serious hematomas outside the intracranial compartment. A hairline orbital roof fracture can be associated with underlying subperiosteal hematoma of the orbit [102]. An example of a fracture involving the orbital roof is shown in Fig. 3.7.

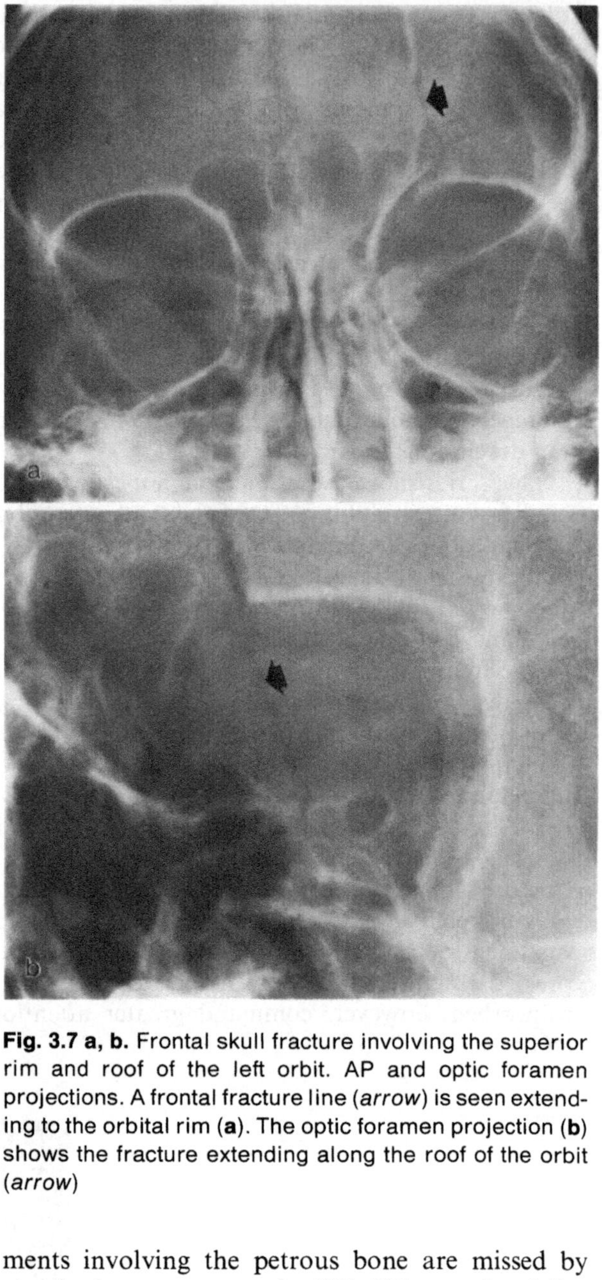

Fig. 3.7 a, b. Frontal skull fracture involving the superior rim and roof of the left orbit. AP and optic foramen projections. A frontal fracture line (*arrow*) is seen extending to the orbital rim (**a**). The optic foramen projection (**b**) shows the fracture extending along the roof of the orbit (*arrow*)

3.2.2 Fractures Involving the Skull Base, Paranasal Sinuses, and Petromastoid Structures

Basilar skull fracture may be suspected clinically but may not be demonstrated roentgenographically. The presence of blood behind the tympanic membrane does not necessarily mean that the patient has a basilar skull fracture. Obviously, CSF leaking through a torn tympanic membrane or external auditory canal would indicate the presence of such. Many such fractures are very difficult to demonstrate radiographically, and in the majority of cases they need not be so. If there is no CSF leak, or if there was one earlier but it has stopped, further radiologic investigation would have little clinical bearing. If there is evidence of damage to the facial nerve or of the inner or middle ear, tomography may be indicated since most fractures and traumatic displacements involving the petrous bone are missed by standard roentgenography [39]. CT may also delineate fractures unidentified by standard roentgenography [68].

In other patients with basal skull fractures, films taken with a horizontal beam while the patient is supine may demonstrate an air-fluid level. This indicates blood or CSF in the sphenoidal sinus, an important sign of fracture of the sphenoid bone. If there is evidence of obvious CSF leak, then this would favor the air-fluid level to be CSF in origin. If the air-fluid level persists, then it is more likely that it is CSF, as blood in the sinuses will resolve with time. The vast majority of CSF leaks will spontaneously abate after the first few days. Debate exists

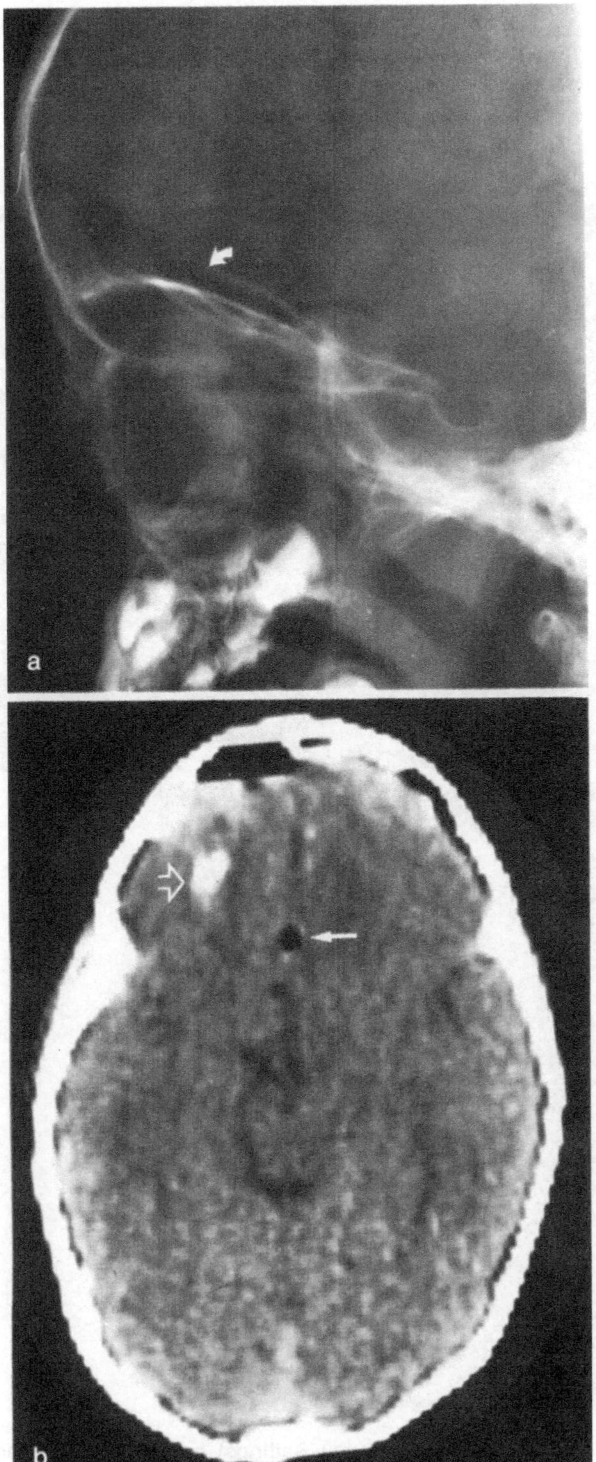

Fig. 3.8 a, b. Orbital roof fracture with pneumocephalus. A lateral skull film (**a**) shows supraorbital air above the site of the fracture fragment (*arrow*) projecting from the left orbital roof. **b** CT scan of the same patient. Note the air under the inner table of the skull and also in the interhemispheric fissure (*closed white arrow*). The tip of the left-sided bone fragment is noted (*open white arrow*)

as to whether or not a CSF leak immediately after trauma need be treated with antibiotics. Some, indeed, advocate such treatment. On the other hand, clinical studies have shown that the use of prophylactic antibiotics does not decrease the incidence of meningitis. If the CSF leak persists for more than a week, or is associated with an obvious infection, then there is no question that antibiotics would be advocated by most clinicians. The majority of CSF leaks occur in the frontal fossa, fluid draining via the frontal, ethmoidal, or sphenoid sinuses. Persistent CSF leaks from the middle and posterior fossae are much less common. Thus, CSF fistulas may result in either CSF rhinorrhea or otorrhea.

Since CSF leaks are symptomatic of bony defects in areas that are anatomically intricate and difficult to assess by plain roentgenography, tomography is often required to delineate the causative fracture. Even with complex motion tomography in AP and lateral projections, it may be difficult to outline the appropriate fracture when it is present. Intrathecal radionuclide has also been used to identify the site of a leak. Positive contrast medium studies have been used in the evaluation of acquired CSF fistulas; they

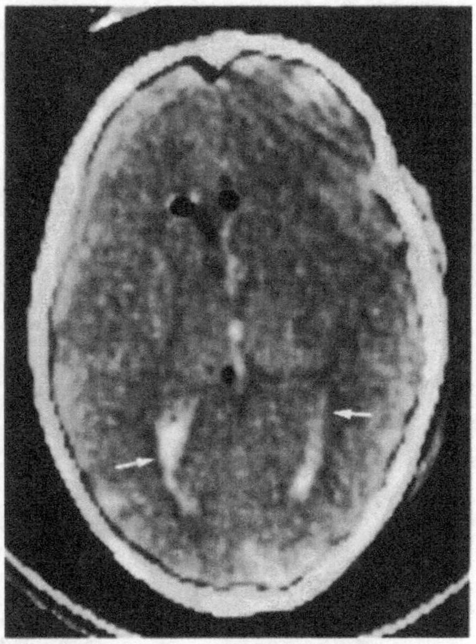

Fig. 3.9. Intracranial air and blood shown by CT. Note air within the tips of both frontal horns, as well as in the upper quadrigeminal cistern appearing as small rounded black areas. A small amount of air is also situated under the frontal bone. The smaller collections of air could not be appreciated on concomitant skull films in this case. Blood within the ventricular system, principally in both occipital horns (*white arrows*), is also noted. There is a right to left shift of the frontal horns due to cerebral edema and possibly contusion on the right

are not considered indispensable, however, and sometimes they are fruitless [49]. We have had no occasion to use positive contrast material in diagnosing CSF fistula since this is a relatively uncommon complication of trauma in childhood.

It should be remembered that infection may occur through fractures at the base of the skull even in the absence of a clinically evident CSF leak [95].

Fractures involving the posterior table of the frontal sinus may result not only in CSF rhinorrhea

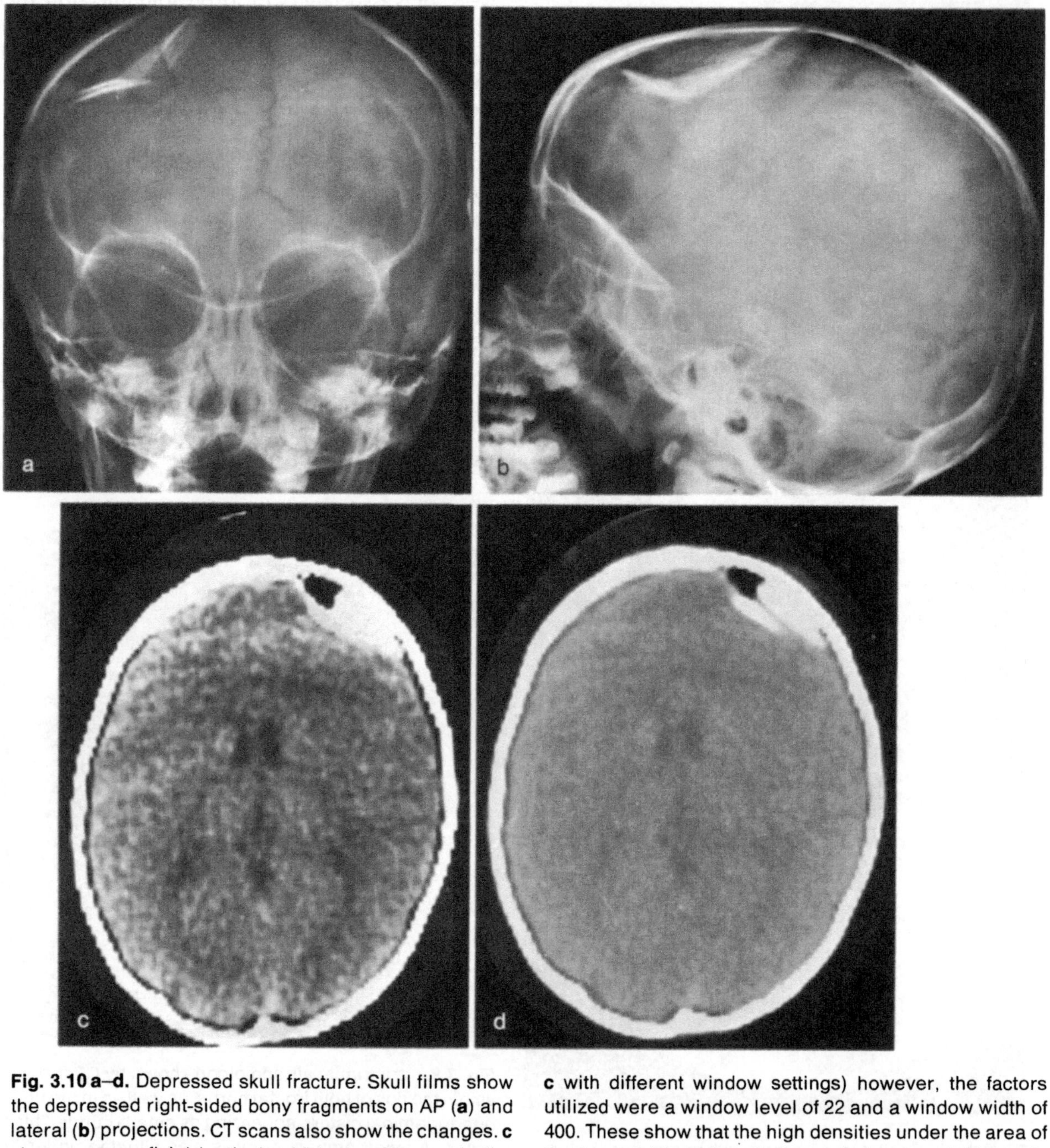

Fig. 3.10 a–d. Depressed skull fracture. Skull films show the depressed right-sided bony fragments on AP (**a**) and lateral (**b**) projections. CT scans also show the changes. **c** shows a superficial lenticular high density area in the right frontal region with a small collection of air (in peak black) anteromedially. This slice was performed with a window level of 22 and a window width of 100. Using these factors, it would not be possible to exclude an epidural hematoma (with air entering via an associated fracture) when interpreting the CT scan alone. On **d** (same slice as **c** with different window settings) however, the factors utilized were a window level of 22 and a window width of 400. These show that the high densities under the area of the inner table of the skull are, in fact, much higher in attenuation values (still in peak white) and therefore represent bony fragments rather than blood. The air collection is recognized in addition; note that the air now appears much darker than the fluid in the frontal horns of the lateral ventricles – this is also due to the use of an expanded window width

but also in mucosal ingrowth into the anterior fossa. Fracture of the frontal sinus is unusual in children [76, 100]. The frontal sinus may start to develop as early as 2 years of life, but the frontal sinus seldom reaches clinical significance until the age of 10. It does not reach adult size until the age of 16. With fractures involving the nasofrontal duct, later development of mucocele or pyocele may develop. Therefore, roentgenographic examination, including tomography, should enable evaluation of the area of the nasofrontal duct, as well as the posterior table of the frontal sinus since treatment depends on whether or not these structures are involved [76, 100].

Fracture with pneumocephalus [5, 78] can occur in childhood but it is uncommon. Fracture associated with pneumocephalus usually involves the paranasal sinuses or mastoids, but fractures associated with a laceration involving the entire thickness of the cranial vault may permit air to enter the intracranial compartment. Air may be found within the subarachnoid, subdural, or extradural spaces or within the brain or ventricular system [16] (Figs. 3.8, 3.9, 3.10).

Pneumocephalus may be readily detected by plain skull films but very small amounts of intracranial air may be detected only by CT (Fig. 3.9). In the majority of cases, the air is absorbed with time. If pneumocephalus persists (indicating a persistent CSF leak), further investigation is warranted with the intention of surgically repairing the defect. Surgical repair is aimed at preventing the complication of meningitis.

3.2.3 Depressed Skull Fractures

3.2.3.1 General Comments

In a series of childhood skull fractures studied by Harwood-Nash et al. [40] it was shown that depressed fractures most commonly involve the parietal bones (Fig. 3.11). Underlying dural tears are fairly common in children, occurring in 33% of depressed fractures. On the other hand, extradural hematomas (3%) and subdural hematomas (1%) are uncommon major complications. Brain abscess or meningitis may complicate compound depressed fractures as well as fractures of the base that involve the paranasal sinuses [95].

Nowadays, it may be easy to miss minor depressions in the contour of the skull underlying large masses of scalp hair on physical examination. Therefore, if a depressed skull fracture is suspected, careful manipulation and examination of the whole head should be carried out by the clinician. Depressed skull fractures beneath scalp lacerations may be undetected clinically but require debridement in order to prevent infection [95]. Depressed fractures of the skull will require X-ray examination to allow the operating surgeon to determine the extent of the fracture and the depth to which the fracture fragments have penetrated the brain [42].

In general, it is thought that if a fracture is depressed less than 5.0 mm surgical elevation is not necessary. On the other hand, if a fracture is depressed more than 10.0 mm, elevation is indicated. Those fractures that are depressed between 5.0 and 10.0 mm may or may not need surgical attention. If a depressed fracture is open, it should ideally be elevated as soon as possible (in general within the first 6 h). A closed depressed fracture can be elevated within 1 to 2 days following the injury. However, once a fracture is 10 days to 2 weeks old, the bone tends to be difficult to elevate [42]. Elevation is thought to decrease the chance of further local injury to the brain, especially if a fragment has been driven through the dura. The so-called double-bone density on skull X-rays (Figs. 3.10, 3.11, 3.12) indicates that one thickness of bone has come to lie beneath another thickness of bone. In general, this would tend to indicate that the fracture is significantly depressed, and therefore requires surgical elevation. If there is any doubt as to the extent of the depression, tangential views (Fig. 3.11) and possibly tomography, may be indicated for fuller delineation. CT may also be very effective (Fig. 3.10).

3.2.3.2 In Infancy

Depressed skull fractures may also occur in infants (Fig. 3.12). Gresham observes that many of these depressed fractures are seen in only one view of the skull so that multiple radiographic projections may be necessary to confirm the diagnosis [32].

Intrauterine depressed fractures of an infant's skull, unrelated to the birth process, may occur. Alexander and Davis [1] show one case of an infant's left parietal bone being depressed by the maternal sacral promontory in utero. They describe six infants with depressed skull fractures at birth and consider five of these to be caused by contact of the skull against the promontory of the maternal sacrum (including one case where the mother had sustained extensive pelvic trauma).

Localized depressions without actual break in the continuity of the bone may occur in infants (Fig. 3.12) and these may have to be elevated by a surgical procedure. It may be possible, however, to elevate such fractures by applying corrective pressure with

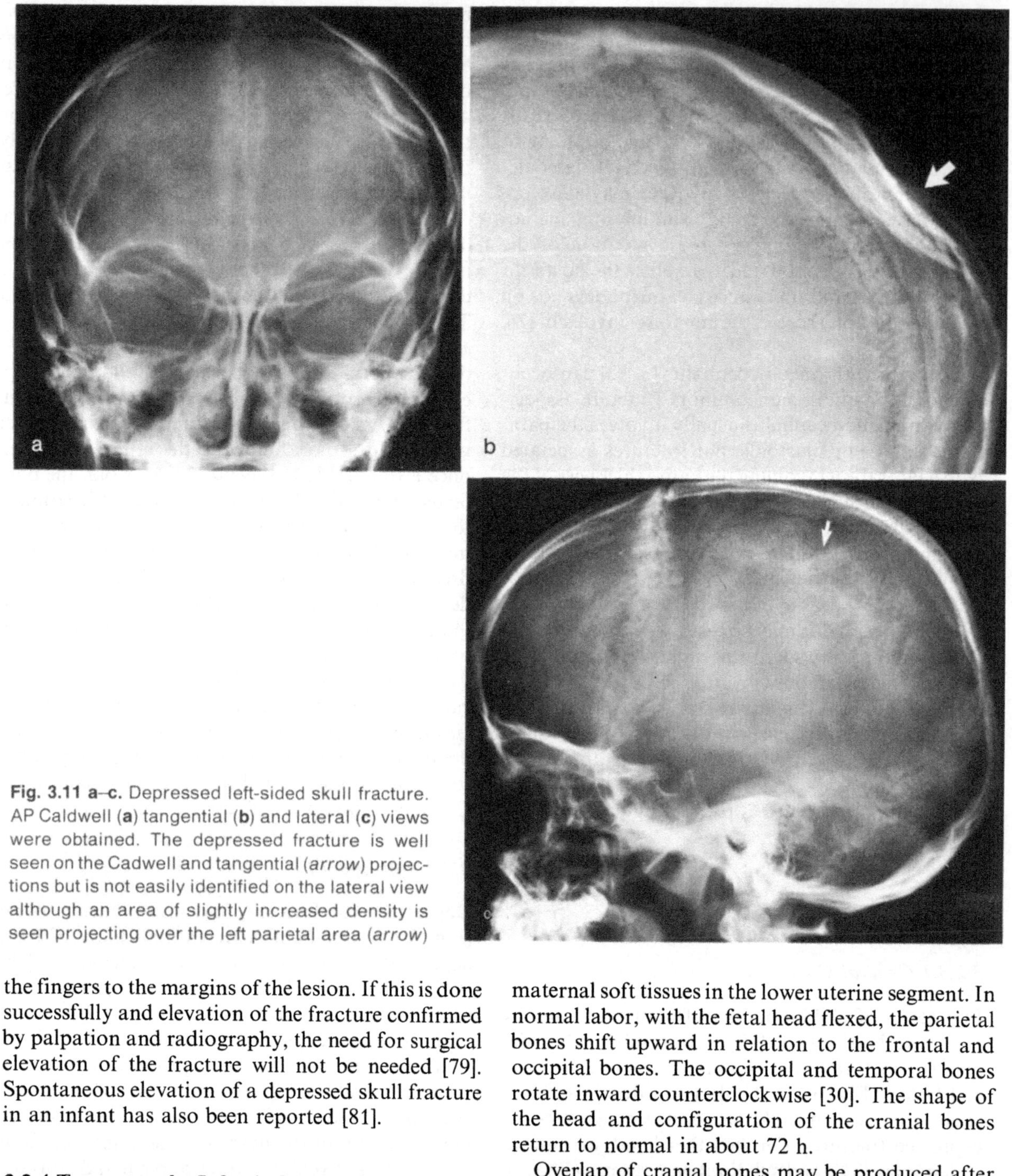

Fig. 3.11 a–c. Depressed left-sided skull fracture. AP Caldwell (**a**) tangential (**b**) and lateral (**c**) views were obtained. The depressed fracture is well seen on the Cadwell and tangential (*arrow*) projections but is not easily identified on the lateral view although an area of slightly increased density is seen projecting over the left parietal area (*arrow*)

the fingers to the margins of the lesion. If this is done successfully and elevation of the fracture confirmed by palpation and radiography, the need for surgical elevation of the fracture will not be needed [79]. Spontaneous elevation of a depressed skull fracture in an infant has also been reported [81].

3.2.4 Trauma to the Infant's Skull

Molding and cephalohematoma are discussed below; depressed skull fractures in infants were discussed in Sect. 3.2.3.2.

3.2.4.1 Molding

Molding occurring during "normal delivery" is the result of pressure exerted on the fetal head by the maternal soft tissues in the lower uterine segment. In normal labor, with the fetal head flexed, the parietal bones shift upward in relation to the frontal and occipital bones. The occipital and temporal bones rotate inward counterclockwise [30]. The shape of the head and configuration of the cranial bones return to normal in about 72 h.

Overlap of cranial bones may be produced after disappearance of initial molding when an infant is merely placed on its back with the head resting on the occiput [71]. This overlap is accentuated when the supine position of the head is prolonged (particularly on a firm surface) or when the head is immobilized by a compression band (or when dilated ventricles are drained.) In premature infants, lying supine for a prolonged period, the weight of the head tends to be supported by the occipital bone which

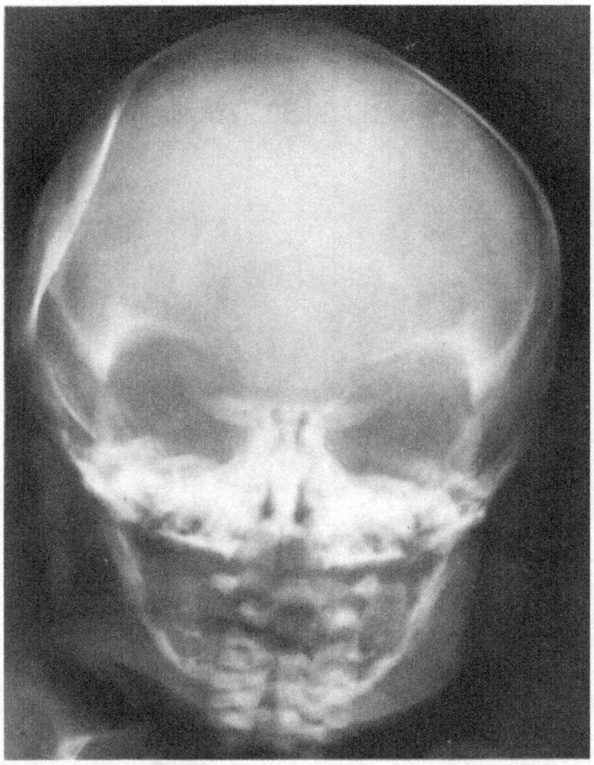

Fig. 3.12. Depressed "Ping-Pong ball" fracture. AP skull projection in a 1-day-old infant. Note the double density and alteration of skull contour produced by the right-sided depressed skull fracture

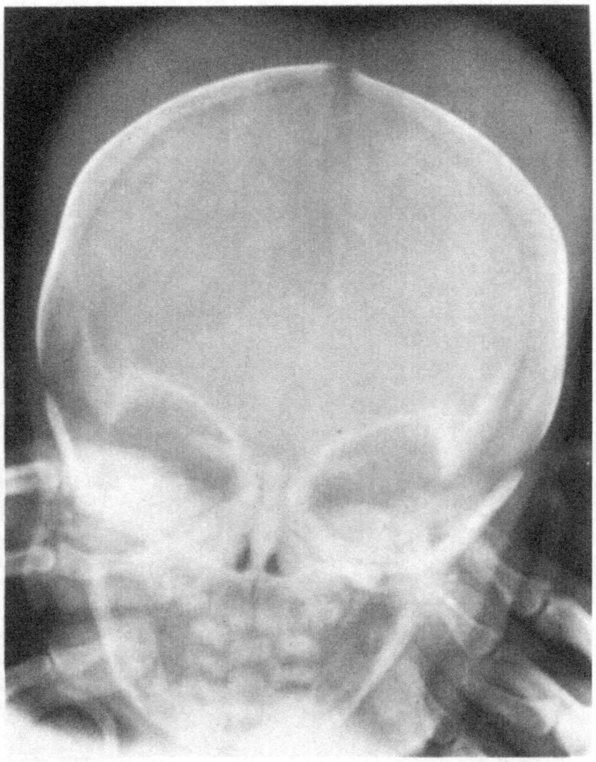

Fig. 3.13. Bilateral parietal cephalohematomas. An AP projection of an infant's skull shows mounds of soft tissue swelling over both parietal bones. The swelling is not as extensive over the sagittal suture. This feature is characteristic of cephalohematoma because parietal cephalohematomas do not cross the midline

moves inward relative to the parietal bone, resulting in parieto-occipital overlap. Newton and Gooding [71] have shown that when this overlap does occur, there may be compression of the superior sagittal sinus [71].

It is interesting that this overlap promptly disappears in most instances when the child's head is rotated to one side.

3.2.4.2 Cephalohematoma

Cephalohematoma may be defined as an encapsulated extravasation of blood between the periosteum (pericranium) and the external surface of one or more bones of the calvarium [9, 24]. Cephalohematoma is commonly observed in the newborn. Since the hematoma is subperiosteal and is limited by periosteal attachments, it does not extend across suture lines (Fig. 3.13). This characteristic clinically differentiates it from the more innocuous caput succedaneum, a benign, self-limited collection of fluid or blood in the loose subcutaneous tissues of the scalp which may extend over considerable areas of the skull, unlimited by the bony sutural margins [30] (Fig. 3.14).

Cephalohematomas may be unilateral or bilateral. They occur in 0.2% to 2.5% of all live deliveries [30, 32, 104].

Fractures associated with cephalohematomas are mainly found among infants delivered by forceps [30, 104] and also occur in breech and cesarean deliveries, but fractures are not likely to be present in children with cephalohematomas who have had normal spontaneous deliveries.

While there is a high incidence of skull fractures (18%) among infants with bilateral cephalohematomas, only 6 of 111 children (5.4%) had linear fractures underlying cephalohematomas in the series reported by Zelson et al. [104]. Zelson states that four of the six recognized skull fractures were in children delivered by forceps; one had a cesarean section, another had a breech extraction, but no fractures occurred in infants born by spontaneous normal delivery. The lower incidence of fractures, 5.4%, was considered to be related to the less frequent use of forceps delivery currently when

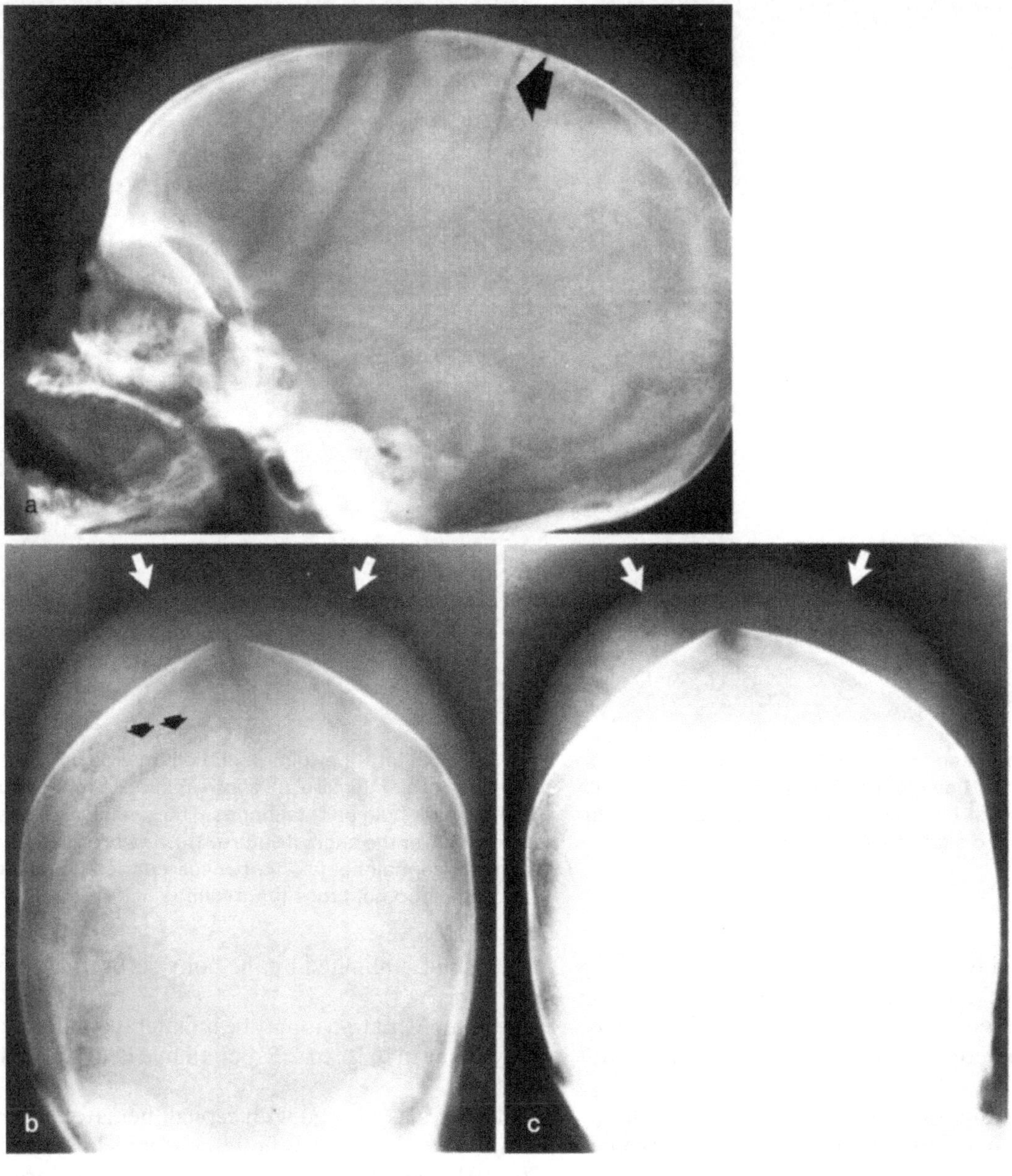

Fig. 3.14 a–c. Caput succedaneum. Lateral (**a**) and Towne (**b, c**) skull views. **c** is identical to **b** but is reprocessed to emphasize the scalp soft tissue swelling. Note that the soft tissue swelling extends uniformly over both parietal bones and above the level of the sagittal suture (*white arrows*). It is not restricted at the sagittal suture. This feature distinguishes this scalp swelling from cephalohematoma. Note also the underlying right parietal fracture (*black arrows*) in this 3-day-old infant (**a, b**)

compared with the more frequent use of forceps in earlier times and a fracture incidence of 25% [30, 104].

Radiographically, in cephalohematoma, soft tissue masses are seen on either side of the head; since the hematoma does not cross the sagittal suture, the radiographic appearance is characteristic and can be differentiated from caput succedaneum (Figs. 3.13, 3.14). The blood collections overlie the parietal bones in most cases but lesions overlying the occipital and frontal bones are observed occasionally.

Ten to fourteen days after cephalohematoma develops, a faint rim of periosteal calcification may be seen at its outer margins. The calcification can be seen as early as 2 days [41] and it gradually extends over the hematoma (Fig. 3.15).

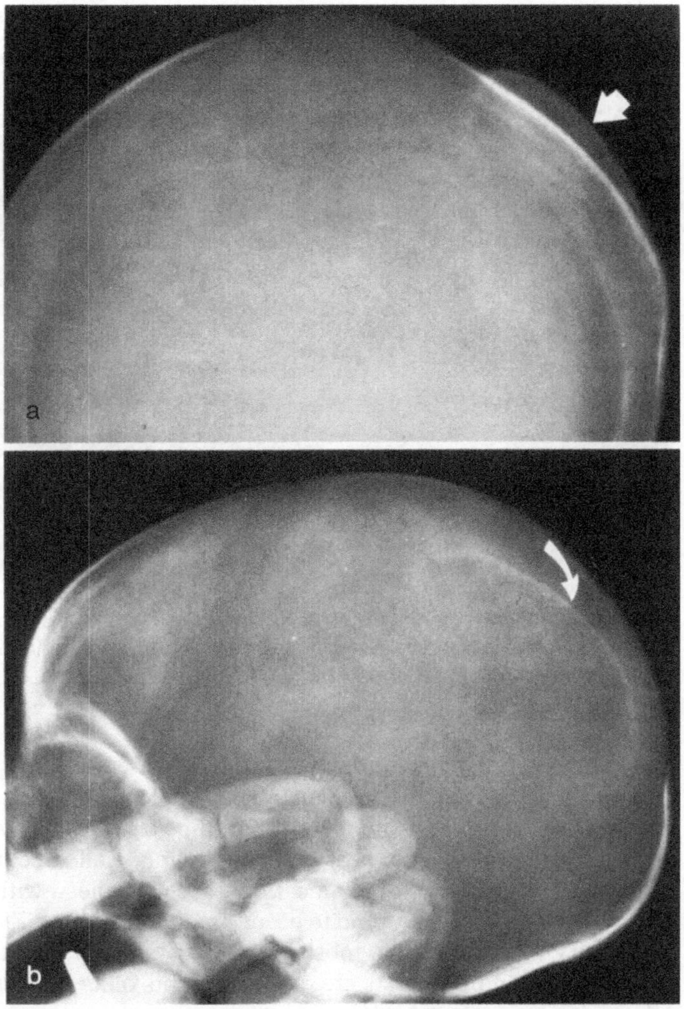

Fig. 3.15 a, b. Calcified cephalohematoma. Infant's skull, AP and lateral projections. In **a** (AP projection) note the curvilinear calcification (*arrow*) extending over the superior surface of the left-sided hematoma. In **b** a curvilinear calcification (*arrow*) is evident over the parietal bone on the lateral skull film

Resorption or shrinkage of the hematoma takes about 6 to 10 weeks depending upon its size but the radiographic signs persist much longer. The cephalohematoma may totally disappear; occasionally, however, there may be a residual area of hyperostosis involving the outer table of the skull. Sometimes a prominent lump may persist, appearing as a wide and thickened diploic space with irregular tables at the site of prior calcification and subsequent ossification. According to Caffey [9], the space between the new shell of bone and the inner table, in some cases remains widened for many years and the space originally occupied by the hematoma becomes filled with normal diploic bone. In other cases, large and small cystlike defects persist at the sites of cephalohematomas for months and years [9].

3.2.5 Enlarging Skull Fractures

Enlargement or growth of a skull fracture is a traumatic sequel seen primarily in children [30, 33, 36, 53, 82]. Enlarging skull fractures may be associated with underlying abnormalities of the dura, brain, and vessels. Such a fracture has been most commonly attributed to leptomeningeal cyst formation. Other causes such as herniation of the brain through the bony defect and porencephaly have, however, been reported. Surgical correction of the bony defect and underlying lesion is generally required but Rothman et al. [82] have observed one case of spontaneous healing of growing skull fracture.

A leptomeningeal cyst is a possible complication of skull fracture (Fig. 3.16). When the dura underlying a fracture is torn, herniation of the arachnoid into the area of the fracture may result. Fluid then collects under the arachnoid, adhesions develop, and a leptomeningeal cyst is formed. Pulsations from the underlying brain exert pressure on the developing cyst and the width of the fracture increases to a sizeable bony defect. This process of growing skull fracture may be rapid and take as little as 6 weeks, although in other cases development

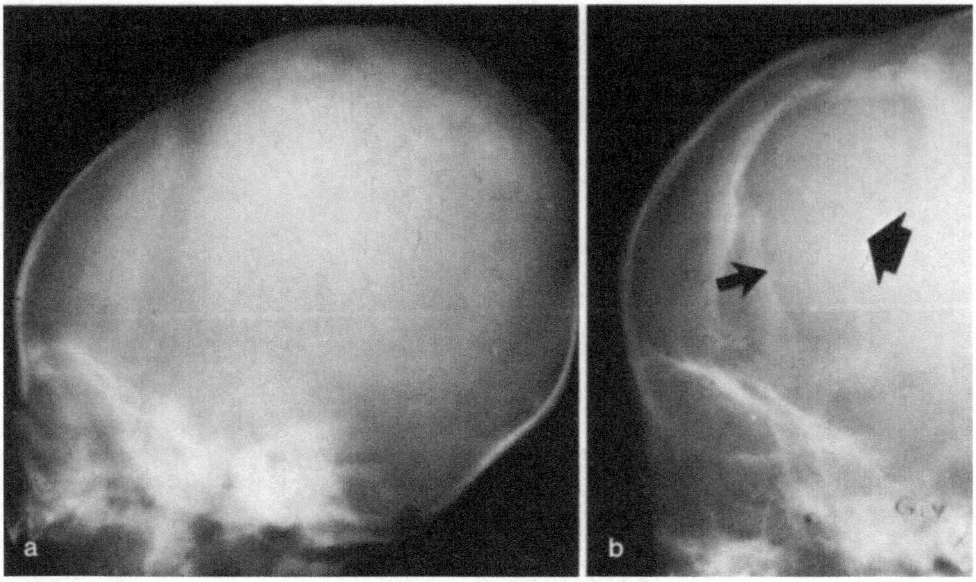

Fig. 3.16 a, b. Leptomeningeal cyst. A lateral skull film (**a**) shows a diastatic fracture involving the coronal suture in a 1-day-old infant. *b*, also a lateral projection, obtained 5 months later, shows enlargement of the fracture resulting in a large bony defect (*arrows*). (Films courtesy of Fred A. Lee, MD)

may take place over a number of years. Most cases of leptomeningeal cysts are in the parietal bone, which is also the commonest site for ordinary linear skull fractures. However, it is possible for growing skull fractures to occur in other locations such as the occipital bone [43]. They tend to occur predominantly in very young children, most by under 3 years of age. Leptomeningeal cysts are rare in patients older than 3 years of age [36]. Front, however, has reported a number of cases above this age group [49].

Some have suggested that children with skull fractures should be followed by clinical and radiological evaluation 4–6 weeks after injury and then 3, and possibly 4 months after the original trauma [82]. It seems difficult to justify this practice as growing fractures are very infrequent and more often than not brought to the clinician's attention by the family who have noted an increasing pulsatile mass at the site of a previous fracture. Palpation alone is frequently all that is needed to determine if a significant growing fracture has developed.

It generally takes 4 months or longer for roentgenographically demonstrable bone erosions to occur, but widening of the fracture line may occur as early as 1 month following trauma, as demonstrated in a reported case of a 1-year-old patient [36].

A leptomeningeal cyst should be suspected in a child who has a fluid collection under the scalp, which remains soft and compressible. This suggests a dural and arachnoidal tear with CSF leakage. For this reason, periodic observation and palpation of the scalp in the area of the injury is indicated. If a leptomeningeal cyst is to develop, it will generally do so within 4–6 months and the diagnosis can usually be made by roentgenograms taken at this time, without an earlier one for comparison [36].

The patient may be asymptomatic except for a soft, pulsating cranial defect, but headache may develop as well as neurological complications such as hemiparesis, hemiatrophy, epilepsy, or visual disturbance. Neurological sequels may be secondary to compression and atrophy of the underlying brain [86]. Low and Correll [56] report a case of very severe head pain associated with a leptomenigeal cyst; their case was unique in that the patient's only symptom, head pain, had not previously been recorded as a feature of leptomeningeal cyst. Lende [53] states that local cerebral injury is always present beneath the enlarging fracture and he indicates that as a result of this underlying trauma to the brain, local cerebral atrophy and formation of porencephalic cysts and focal ventricular dilatation may result. These findings may be demonstrated by CT.

The development of these changes is probably due to either compressed cortical vessels underneath the fracture (leading to cerebral infarction), or associated cerebral contusion or hematoma at the time of fracture [82]. Pseudoaneurysm formation underneath the fracture site may occur and may be shown at angiography [82].

Growing skull fracture is prone to develop when the original fracture is prominent (greater than 4.0

mm wide) [36]. Roentgenographically, the bone defect in growing skull fracture appears as an elongated area of lucency tapering at the ends of an old fracture. The margins of the growing fracture are usually scalloped and may be sclerotic. The margins may also turn outward. When leptomeningeal cyst is found, the repair of the dural tear is essential since it is through this tear that arachnoidal herniation and cyst formation result and provoke the development of enlargement of the fracture.

Leptomeningeal cysts are not true cysts since they communicate with the subarachnoid space. They usually do not fill with air at pneumoencephalography because of the many associated adhesions. Scinticisternography performed following intrathecal injection of radionuclide may show the cyst, which appears as an abnormal collection of radioactive tracer, best seen at 48 h when most other radioactivity has disappeared from the CSF spaces [29]. However, scinticisternography is not needed for diagnosis since plain X-rays and clinical findings are, in general, sufficient.

Tenner and Stein [96] have reported on another cause of growing skull fracture, cerebral herniation. Preoperative angiography made the diagnosis possible by showing the presence of cortical cerebral vessels that extended through the bony defect and beyond the outer table of the skull, giving evidence that brain had herniated. Two of the children in this report had neurological deficit related to the area of injury. At surgery, encephalomalacic brain without leptomeningeal cyst was found.

3.2.6 Roentgenographic Changes in Head Bangers

Head-banging is sometimes seen in normal children under 3 or 4 years of age, but head banging may persist until adulthood. Such adults are psychiatric patients or are mentally retarded.

Williams et al. [101] described radiographic skull features of children who are headbangers. The findings on skull films consist of scalp hematoma, "cauliflower ears," intraocular calcifications, calvarial thickening, and sutural diastasis; all are the result of self-inflicted abuse.

Fragmentation and calcification of the cartilage of the ear were also demonstrated roentgenographically on films of the cauliflower ear. Calcification of the eye in one case was the residue of panophthalmitis. Fractures directly attributable to head banging were not found, but sutural diastasis did occur. Thickening of the calvarium was believed to be due to repeated subperiosteal hemorrhage with resulting calcification. In these patients, a distinct layer of periosteal bone formation, not unlike the incompletely calcified cephalohematoma seen in newborns, was noted. In one instance, osteomyelitis of the calvarium resulted from secondary scalp infection in the series described by Williams [101].

3.2.7 Intracranial Foreign Bodies

It is convenient to classify intracranial foreign bodies in the section dealing with trauma involving the skull since most of them have indeed penetrated the bone of the skull. Occasionally, however, a foreign body can enter the cranium without piercing bone. We have, for example, seen a case where a metallic foreign body entered the intracranial compartment via the superior orbital fissure without producing a fracture (see Fig. 3.47).

Due to the thinness of the incompletely ossified pediatric skull, seemingly minor injuries may be associated with dural violation and brain injury. Penetrating wounds of the pediatric skull may occasionally result in gross impalement of the brain. This is particularly so in the instance of the orbital roof, which is quite thin and fragile [22].

Every effort should be made to locate foreign bodies or indriven intracerebal bone fragments since these can unquestionably be associated with delayed CNS abscess.

Intracranial penetration of certain objects may occur through the orbital roof. Entry through this site may occur with considerably less force than that required to cause significant injury elsewhere in the skull, due to fragility of the orbital roof. It may be difficult or impossible to detect on plain skull films the site of the bony dehiscense and the indriven foreign body may also be impossible to appreciate. Wooden pencils or sticks, for example, might not be seen on ordinary X-rays.

Many foreign bodies are metallic [37, 63] and are easily identified roentgenographically (Figs 3.47, 3.48). Every effort should be made to locate indriven intracerebral bone fragments or foreign bodies because of the threat of delayed CNS abscess. Sometimes, tomography may be useful in delineating indriven bone fragments [22].

Penetrating intracranial foreign bodies require prompt neurosurgical and ophthalmological attention. In addition to infection as a complication of intracranial foreign body, intracerebal hemorrhage, contusion, and major vessel injury may contribute to posttraumatic mortality. Carotid cavernous fistula, epilepsy, CSF rhinorrhea, ophthalmoplegia, pneumoencephalocele, and neurological deficit are all possible complications [22].

Persistent CSF drainage, when associated with a known anterior fossa fracture warrants surgical exploration and repair of the dural defect. A conservative policy is justified when the leakage is dubious or very transient and skull films show no fracture. Many neurosurgeons believe that every penetrating orbitocranial injury with a foreign body should undergo emergency craniotomy and exploration [22, 25].

3.3 Intracranial Hemorrhage and Cerebral Trauma

3.3.1 Fundamental Considerations

Since its introduction, CT has become the primary imaging modality used in children suffering from head trauma. Clearly, CT examinations of the head in traumatized children can be performed with great speed, particularly on scanners with fast slice times. Another advantage is well known: CT can be performed with unparalleled safety.

One problem with CT, however, is that motion can seriously degrade the images, and this is difficult to control when scanning trauma patients, particularly when scanners that require lengthy slice times are employed. Fortunately, however, it is usually possible to get quite an adequate examination of the child suffering from head trauma: often this can be accomplished satisfactorily without sedation, merely by keeping the patient comfortable and immobilizing when necessary. Sedation should be used sparingly; when it is needed to help control patient movement it can depress the patient and may impair assessment of neurological status as well. When sedatives are given, short-acting agents are preferable. A patient who is already on a respirator can be given a paralytic agent such as Pavulon (Pancuronium Bromide) to control movement and improve the CT examination.

One of the major reasons CT scanning is so helpful in head trauma patients is that it is possible to identify collections of blood in a manner previously not possible. Freshly extravasated blood can be readily discriminated, not only within the brain but also within the ventricles, the subarachnoid space, the subdural space or the extradural space. These blood collections are readily identified because they attenuate X-rays to a greater extent than normal cerebral tissue. New and Aronow [70] have shown that whole blood with a hematocrit of 45% has an attenuation value of 28 EMI units (old scale) which is greater than that for normal brain tissue. Thus, the"density" of blood is greater than the "density" of normal cerebral tissue.

Furthermore, New and Aronow have made the intresting observation that high attenuation values of blood are due largely to the protein fraction of hemoglobin, whereas the iron content contributes only 7%–8% of the attenuation. On the other hand, the attenuation contributed by calcium in serum or red blood cells is negligible. Because it lacks the essential hemoglobin elements, a platelet-fibrin thrombus (white clot) has only half the attenuation of a similarly retracted red blood clot.

In addition, it has been established that there is a linear relationship between hematocrit levels in the blood and radioattenuation. Theoretically, extravasated fresh blood at very low hemoglobin levels (i.e., extravasated blood with a hemoglobin concentration of approximately 9–11 g%) could be of the same density as the brain (i.e., "isodense") or even less dense.

CT provides excellent anatomical localization. Usually it is possible to localize clots accurately in various locations within the brain without difficulty. Extracerebral blood collections can usually be correctly identified as being subarachnoid, subdural, or extradural (Figs. 3.27, 3.28, 3.30, 3.32–3.38, 3.41–3.44). High density collections conforming to the ventricular system are readily identified as intraventricular hemorrhage (Figs. 3.9, 3.26). While the diagnosis of intracranial hemorrhage can be made with great confidence by CT, there are pitfalls the neuroradiologist must avoid; for example, high density artifacts can occur and simulate acute intracranial hemorrhage (for example, Fig. 3.18).

It is possible for a partially calcified lesion to have a density that is within the blood range and thus confuse a homogeneous area of partial calcification with an area of hemorrhage. Usually, the clinical data as well as accessory findings on CT will enable differentiation. While dual-kilovoltage studies can be undertaken to help differentiate calcification from blood, it is usually possible to resolve the matter by obtaining follow-up CT scans at a later date. Sequential CT studies will show no change in the appearance of the calcified lesion or structure whereas the blood density will subside with time.

A very small clot can be missed by CT because of the "partial volume effect"; fortunately, such a tiny lesion has little surgical import as a rule. The higher density of a tiny clot averaged in with adjacent normal brain can result in an isodense area on the CT scan.

When there has been intracranial hemorrhage the possibility of a primary underlying aneurysm, arteriovenous malformation or even neoplasm, must be considered. Such a primary lesion may bleed intracranially, thereby precipitating the event which leads to head injury. This sequence of events is more common in adults but could happen in childhood and adolescence.

When bleeding has occurred and there is not a clear-cut history of trauma, skull films will occasionally reveal the presence of fracture, providing evidence for the previously unsuspected head trauma.

With CT, not only is it possible to identify intracranial hemorrhage in head trauma, but other alterations in density resulting from trauma can also be identified. Mass effect resulting from trauma and the changes of herniation may also be readily appreciated on CT scans in patients with head injuries [74, 91].

The earliest sign of descending tentorial herniation on CT [91] is encroachment on the lateral aspect of the suprasellar cistern caused by medial herniation of the uncus. Seen next is widening of the ipsilateral crural, ambient, and lateral pontine cisterns. This is usually associated with brainstem rotation. (The direction of rotation depends on whether uncal or posterior hippocampal hernia predominates.) With more advanced herniation, effacement of cisternal spaces at the tentorial level is evident.

When herniation is sufficiently severe, partial hydrocephalus results, with contralateral widening of the temporal horn, which is shielded by midline bony structures, and atrium and occipital horn, which are shielded by the posterior falx. Hydrocephalus involving portions of the ventricular system not directly exposed to mass compression is believed to be due to obstruction at the aqueductal level [91].

Infarction in the posterior cerebal distribution resulting from herniation may be appreciated by CT. Infarction is secondary to kinking of a depressed ipsilateral posterior cerebral artery over the free margin of the tentorial hiatus [91].

Intravenously injected contrast materials may be useful in the CT evaluation of head trauma [97], contrary of the earliest reports on the use of CT in head trauma. Contrast medium injection is perhaps more useful in adults in whom isodense subdural hematomas seem to be more common. However, children occasionally can present with isodense subdural collections of blood, and contrast-enhanced CT will assist in the diagnosis (see Sect. 3.3.5). Contrast studies will also help delineate areas of cerebral contusion appearing isodense on non-contrast scans [97].

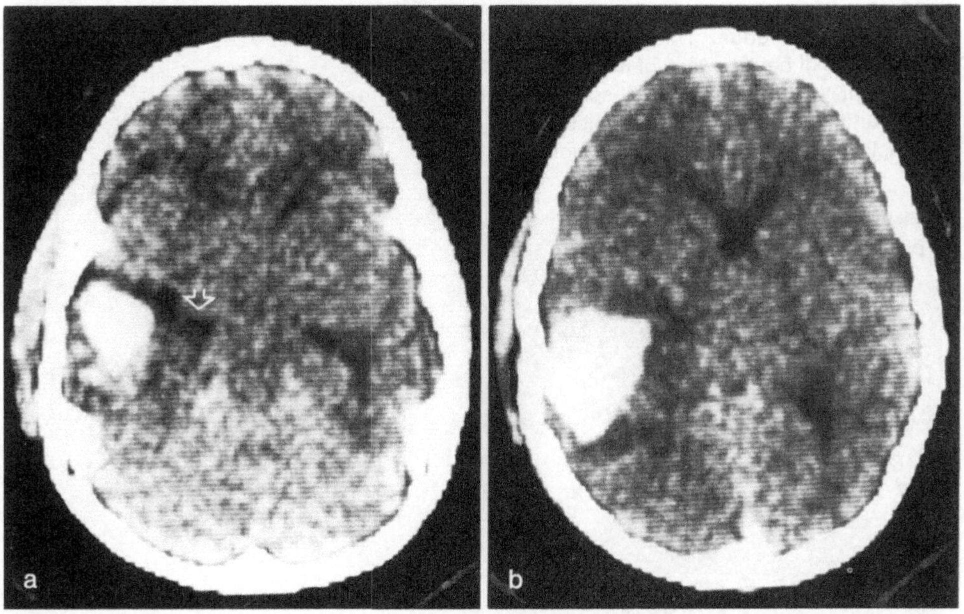

Fig. 3.17 a,b. Left temporal lobe hematoma. Note the high density lesion representing a hematoma with surrounding edema in the left temporal lobe shown by CT scans (**a, b**). Outside of the vault is a scalp hematoma. The left temporal lobe hematoma is shown to compress and displace the left temporal horn (*open arrow*) medially in **a**. The right temporal horn tip is also seen on the same slice. It is more generous than usual but has a perfectly normal configuration for comparison. There is also a left to right shift of the frontal horns and septum pellucidum (**b**). Because of the mass effect from the hematoma, the quadrigeminal cistern was obliterated. If one were to draw a line representing the sagittal diameter of the hematoma, its ends would be deep to the inner table of the skull (in contrast to extracerebral hematomas)

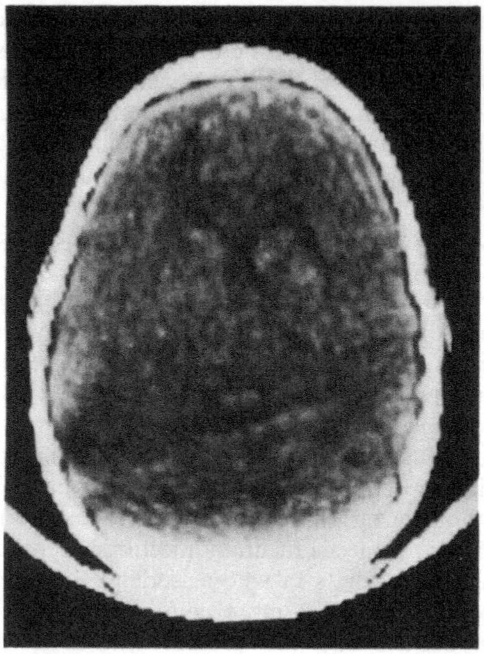

Fig. 3.18. Artifact simulating subdural hematoma. A CT scan shows an apparent high density area under the occipital bone. This is an artifact seen with the EMI CT 1010 scanner when the head is close to the margin of the gantry. This apparent high density zone simulating subdural hematoma was no longer seen when the head was placed more centrally within the scanning gantry and away from its edge. This example emphasizes the importance of being aware of the various artifacts which can occur with each individual scanner. Repetition of a slice under different circumstances may elimate an artifact whereas a pathological lesion will remain

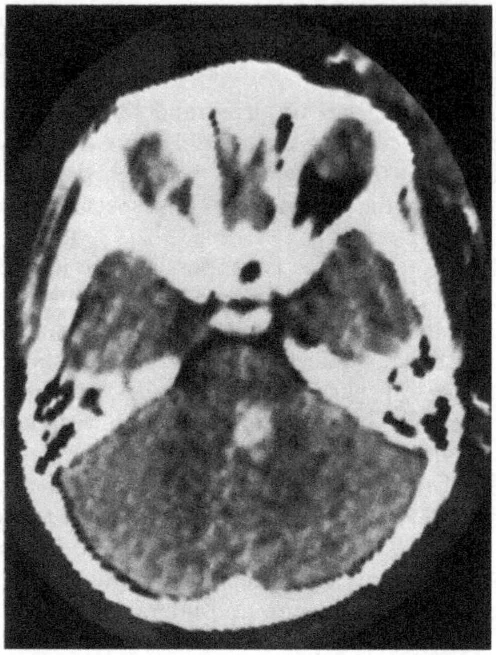

Fig. 3.19. Brainstem hematoma. A high density zone is seen within the posterior part of the pons following head trauma. Some surrounding lucency is seen. Due to the mass effect of the hematoma, the fourth ventricle is largely obliterated

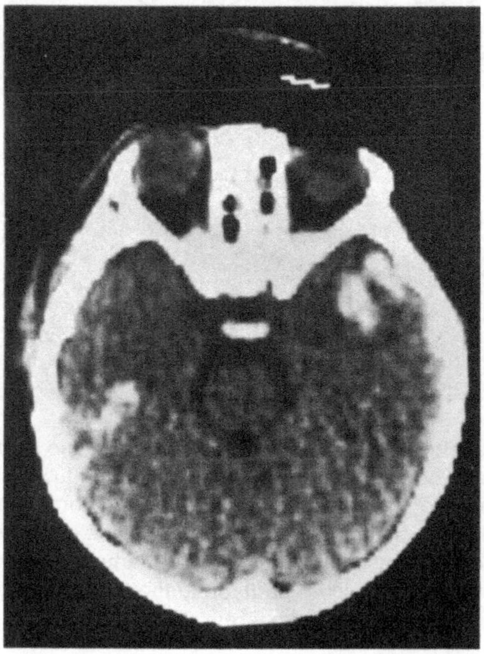

◁ **Fig. 3.20.** Contusional hemorrhages right temporal lobe tip. Two distinct high density foci representing blood are seen on a CT slice just behind the right greater sphenoid ridge. These high density foci come into contact anteriorly and there is a small area of surrounding lucency

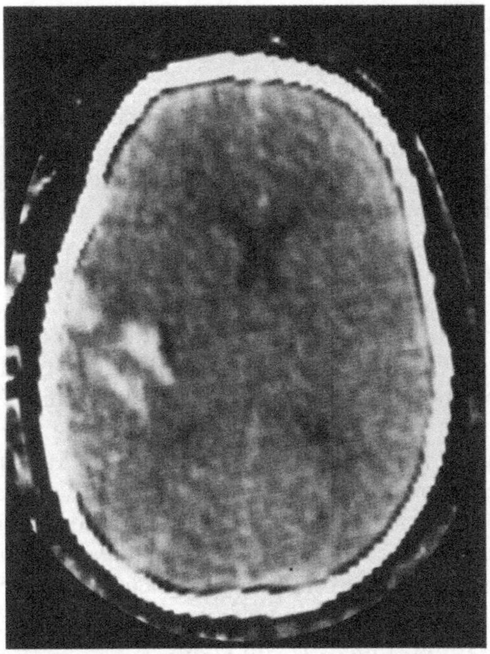

Fig. 3.21. Intracerebral hemorrhage. Note two linear areas and other foci of increased density within the brain representing posttraumatic hemorrhage. Note the surrounding cerebral lucency and mild left to right shift shown by CT

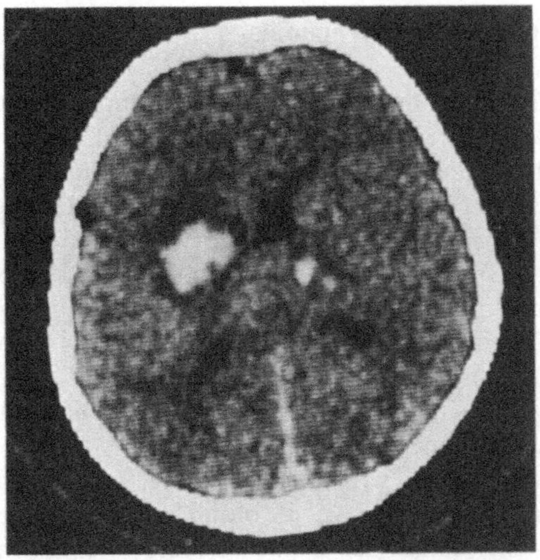

Fig. 3.22. Bilateral deep posttraumatic hematomas. Note the large high density hematoma in the left lenticular nucleus with surrounding edema. Two smaller contusional hemorrhages in the right thalamus are seen by CT. Lucency is seen around all hemorrhagic areas. Note also the compression of the left frontal horn associated with the left centrosylvian hematoma. This was a noncontrast scan in a small boy. The area of increased density in the interhemispheric fissure represents subarachnoid blood

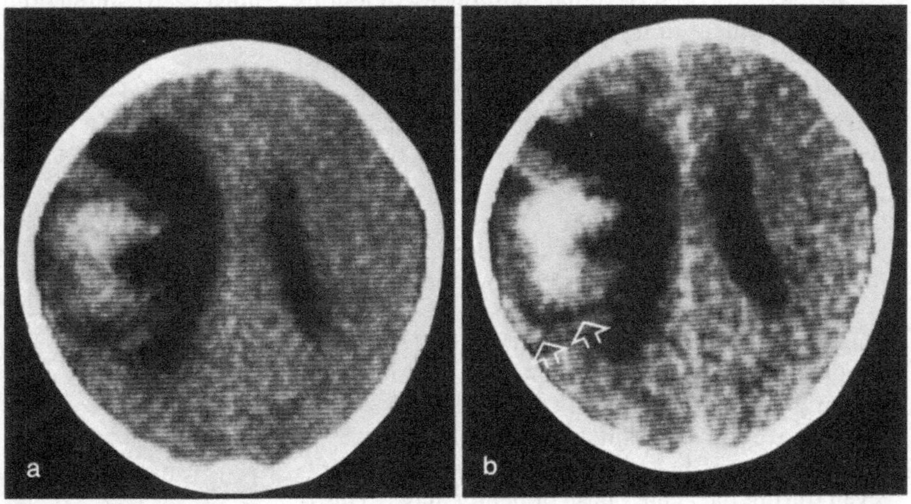

Fig. 3.23 a, b. Enhancement around intracerebral hematoma. CT scans were performed before (**a**) and after (**b**) intravenous contrast injection in a young child who sustained head injury 3 weeks prior to these scans. Earlier scans had shown a high density intracerebral hematoma. On the precontrast scans (**a**) a high density area with some surrounding lucency is seen adjacent to the left lateral ventricle representing intracerebral hemorrhage. Following intravenous contrast injection (**b**) enhancement is seen around the posterior margin of the intracerebral hematoma (*open arrows*)

3.3.2 Intracerebral Hematoma

Prior to the CT era, it was frequently impossible to make a definite diagnosis of intracerebral hematoma. Clearly, skull films in children with traumatic intracerebral hemorrhage provide no specific diagnostic information, although in two-thirds of the subjects a fracture can be found on skull films or on postmortem examination [40]. Even angiography in cases of hematoma usually shows only a mass lesion that is impossible to differentiate from other space-occupying lesions involving the brain such as contusion, abscess and neoplasm.

Now, however, with the availability of CT, it is quite easy to identify an acute blood collection which makes the diagnosis of intracerebral hematoma quite easy. Since surgery may be indicated for such a lesion but not for an area of cerebral edema on contusion, this is obviously of great importance.

Acute traumatic hematomas appear within the brain as areas of increased density which tend to be more irregular and poorly marginated than the usual "spontaneous" hemorrhage (Figs. 3.19, 3.21). French [28] attributes the fluffy margins of the traumatic hematomas to areas of confluence of smaller contusional hemorrhages with a larger area of major bleeding.

We have also observed that multiplicity of lesions is quite frequent in traumatic cerebral hemorrhage (Figs. 3.20, 3.21, 3.22). On the other hand, most spontaneous (nontraumatic) hemorrhages are solitary and do not tend to be scattered in various arreas within the brain as they do with the traumatic lesions.

New and Aronow [70] point out that serial scans of patients with intracerebral hemorrhages show that the attenuation values rise by approximately 7–14 EMI units in a very short time, consistent with the formation of clot and clot retraction. Thereafter, at a variable rate, there is progressive diminution of the original high absorption values. These investigators also point out that it is possible to have an isodense hemorrhage in a severely anemic patient, even during the acute phase of hemorrhage. This is because there is a linear relationship between attenuation values and hematocrit levels. Extravasated blood with a hemoglobin concentration of approximately 9–11 g% would have approximately the same attenuation value as normal brain tissue.

The area of increased density within a hematoma usually persists for 1–3 weeks, and in larger hemorrhages the high density may remain elevated even longer. The progressive reduction in density that is found in intracerebal hemorrhages is visible first at the periphery and then gradually moves centrally. Also, the progressive diminution of the originally high absorption proceeds at a variable rate, comparing one case with another.

Generally, one expects to find a halo of low absorption around a traumatic hematoma (Figs. 3.17, 3.22, 3.23), due to edema or to cerebral contusion. With time, this low density area may come to occupy a larger part of the area of abnormality with a decrease in volume of the dense component of the hematoma.

Eventually, areas within the hematoma may become isodense with normal brain. Ultimataly, the clot appears as an area of low density within the brain (Fig. 3.25). Usually, the density appears less dense than normal brain after about 4 weeks. One may be tempted to interpret the low density area as one of clot resorption with cystic residue, but delayed postmortem examinations on these patients nevertheless show residual "old" hematoma [65]. Thus, the low-density area seen on CT is not a fluid-filled cyst but, rather, is still a clot.

It may be very difficult to distinguish with CT a posttraumatic hematoma from hemorrhage into a neoplasm; blood density centrally, with surrounding lucency, can be present in both, and intravenous contrast cannot be relied upon to assist in the differentiation. Furthermore, the neuroradiologist must keep in mind (and so must the neuroclinican, of course) that, occasionally, trauma may result after

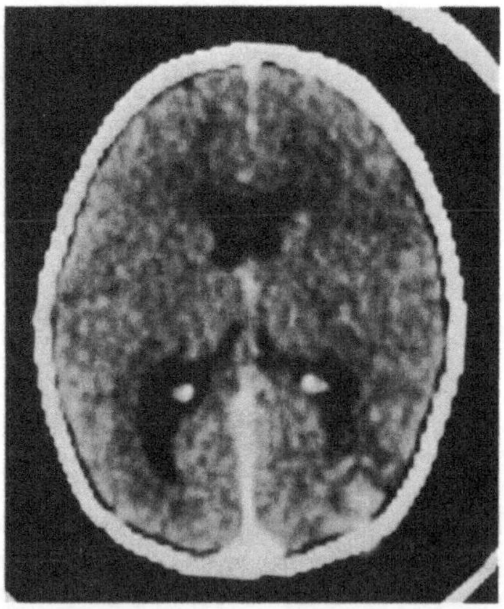

Fig. 3.24. Ring enhancement surrounding intracerebral hematoma. This is a postcontrast CT scan in a 9-month-old child with recent head trauma. Note the rounded high density area behind the right occipital horn representing a hematoma. This was seen on precontrast scans. On this postcontrast scan, a ring of enhancement is seen around the hematoma following intravenous injection of contrast material

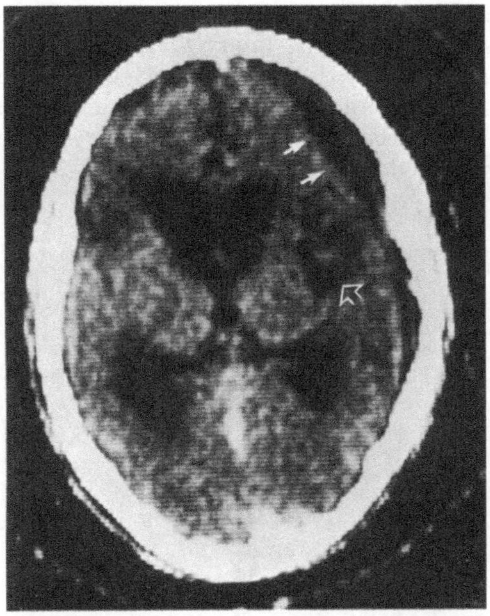

Fig. 3.25. Multiple posttraumatic changes shown by CT scanning. A low density area is seen in the opercular region on the right (*open white arrow*). This lucent area is a residue of a previous posttraumatic hematoma. Note also bilateral ventricular dilatation due to hydrocephalus. There is also a low density extracerebral zone on the right side representing a chronic subdural hematoma (*two closed white arrows*). Note the mild right to left shift of the ventricular system

the patient has suffered intracerebral hemorrhage from a berry aneurysm. A confusing sequence of events such as this, however, is more likely in adulthood (where the incidence of arterial aneurysm is greatest) than in childhood.

Usually, there is little difficulty in distinguishing a peripheral intracerebral hematoma from an extracerebral blood collection. The intracerebral hematoma tends to have its maximum diameter at some distance from the inner table of the skull (see Fig. 3.17) whereas a subdural or epidural hematoma's greatest linear dimension will have its edges in contact with the inner table of the skull (see Fig. 3.43). Cortical and subcortical hematomas could appear as a peripheral band of increased density which might simulate subdural, epidural, or subpial hemorrhages. A surrounding halo of edema on the medial aspect of the cortical and subcortical hematomas was originally believed to help differentiate these intra-axial blood collections from extracerebral hematomas [61]. However, it is possible for there to be cerebral contusion and edema underlying subdural and epidural hemorrhages, hence the presence of this area of lucency cannot always be relied upon for differentiation.

If patients with intracerebral hemorrhage are scanned some time after the traumatic event and if contrast enhancement is used, a ringlike area of enhancement circumscribing the area of hematoma may be seen (Figs. 3.23, 3.24). This ring first appears from 6 days to 6 weeks after the bleed and disappears roughly 2–6 months after the initial hemorrhage [52, 106]. This ringlike area of enhancement appears to be a characteristic reponse of the brain to the hemorrhage and should not be misinterpreted as being due to an underlying tumor or a complicating abscess.

Most intracranial hematomas will be identified on initial scans obtained following hospitalization for intracranial hemorrhage. However, occasionally, the occurrence of a hematoma may be delayed, appearing first days or weeks after the precipitating traumatic event. In the patient who deteriorates following head injury, delayed hemorrhage is one of the possibilities that should be kept in mind [28, 61, 94].

3.3.3 Intraventricular Hemorrhage

Intraventricular hemorrhage may occur following head trauma. It may also occur in newborns during delivery; it is more likely to happen when there is a difficult delivery. The appearance on CT is characteristic since high density blood is shown on scans conforming to the ventricular configuration (Figs. 3.9, 3.26). The location of the blood may shift with changes in the patient's head position. Fluid levels between blood and CSF are often apparent. Following an episode of trauma with intraventricular hemorrhage, the blood may be seen to clear rapidly from the ventricular system within a matter of days. Usually, blood is not apparent within the ventricular system by CT longer than 1 week following injury.

Usually, intraventricular hemorrhage is associated with other traumatic intracranial lesions such as intra- or extra-cerebral hemorrhage or cerebral contusion. Occasionally, however, traumatic intraventricular hemorrhage may be isolated without other lesions being found.

Ventricular enlargement may develop following intraventricular hemorrhage due to intraventricular or extraventricular obstruction of CSF flow. This may take place rapidly within a matter of hours, but may take weeks or months to develop. Ventricular enlargement seems to be more likely to develop following larger bleeds.

In traumatic intraventricular hemorrhage, scans obtained following contrast injection may demonstrate irregular subependymal enhacement. This indicates damage to the supependymal vessels with leakage of contrast into the areas. Patients with intraventricular hemorrhage and marginal enhancement have a worse prognosis than those without enhancement [97]. In general, with intraventricular hemorrhage the prognosis is poor. Obviously, as indicated in a preceding paragraph, many of these patients have additional injury to the brain. The prognosis, however, is not uniformly grim. Some patients do well following intraventricular hemorrhage; good recovery occurred in four of nine patients studied by French and Dublin [28].

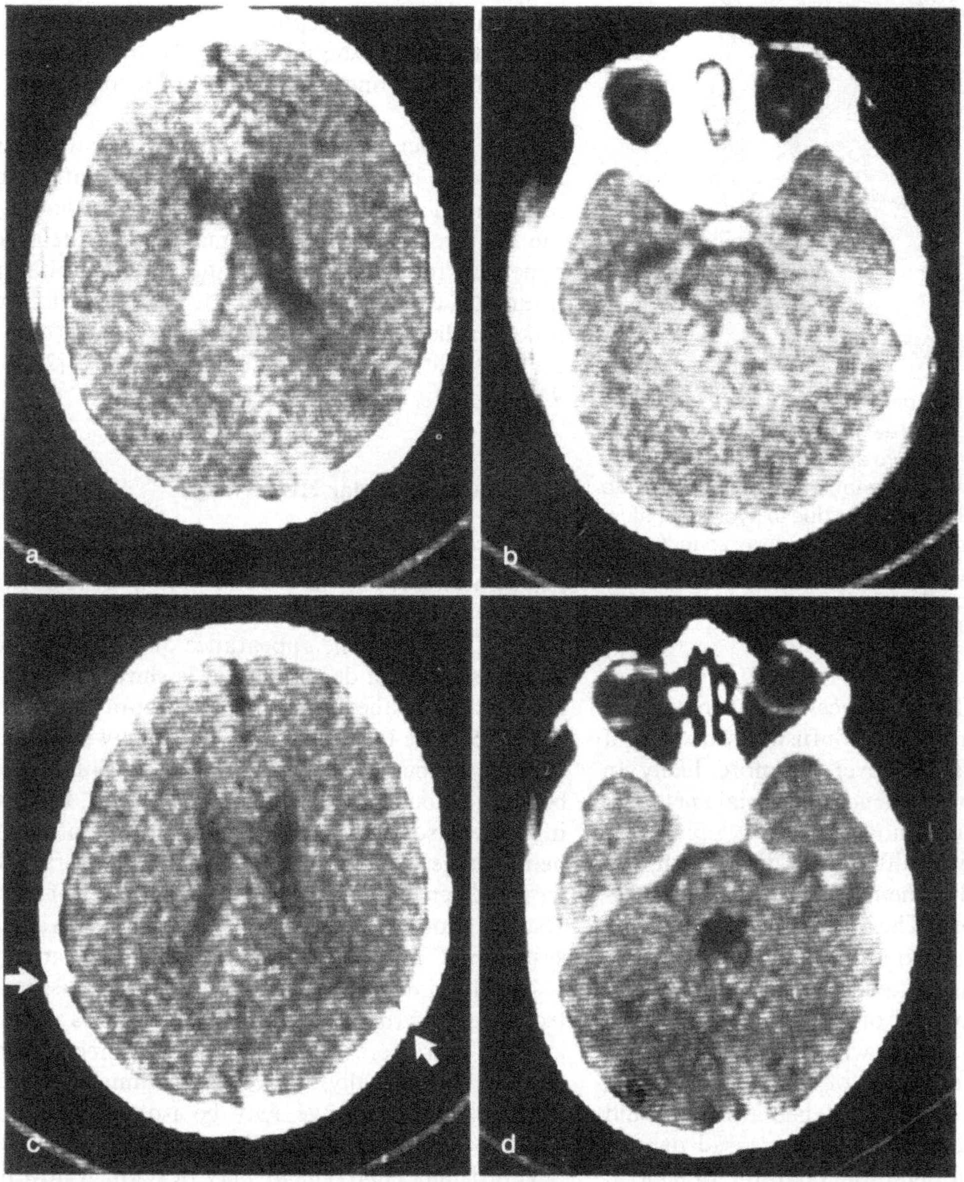

Fig. 3.26 a–d. Posttraumatic intraventricular hemorrhage. Blood is seen within the left lateral (**a**) and fourth ventricles (**b**). A left-sided scalp hematoma is also shown. Repeat scans 1 week later show no blood within lateral (**c**) or fourth ventricles (**d**) when **a** and **b** are compared with **c** and **d**. Note bilateral discontinuity of the parietal bones due to skull fractures (*white arrows*) on **c**

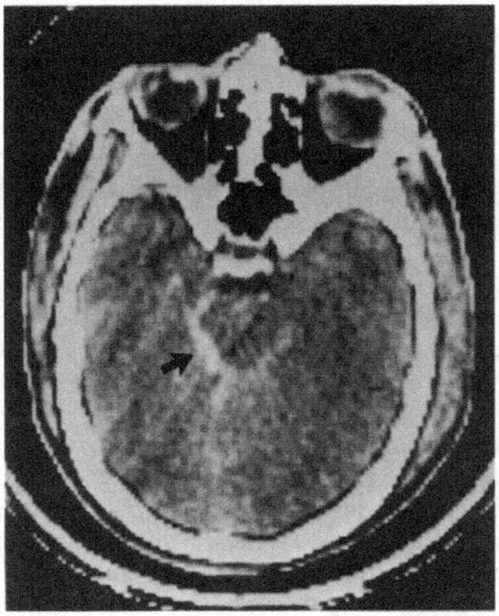

Fig. 3.27. Posttraumatic subarachnoid cisternal hemorrhage. Note the blood within the perimesencephalic cisterns, particularly pronounced on the left (*arrow*) on scans obtained shortly after head trauma

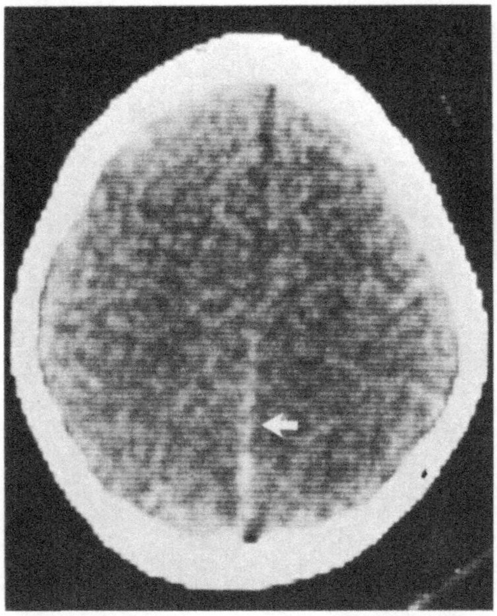

Fig. 3.28. Interhemispheric bleeding. A high density area representing blood in the subarachnoid space is seen posteriorly in the interhemispheric fissure (*aroww*). This is not uncommonly found in children after head trauma

3.3.4 Subarachnoid Hemorrhage

The CT appearance of subarachnoid hemorrhage is characteristic since blood conforms to the configuration of the cisternal spaces (Figs. 3.27, 3.28). When there is sufficient dilution of blood within the cisternal CSF, the basal cisterns may be rendered isodense with brain and, hence, will not be visualized on CT.

The finding of subarachnoid hemorrhage is quite frequent in severely head-injured children [19]. Bleeding into the interhemispheric fissure may produce a linear area of increased density (Fig. 3.28). This may have a similar appearance to falx calcification which we have seen occasionally in the pediatric age group. With time, differentiation is not difficult since the increased density produced by blood eventually disappears. However, in the initial phase after trauma, differentiation may be difficult by ordinary methods since numbers in the blood range can be produced by a dense (probably calcified) falx. A densely calcified falx with numerical values above the blood range, on the other hand, could easily be distinguished, but a densely calcified falx is quite uncommon in childhood.

3.3.5 Subdural Hematoma

In 1956, Norman [73] categorized the angiographic appearances of subdural hematomas into acute and chronic forms. The acute hematoma was described as being crescent-shaped whereas the avascular area in a chronic subdural hematoma was described as being lentiform or biconvex. This is frequently valid in the adult patient, but in children the appearance of chronic subdural hematoma is often quite different [34, 35]: the internal surface of the hematoma is often concave to the surface of the brain and very frequently it is bilateral (Fig. 3.29). Separation of vessels on the medial side of both hemispheres often occurs due to interhemispheric extension of blood. On occasion, however, even in childhood, a lentiform configuration to subdural hematoma may be recognized.

When CT is unavailable or inoperative, it still may be necessary to resort to cerebral angiography for a diagnosis of subdural hematoma. Even in a moderately uncooperative patient, it is generally possible to demonstrate displacement of cortical vessels inward from the skull's inner table. The injured patient, who is restless and moving even for intermittent periods, may be a difficult candidate for CT examination. The recognition of a small extracerebral collection (which, fortunately, is not as vital as the findings of a large one) in a patient who is

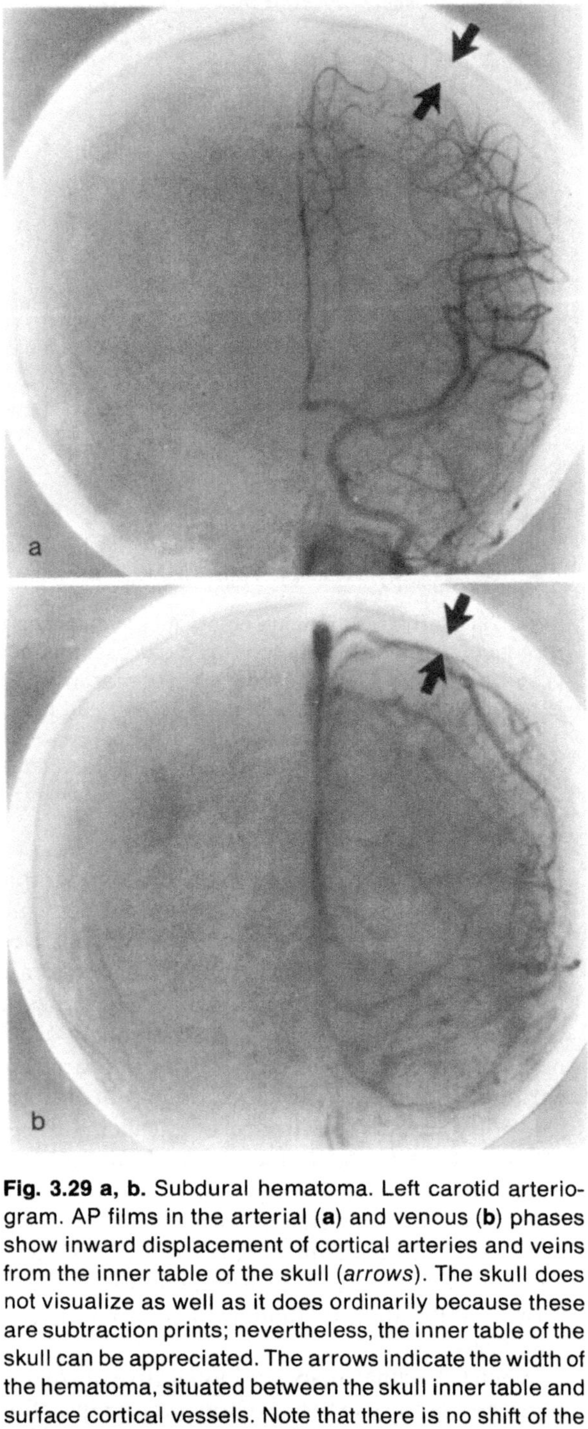

Fig. 3.29 a, b. Subdural hematoma. Left carotid arteriogram. AP films in the arterial (**a**) and venous (**b**) phases show inward displacement of cortical arteries and veins from the inner table of the skull (*arrows*). The skull does not visualize as well as it does ordinarily because these are subtraction prints; nevertheless, the inner table of the skull can be appreciated. The arrows indicate the width of the hematoma, situated between the skull inner table and surface cortical vessels. Note that there is no shift of the midline vessels because a subdural hematoma of similar size was found on the opposite side; thus the usually midline vessels remained in the midline

moving during a CT examination may be very difficult, if not impossible.

Despite this, CT is usually particularly valuable in the detection and delineation of subdural hematomas. In addition to showing the presence and size of hematomas in the subdural compartment, CT may be very useful in helping to estimate the age of the lesion.

It should be remembered that in addition to the extra-axial mass, involvement of the underlying brain may also result from the injury producing the subdural hematoma. One of the advantages of CT is that it is able to show alterations in density of the cerebral tissue from lesions such as hematomas and cerebral contusions for example. The presence of these lesions within the brain itself is of obvious significance in regard to the patient's clinical outcome.

Another advantage of CT is its ability to delineate ventricular size. Hydrocephalus may be found in children with subdural hematoma. Posterior fossa subdural hematoma may cause hydrocephalus by compressing the fourth ventricle [31]. This has been observed infrequently in newborns. Hydrocephalus associated with subdural hematoma, however, is much more frequently of the communicating type [11, 31].

In many cases of childhood subdural hematoma, a prior history of trauma may not be obtainable. Also, in certain bleeding diatheses such as in patients with hemophilia, the traumatic episode may be unrecognized or, in fact, the hematoma may have occurred relatively spontaneously. Because of the possibility of associated skeletal fractures in infants with post-traumatic subdural effusions, X-rays of the long bones should be taken in babies suspected of being battered [44, 89].

3.3.5.1 Timing and Density of Subdural Hematoma

The subdural hematoma is most frequently situated extracerebrally underneath the inner table of the skull. The collection can usually be readily recognized by CT due to its difference in density from the adjacent brain [92].

Subdural hematomas have been shown to lose their initial high attenuation coefficient after 2 or 3 weeks and tend to become less dense than brain after 4 weeks [88].

Scotti et al. divided subdural hematoma cases into three groups based on the time interval between trauma (or onset of symptoms) and date of CT scanning [88]. All acute subdural hematomas in the 0–7 day group were increased in density. Those in the 7–22 day interval were termed "subacute"; 70% of them were isodense. Those with an interval of more than 22 days were called "chronic." In 76% of the chronic variety, the hematomas were hypodense. In Scotti's series, one hematoma was found to be hyperdense, and two were hypodense in the subacute group; two hematomas were hyperdense and three isodense in the chronic group.

In some cases, an area of increased density within a low-density subdural fluid collection may be seen. This is usually interpreted as a recent bleed into an old subdural hematoma (Fig. 3.31). A "rebleed" may be homogeneously mixed with preexisting fluid, and this could result in an isodense collection.

The initial high density of the subdural hematoma usually persists for approximately 2–3 weeks. After about 2 weeks, subdural hematoma may be of mixed density (with areas of increased and decreased attenuation) or isodense.

French and Dublin [28] estimated the age of their isodense subdural collections to be between 2 and 6 weeks [28]. Davis et al. [17] observed that isodense subdurals usually occur 15–90 days after onset as well as in patients with marked anemia.

After about the 2nd month, the subdural hematoma is usually uniformly lucent [88].

CT can be misleading in evaluating the age of a subdural collection. It is not possible to distinguish an acute or subacute hygroma from a chronic subdural hematoma by the usual noncontrast CT scan. Subdural hygroma will always appear as a lucent extracerebral collection regardless of the time after injury [28]. Furthermore, recurrent bleeding into a chronic lesion will alter the density of that lesion (Fig. 3.31). Thus a collection of blood in a subdural space may have a density that is independent of the length of time from injury [28].

3.3.5.2 Acute Subdural Hematoma

The acute subdural hematoma has a high CT density. This initial high density may persist for approximately 2–3 weeks. Convexity subdural hematomas are situated under the inner table of the skull and have an internally concave inner margin (Figs. 3.30, 3.33–3.35). With window settings that include a narrow window width and a relatively low

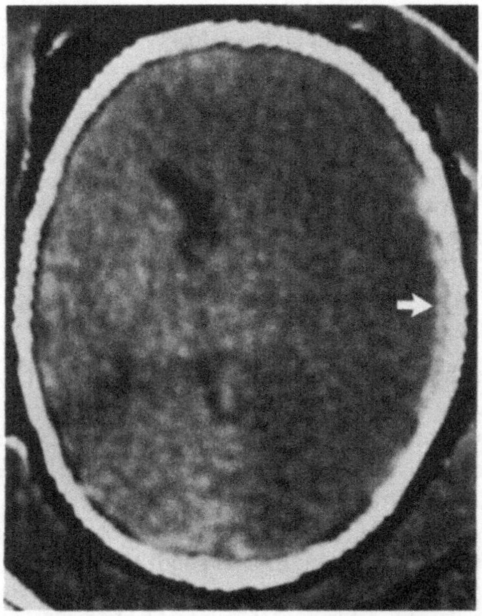

Fig. 3.30. Small acute right subdural hematoma with extensive cerebral edema involving the right hemisphere. Note the small high density area (*arrow*) immedialy beneath the inner table of the skull on CT. This represents a small acute right subdural hematoma (*arrow*). Note the marked low density area involving virtually the entire right hemisphere due to edema. Because of the cerebral swelling, there is fairly marked displacement of the frontal horns from right to left with compression of the right lateral ventricle. Note the difference in density between the right and left cerebrum due to low density right-sided edema

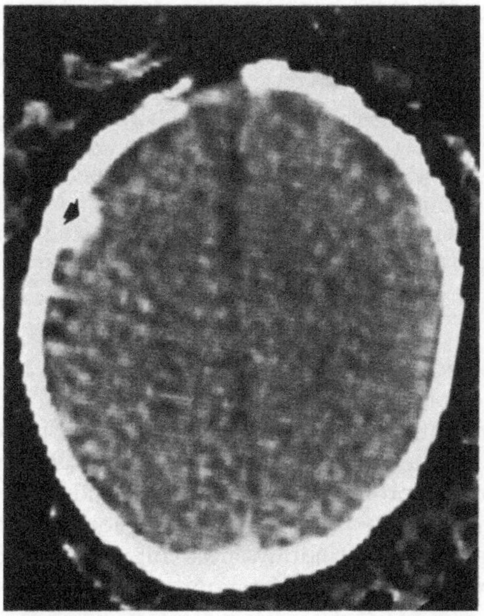

Fig. 3.31. Rebleeding into a left chronic subdural hematoma. In this infant, note the narrow low density areas under the frontal bones bilaterally, representing chronic subdural hematomas. On the left side, there is a focal high density collection (*arrow*) representing an acute rebleed into a chronic subdural hematoma

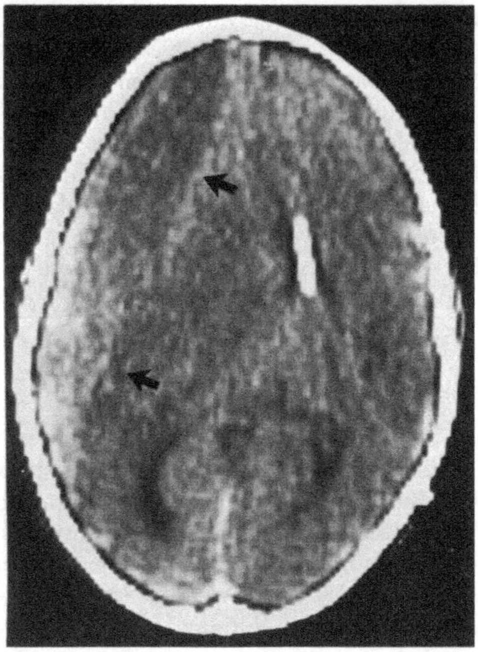

Fig. 3.32. Left subdural hematoma. Note that the large left subdural hematoma has different CT densities. At the upper portion of the hematoma, low density elements predominate so that the collection is lower in density (*upper arrow*) than the adjacent brain. The higher density elements are situated in the more dependent (posterior) portion of the collection (*lower arrow*). Between the high and low density zones the extracerebral collection is similiar in density to brain. Due to this subdural collection, note the marked left to right shift of the frontal horns. The tip of a (high density) shunt tube is noted in the region of the septum pellucidum between the frontal horns

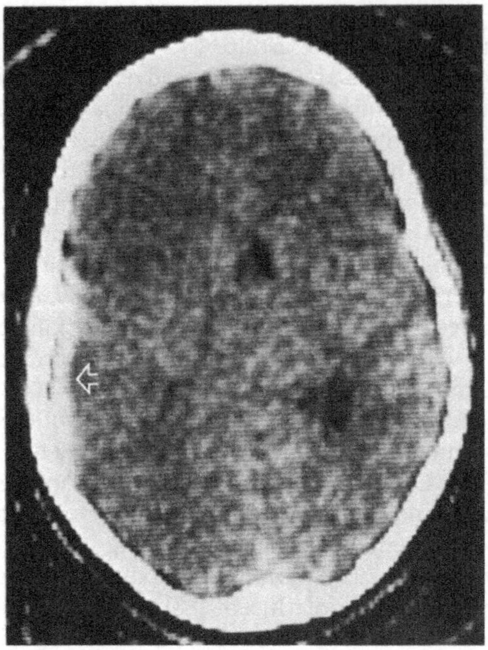

Fig. 3.33. Small high density acute subdural hematoma. Note under the inner table on the left side a high density acute subdural hematoma (*open arrow*). This CT slice was recorded at conventional window level and window width readings. Because of the use of the conventional window settings, the acute blood collection is similar in density to the adjacent bone. Therefore, collections such as this could be easily missed because of similar density and configuration compared to the overlying bone. Note the mild left to right shift of the frontal horns due to the small hematoma and associated cerebral swelling

window level,[2] the density of the hematoma may appear peak white, and similar in density to the overlying calvarium (Fig. 3.33). It is possible, therefore, to miss a small or even moderate-size subdural hematoma. For this reason, we recommend observing all acute trauma cases on the television monitor utilizing expanded window widths (Fig. 3.34) so that the density of an acute hematoma may be easily distinguished from the overlying denser calvarial bone.

Although the configuration of acute subdural hematoma usually consists of a concave inner margin, in some cases the lesion is lenticular, occasionally simulating an extradural hematoma. Not infrequently in childhood, subdural collections may extend into the interhemispheric fissure (Fig. 3.35). A wide blood density between the hemispheres indicates a subdural collection rather than subarachnoid blood which is ordinarily quite thin (cf Fig. 3.28 with Fig. 3.35). In childhood as well as in adults, most subdural hematomas are supratentorial although they occasionally may be infratentorial.

The sedimentation effect may be observed on CT, denser elements settling to the dependent portion of the hematoma with a less dense area of the hematoma seen above.

Arterial aneurysms are quite uncommon in childhood. Occasionally they can bleed into the subdural

---

[2] "Window width" refers to the range of attenuation values represented by the shades of gray between the extremes of the gray scale. Any value above the window width appears pictorially in peak white; anything below it appears in peak black. Thus, a narrow window width will have a smaller range of numerical absorption values between peak white and black, whereas a wide window will have a larger range of attenuation values.

The "window level" is the point on the numerical scale of attenuation values representing the center of the range occupied by the window width. Like the window width, the window level may be adjusted by machine controls.

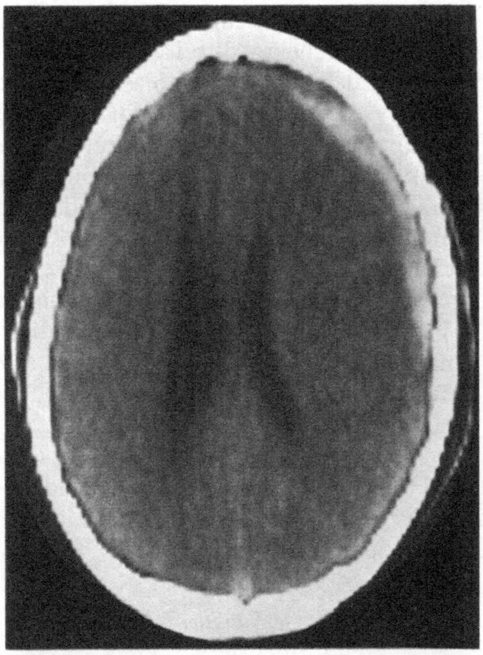

Fig. 3.34. Acute right subdural hematoma demonstrated, ▷ utilizing a wide window width. Note the crescentic collection shown in light gray under the inner table of the skull in the right frontal region. This lesion is greater in density than the adjacent brain (which appears in dark gray) but is less dense than the overlying bone which appears in peak white. This is because of the use of high window width. The window width used to obtain this picture is 200, the window level was 35. Utilizing these windows, it is easy to distinguish the acute blood collection from the higher density overlying bone

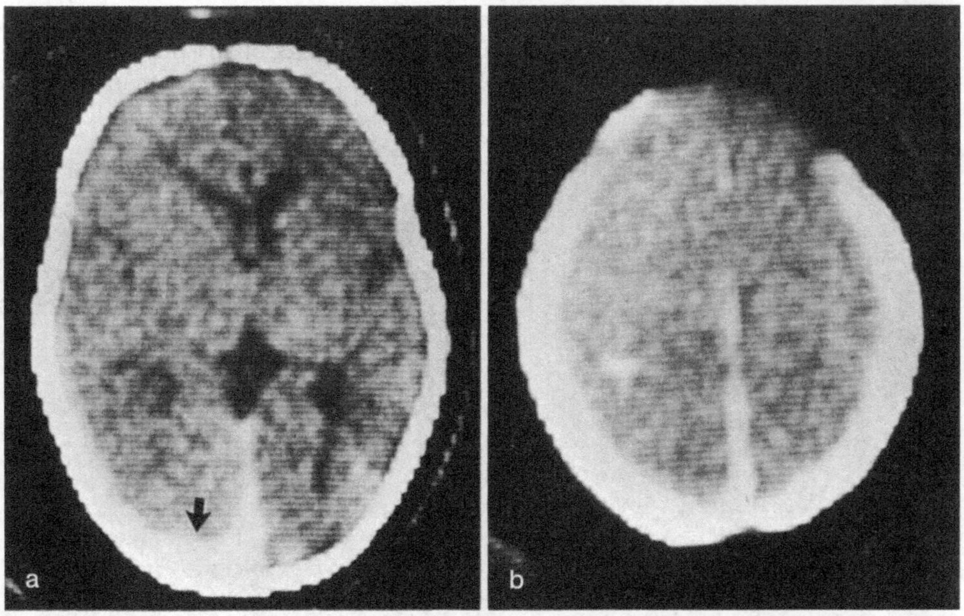

Fig. 3.35 a, b. Acute subdural hematoma overlying the left parietal and occipital lobes with extension into the interhemispheric fissure. The lower slice (**a**) shows the subdural hematoma (*arrow*) extending over the convexity on the left side. Its CT density is similar to that of overlying bone due to the use of conventional window widths. Note extension of the hematoma into the interhemispheric fissure adjacent to the falx on the left side. A CT slice obtained at a higher level (**b**) shows extension of the subdural hematoma into the interhemispheric fissure on the left side in this baby. It is greater in width than the interhemispheric subarachnoid hemorrhage depicted in Fig. 3.28

space and this bleeding can be appreciated by CT scanning. The subdural blood collection may be identified by CT but it may fail to delineate the aneurysm. Angiography, however, will generally confirm the presence of an aneurysm if there is one. It is wise, therefore, to keep in mind the possibility that subdural blood can be secondary to a bleeding aneurysm. Fortunately, this is most uncommon in childhood.

We do not yet have experience with coronal CT. This additional plane of visualization should be most useful, when time permits, in evaluating hematomas in certain locations, e. g., subtemporal hematomas.

Mass effect may occur secondary to acute subdural hematoma. Mass changes secondary to subdural collections will be discussed in greater detail in subsequent paragraphs.

3.3.5.3 Isodense Subdural Hematoma

Subdural hematomas having the same density as the adjacent brain [21] are not particularly common in childhood, but they can occur and must be recognized. As indicated above, isodense subdural hematomas are usually at least 2 weeks old and the isodense component of the hematoma may persist as long as 90 days.

When subdural hematomas are bilateral, there may be little in the way of midline shift. When unilateral, marked shift away from the side of the lesion will be apparent, particularly in larger lesions.

The use of intravenous contrast material has proved very helpful in the demonstration of an isodense subdural collection. Contrast enhancement may demonstrate the interface between the interior of the isodense subdural collection and the brain surface. It is well known from our earlier angiographic experience that cortical vessels may be displaced away from the inner table of the skull by a subdural collection. On CT, these cortical vessels will appear as a group of punctate areas of enhancement separated from the inner table of the skull but roughly parallel to it (Fig. 3.36). In other cases of isodense subdural collection, a curvilinear continuous line rather than punctate dots of enhancement may be seen on the inner surface of an isodense collection. This represents enhancement within subdural membranes [97].

The finding of enhancement on the interior surface of an isodense subdural collection has proved so reliable that angiography is now rarely required to

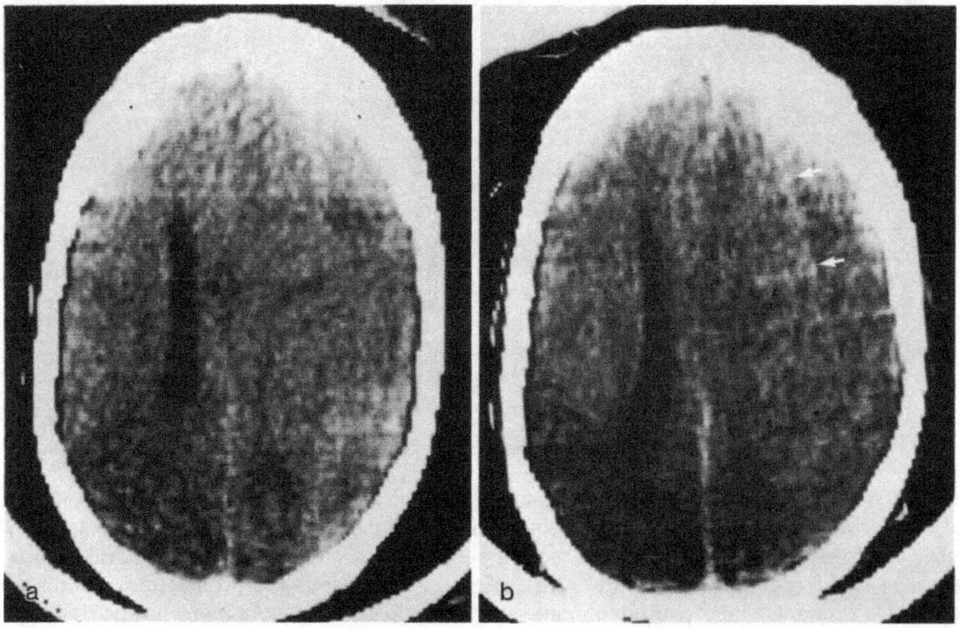

Fig. 3.36 a, b. Largely isodense subdural hematoma. Precontrast (**a**) and postcontrast (**b**) scans were obtained at the same level in this patient. The patient had a large subdural collection which was largely isodense in comparision with the adjacent brain. Precontrast scans (**a**) show compression of the right lateral ventricle and shift of the lateral ventricles from right to left. In most areas, the subdural hematoma is similar in density to the adjacent brain. Postcontrast scans (**b**) show the inward displacement of cortical vessels by the subdural collection (*arrows*). Several small dots seen following contrast injection may be correlated angiographically with vessels on the surface of the brain

show the extra-axial location of such a lesion. However, in order to appreciate these occasionally subtle areas of enhancement, a scanner with good resolution is required and the patient must be reasonably still during the course of the examination.

Messina has shown accumulation of contrast *within* isodense subdural hematoma on scans performed 4–6 h after the intravenous injection of contrast material. He suggested that delayed scans could be of value in such cases of subdural hematoma [64]. In our experience, however, the diagnosis of isodense subdural hematoma is virtually always possible on noncontrast and early postcontrast scans. Thus, it is not ordinarily necessary to obtain delayed scans in arriving at a diagnosis of extra-axial hematoma.

Möller and Ericson [66], in fact, have described a series of changes on *noncontrast* scans which should enable diagnosis of, or at least a strong suspicion of, an isodense subdural hematoma. An extracerebral hematoma must be suspected in any patient in whom a midline shift is found in the absence of changes in attenuation. In two-thirds of patients with an isodense subdural hematoma, a combination of three or four of the following signs may be found: (1) posterior displacement of the ipsilateral frontal horn, (2) anterior displacement of the ipsilateral choroid plexus glomus, (3) compression of the ipsilateral posterior and temporal horns, and (4) widening of the contralateral lateral ventricle. In subdural hematomas, herniation under the falx readily explains the posterior shift of the ipsilateral frontal horn as well as the anterior shift of the trigone.

In the series reported by Möller and Ericson, 12 patients had bilateral subdural hematomas. In these cases, the frontal horns were moderately compressed and displaced medially, and the lateral corners were angled.

The characteristic ventricular deformity seen in subdural hematomas is not encountered in other types of isoattenuating lesions. Most intracerebral lesions large enough to produce dislocation of the midline structures also produce local deformity of the ventricles. This is not seen in subdural hematomas. Möller and Ericson believe that the diagnosis of isoattenuating hematoma can be made on the basis of the characteristic ventricular deformity in 70%–80% of cases and that in these cases other diagnostic procedures are not necessary. In 20%–30% of isoattenuating subdural hematomas, the ventricular deformity is small and uncharacteristic. Most of these hematomas are small and there is little midline shift.

In the presence of subdural hematoma, the cortical sulci may fail to extend to the skull inner table ("amputated" sulci) or they may be compressed and obliterated. The sulci are frequently not visualized in childhood. Thus, they are infrequently of great diagnostic importance since, regardless, density changes are generally present with childhood subdural collections as well.

In some older hematomas, the more cellular (dependent) component of the hematoma may be isodense with a normal brain whereas the fluid (upper) component may appear lucent. Alteration in head position can result in a shift of the fluid and cellular components of the subdural collection; thus, a density gradient between the brain and the posterior portion of the hematoma may be revealed. In some other mixed density subdural collections, the presence of more recent bleeding may render the dependent portion hyperdense. Intermediate between this high density component and the upper fluid density zone may be an intermediate portion which is isodense (Fig. 3.32) compared with brain.

3.3.5.4 Chronic Subdural Hematoma

In childhood, chronic subdural hematomas [69, 77] are frequently bilateral. In fact, in 152 patients under the age of 2 years seen by Anderson [2], there were 141 bilateral chronic subdural hematomas, whereas only 11 were unilateral.

The fluid in a chronic subdural hematoma has low absorption values. Characteristically, hematomas older than 4 weeks become less dense than brain [88]. Thus, a low density subdural hematoma can be delineated without contrast enhancement (Figs. 3.37, 3.38). However, subdural membranes have been documented clinically within a week after bleeding into the subarachnoid space. The membrane thickness is related to the size and chronicity of the hematoma. The outer membrane is thicker than the usually diaphanous inner membrane which is distinct from the pia-arachnoid covering of the cerebrum. Since they are thin, it is extremely unlikely that inner membranes are constrictive as far as brain growth is concerned under usual circumstances [2]. Both inner and outer membranes are vascular and may contain hemosiderin. Enhancement within these membranes may be appreciated at CT.

Another type of enhancement may also be seen on the inner surface of subdural hematoma: punctate areas of enhancement along the internal surface of the subdural collection, most likely representing contrast within displaced cortical vessels. These areas of enhancement, however, are not as vital diagnostically as they are with isodense subdural hematomas since the extracerebral low density zones can be readily distinguished in chronic subdural hematoma.

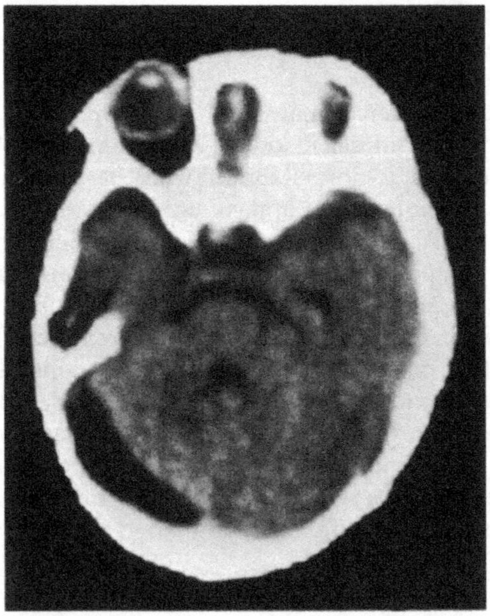

Fig. 3.37. Chronic posterior fossa subdural hematoma. Note the low density collection between the inner table of the skull and the left cerebellar hemisphere. It extends as far forward as the lateral portion of the left petrous bone. This chronic subdural hematoma was not sufficiently large to compress the fourth ventricle or to provide significant compromise of the pontine cistern

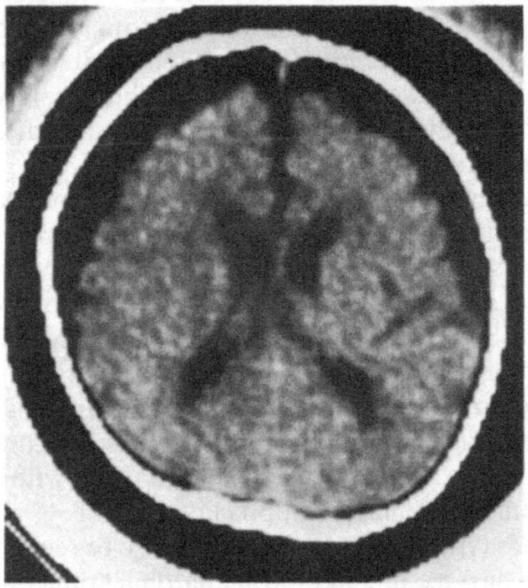

Fig. 3.38. Bilateral frontal chronic subdural hematomas. Note the bilateral low density extracerebral collections with some extension into the frontal interhemispheric fissure. This scan was obtained at the level of the bodies of the lateral ventricles in a small child

Occasionally, a high density area producing a vertical band at the outer aspect of the chronic subdural hematoma can be seen. This suggests a recurrent subdural hematoma superimposed on a chronic subdural (see also Fig. 3.31). French [28], in fact, shows a case with a low density extracerebral lesion 40 days after head injury; 60 days after that another band of increased density was superimposed on the low density area which indicated rebleeding into the subdural lesion at some period between the scans. Furthermore, an acute or recurrent hemorrhage may mix with the fluid within a chronic subdural hematoma and result in a lesion of uniformly increased density or may render it isodense at least in portions (see Fig. 3.32). Such rebleeds may lead to an increase in size of chronic subdural hematoma, but other causes have been proposed for this increase, including osmotic gradients and increased permeability of newly vascularized portions of outer membranes and adjacent dura (these are disputed mechanisms) [58, 59].

On CT examination, a number of conditions may simulate chronic subdural hematoma. Subdural hygromas (i. e., subdural collections of CSF which enter the subdural space through arachnoidal tears) have low attenuation coefficients and may simulate chronic subdural hematomas on CT. They do not, however, have enhancing membranes. The surgical diagnosis of subdural hygroma is not always easy but should be made when fluid is clear and no membrane formation is found. French and Dublin [28] report ten patients who developed lucent extracerebral collections as a delayed sequel of head injury; these proved to be subdural hygromas at surgery.

Subdural effusions secondary to meningitis (for example, those resulting from *Hemophilus influenzae* meningitis) are also low density collections seen relatively frequently in pediatric institutions.

Low absorption areas may also be seen in subdural empyema. Thick membrane enhancement (thicker than the usual subdural hematoma) is characteristic for subdural empyema.

Fluid in widened subarachnoid spaces may simulate chronic subdural hematoma. Widened sulci and, possibly, focal ventricular enlargement in that area will serve to differentiate atrophy from subdural hematoma. It should be mentioned that merely visualizing sulci underneath a fluid collection does not necessarily exclude chronic subdural hematoma. We have seen small subdural hematomas under which cortical sulci could be visualized by CT.

In children in the first 6 months of life, widened subarachnoid spaces which may simulate chronic subdural hematoma may be seen. Gyral immaturity may be the explanation for these fluid densities capping the frontal lobes. If the patient is placed prone, the frontal lobes may be seen to assume a position adjacent to the inner table of the skull and obliterating the widened subarachnoid spaces. Later, brain growth obliterates the subarachnoid fluid space.

Occasionally, calcification may occur within chronic subdural hematomas. This may be appreciated at CT and occasionally there will even be sufficient calcium to be evident on plain skull films (Fig. 3.39).

3.3.5.5 Skull Film in Subdural Hematoma

In older children in whom there is a calcified pineal, a shift away from the side of a unilateral hematoma (or the larger of bilateral hematomas) can be observed. Split sutures may also be seen with subdural hematoma as a reflection of increase in intracranial pressure.

Fractures obviously may occur in association with subdural hematomas but the incidence is surprisingly low. Only 9% to 15% of childhood subdural hematomas have associated skull fractures [40, 57]. According to Harwood-Nash et al. the incidence of fracture associated with subdural hematoma increases with age. Children in the first 6 months of life have an incidence of 7% for fractures with subdural hematomas [40]. In the 6- month to 2-year age group, 22% of children with subdural hematomas have fractures; in the 2- to 14-year age group, one-third have fractures [40].

The site of fracture is not reliable in determining the site of a subdural hematoma. In other words, a subdural hematoma may be on the opposite side of the head from a fracture. Of 24 posterior fossa

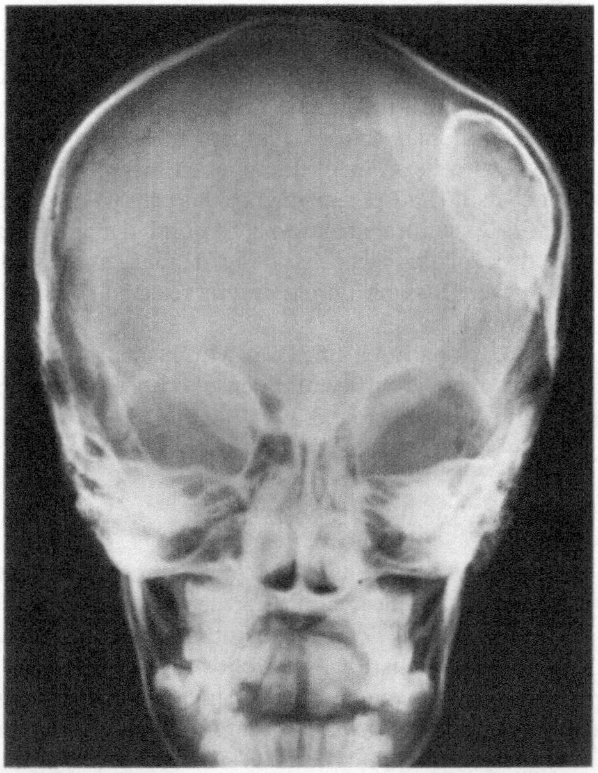

Fig. 3.39. Calcified subdural hematoma. Note the calcified subdural hematoma on the left side on this AP skull view. The overlying skull is thinned with focal depression of the calvarium

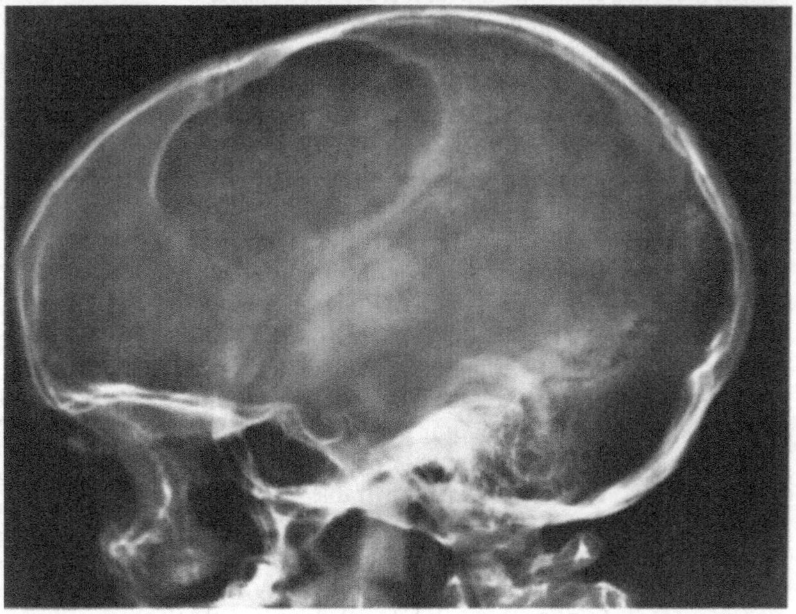

Fig. 3.40. Calvarial thinning due to chronic subdural hematoma. A lateral view of the skull shows a large area of calvarial thinning resulting from an underlying chronic subdural hematoma. A small epidural hematoma due to superimposed recent injury was also found under the defect at surgery in this boy. (Skull film courtesy of William Wright, MD)

subdural hematomas in Harwood-Nash's series, only one was associated with an occipital fracture [40]. Bilateral subdural hematomas occurred in 143 children but only six had bilateral fractures. A subdural hematoma was not uncommonly located contralateral to a fracture when one was present. Therefore, not only is subdural hematoma infrequently related to the presence of a fracture, but also the site of the fracture is not a reliable index to the location of the hematoma when there is one.

In association with chronic subdural hematoma, local bulging and thinning of the vault may occur (Fig. 3.40). In the middle fossa, a chronic subdural collection may cause enlargement of the middle fossa with elevation of the sphenoid wing. In infants and small children, megalencephaly may occur with chronic subdural hematoma – second in incidence to hydrocephalus as a cause of head enlargement [30] – and there may be a unilateral increase in the size of the vault.

Occasionally, calcification within subdural hematomas may be sufficiently dense to be seen on plain skull films [98] (Fig. 3.39).

3.3.6 Extradural Hematoma

As medical students, most of us were taught that there was a typical clinical presentation of epidural hematoma. This clinical picture included an initial state of unconsciousness following injury, with a subsequent lucent interval and increasing stupor and coma. In addition were ipsilateral dilated pupil and contralateral hemiparesis.

In fact, this classical clinical picture occurs in less than 10% of children with epidural hematoma [42]. The only common factors found throughout a series of extradural hematomas were those of a deepening level of unconsciousness and a dilated pupil, not necessarily on the side of the clot [42].

Skull films are used routinely in the evaluation of head-injured children, nevertheless a skull X-ray may be contraindicated in a rapidly deteriorating patient who may have an epidural hematoma. Furthermore, a fracture of the skull may not be present in a child with epidural hematoma; the reported incidence is variable, occurring in as few as one-quarter to nearly three-quarters of children with epidural hematoma, depending on the series [10, 40, 57]. Occasionally, a fracture may be appreciated at surgery but found not demonstrable on skull examination.

A number of posterior fossa epidural hematomas have also been reported without skull fracture [3]. Many skull fractures in childhood involve the occipital bone but less than 1% of occipital fractures are associated with epidural hematomas [4] (Fig. 3.42).

In those cases where skull films are positive, a fracture line may be seen to traverse the region of a meningeal groove, or a fracture may be seen crossing the transverse sinus in cases with posterior fossa clots. The commonest location of bleeding in extradural hematoma is the posterior branch of the middle meningeal artery. In such cases, the site of bleeding may not be detected by a burr hole placed only in the temporal region [18]. Bleeding may also come from the anterior meningeal branch of the middle meningeal artery. Other less comon sites are dural sinuses (superior sagittal sinus or lateral sinus) or veins in the dura. Occasionally, the bleeding site is not found.

Most epidural hematomas develop rapidly and are studied acutely, but at least one case in the literature demonstrates calcification within a chronic extradural hematoma. In this case, the skull films showing the calcification were obtained 10 months after injury [48].

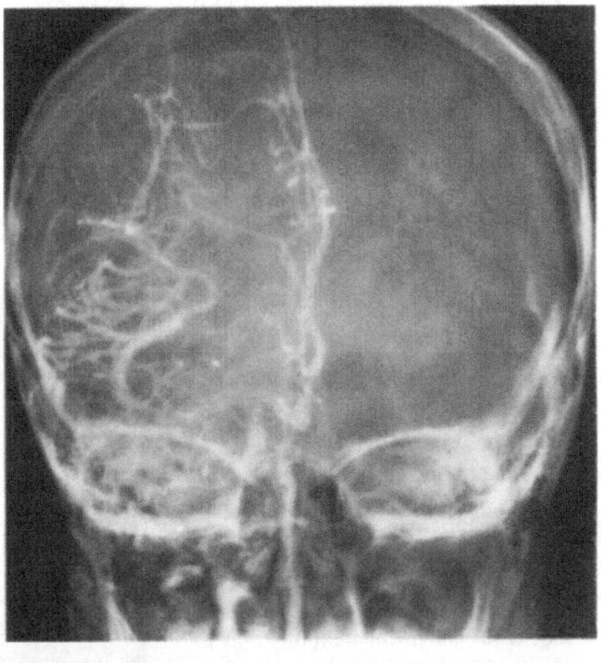

Fig. 3.41. Right epidural hematoma. AP angiogram during the arterial phase shows inward displacement of cortical branches of the right middle cerebral artery due to a lenticular extracerebral collection which proved to be an epidural hematoma at surgery. Note the inward displacement of the angiographic sylvian point and right to left shift of the anterior cerebral artery. The angiogram on this child was obtained in the era prior to computed tomography

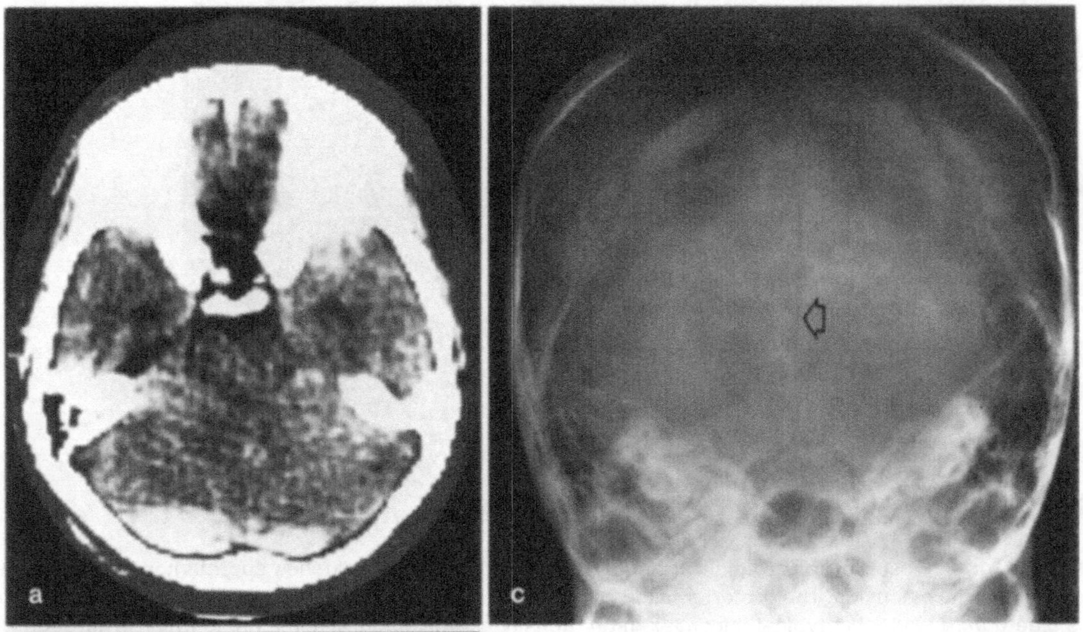

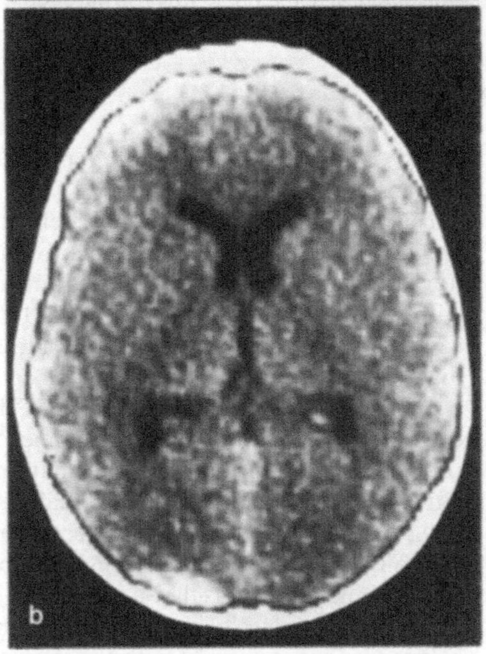

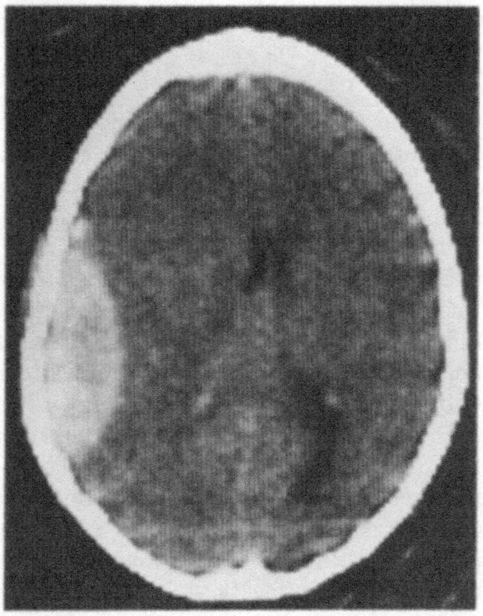

Fig. 3.42 a–c. Acute posterior fossa epidural hematoma. CT scans (**a, b**) were obtained through the posterior fossa (**a**) and higher up (**b**). **a** shows a lenticular retrocerebellar acute epidural blood collection. **b** shows that the high density epidural blood collection has extended supratentorially and is behind the left occipital lobe and left occipital horn. This is a characteristic feature of epidural hematoma and is not seen in subdural hematomas since subdural collections do not traverse the tentorium. **c** shows an occipital fracture (*open arrow*) on a Towne skull projection in the same patient. Note that the fracture extends to the posterior lip of the foramen magnum

Fig. 3.43. Acute extradural hematoma. Note the lenticular extracerebral blood collection on the left side typical of extradural hematoma. The configuration of the hematoma does not suggest subdural hematoma at all. Note that the edges of the extadural collection and the adjacent skull form an obtuse angle facing the underlying brain. The ends of a line joining the anterior and posterior limits of this hematoma would be in contact with the inner table of the skull, unlike most peripheral intracerebral hematomas. Note the marked left to right shift of the bodies of the lateral ventricles

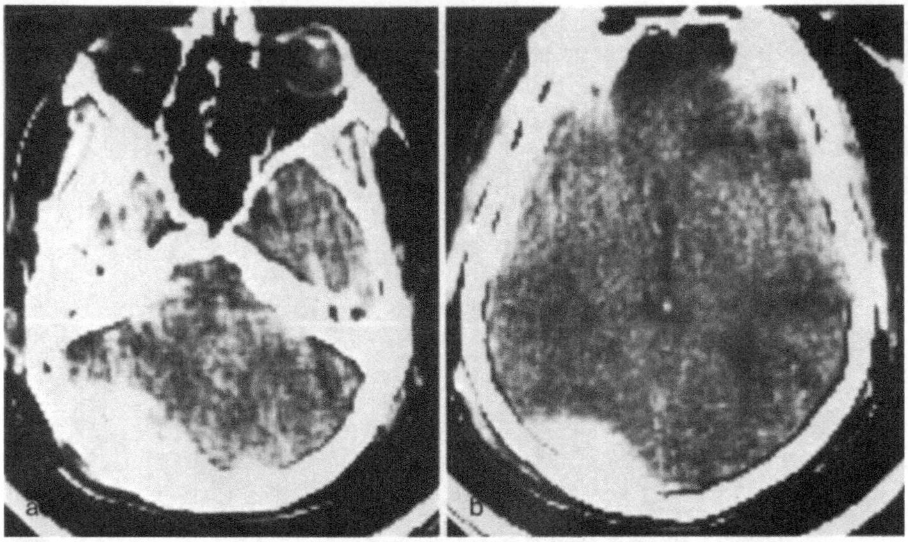

Fig. 3.44 a, b. Posterior fossa epidural hematoma with supratentorial extension. The posterior fossa component is seen in **a** with the typical biconvex high density collection between the inner table of the skull and the adjacent cerebellum. Note in **b** that the high density collection extends supratentorially and appears behind the left occipital lobe. This is a characteristic feature seen with epidural hematomas which is not seen with subdural hematomas

In one series, which included 19 posttraumatic extradural hematomas in infants, plain X-rays of the skull showed a fracture in 14 (two cases had separated sutures); nine of the infants were less than 1 year old [10]. In infants, the dura is firmly adherent to the skull only at the level of the coronal suture. Therefore, the hematoma may be quite extensive; this was so in 12 of 19 cases. In four cases, there was an underlying brain contusion. Death occurred in two [10].

In contradistinction to the usual clinical presentation of extradural hematoma, Di Tullio [18] has reported a case of a 12-year-old boy with a large extradural hematoma who was awake, alert, and had no history of concussion. This patient also demonstrated no calvarial fracture and had an ipsilateral complete paralysis of the oculomotor nerve as the sole neurological deficit. We have had an almost identical case in a 13-year-old boy at the Childrens Hospital of Los Angeles.

Prior to the CT era, angiography was utilized to confirm the presence of an extracerebral hematoma. In addition to a biconvex intracerebral collection displacing cortical vessels inward (Fig. 3.41), the demonstration of inward displacement of middle meningeal arteries or dural sinuses on appropriate tangential projections was helpful in the diagnosis of epidural hematoma. Pseudoaneurysm of the middle meningeal artery or an arteriovenous fistula from meningeal arteries into meningeal veins was appreciated fairly frequently in adult patients but was rarely seen in children.

Fortunately, CT is now used very effectively in the diagnosis of extradural hematoma; angiography is now rarely required in the evaluation of children with extradural hematomas. This is fortunate because the CT examination provides a much quicker diagnosis than angiography. This is often vital in patients with extradural hematoma. CT diagnosis of extradural hematoma is very simple, whereas a proper diagnosis of extradural hematoma by angiography often requires expertise, analysis, and time.

At CT, an acute extradural hematoma appears typically as a biconvex high density lesion adjacent to the inner table of the skull (Figs. 3.42–3.44). Typically, the edges of the broadest diameter of the hematoma are in contact with the inner table of the skull in contradistinction to the intracerebral hematoma (its diameter is some distance in from the inner table of the skull).

Most biconvex extracerebral blood collections are extradural hematomas, but occasionally an acute subdural hematoma may have a biconvex configuration. An important differential point is that the edge of an extradural hematoma tends to form a distinct obtuse angle at the inner table of the skull whereas the edge of the subdural hematoma tends to taper over the surface of the brain [51].

An extradural hematoma arising from the transverse sinus can be appreciated as being both supra-

and infratentoral as it extends above and below the transverse sinus (Figs. 3.42, 3.44). This is a feature that is not seen with subdural hematoma since the tentorium separates the supratentorial and infratentorial subdural compartments.

Usually, the CT appeareance of the extradural blood collection is homogeneous, but occasionally differing densities within the hematoma may be appreciated. In fact, a sedimentation phenomenon may be observed with a fluid-fluid level between less dense and denser blood elements. Even though a diagnosis of extradural hematoma may be made early during the course of an examination it may be advantageous to complete the examination while the operating room is being prepared for surgery, provided the patient's clinical condition permits. A complete study from the foramen magnum to the vertex will prevent missing a second potentially significant lesion (such as a subdural hematoma; multiple epidural hematomas are uncommon) provided the examination is adequate. Occasionally, air may be seen within an extradural hematoma entering through a scalp laceration and fracture, or entering the hematoma from a sinus via a fracture defect. We have not yet seen air within a fresh subdural hematoma; theoretically, air could enter a subdural hematoma if there was, in addition, a dural tear.

Of course, there may also be displacement of midline and other structures as a result of mass effect related to the presence of an epidural hematoma.

Following intravenous injection of contrast, subjacent enhancement under an extradural hematoma may be seen due to underlying cortical contusion or necrosis [97].

3.3.7 Cerebral Contusion

Cerebral contusion is a pathological term that implies cerebral laceration (or bruising of the brain) with punctate hemorrhagic foci. Clinically, in uncomplicated contusion, the maximum neurological deficit usually occurs at the moment of injury and from that point on the child remains fairly stable or steadily improves [57].

Pathologically, in contusion, there is bruising or crushing of brain without interruption of physical continuity of cerebral cortex. The bruises or hemorrhagic areas are macroscopically visible and are the result of disruption of small vessels with extravasation of blood insufficient to produce a frank hematoma [55, 61].

Contusions are usually found in closed head injuries, where the dura is not perforated or lacerated. These develop at the moment of impact and develop wherever the stress, particularly a shearing force, exceeds the cohesive strength or the elastic modulus of vessel walls and other tissue components [55].

Contusional hemorrhages occur from torn or ruptured vessels (arteries, capillaries, and/or veins). Damage to the vessel wall occurs at the moment of impact and, if the patient dies instantaneously, hemorrhages pathologically are very small, punctate or hairlike; they may be mistaken for congested vessels. Usually, however, the patient survives long enough after the injury to allow the hemorrhages time to enlarge so that they can be identified grossly without difficulty. Hemorrhages from these arteries and veins may develop within 30–60 min into large hematomas. These are common in the white matter and basal ganglia.

The common denominator in intracerebral hemorrhage, contusion and edema is loss of vascular integrity. In edema there is, at the least, loss of plasma proteins leaking into the extracellular space. In intracerebral hemorrhage and contusion, however, there is actual disruption of vessels with leakage of blood [55]. In contusion, the mechanism is usually blunt trauma but it can also be secondary to perforating forces.

The CT appearance of contusion overlaps with intracerebral hematoma, on the one hand (having areas of blood density) and with cerebral edema on the other. Pure lucency may be seen on CT in cases of contusion when the areas of hemorrhage are smaller than the resolving capacity of the scanner.

As seen on CT, contusion may have a combination of high density areas with a larger area of surrounding prominent low density. Thus, a mottled or "salt and pepper" appearance may be produced by white areas of blood from contusional hemorrhages interspersed with darker lucent areas of contusion necrosis and edema [28]. The blood gradually resolves, leaving further lucency, as in the case of intracerebral hematoma. Smaller areas of blood within contusions resolve rapidly into lucent areas, in contrast to the larger cerebral hematomas which tend to persist as blood density for 10–14 days or longer, depending upon their initial size. An area of contusion originally containing high density zones may eventually appear totally lucent (Fig. 3.45) since the hemorrhagic foci eventually lose their increased density. In some cases, the smaller areas of hemorrhage and contusion may be initially too small to be identified by the resolving capacity of the CT scanner; hence, only the low density areas may be seen, having an appearance such as that seen in Fig. 3.45.

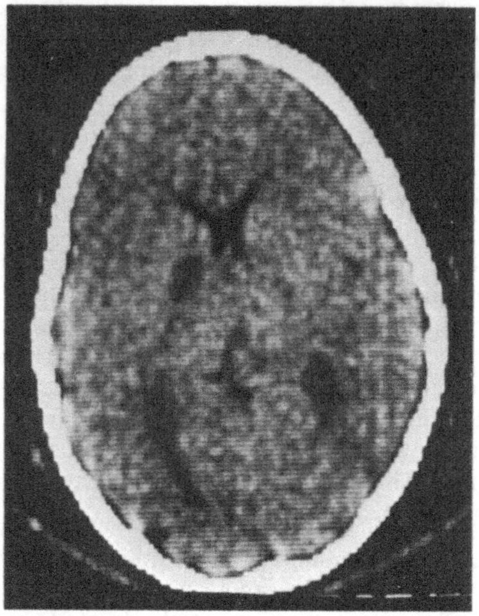

Fig. 3.45. Cerebral contusion. Note the rounded low density area in the region of the left lenticular nucleus adjacent to the junction of the anterior and posterior limbs of the internal capsule at the level of the genu of the internal capsule. Initially, cerebral contusions often contain high density areas, representing small hemorrhages which resolve eventually leaving a purely lucent area. If the hemorrhages are microscopic, they will not be identified even on early posttrauma scans and, thus, the contusion will be purely lucent at the outset

Contusion is, by definition, a focal lesion although more than one area of contusion may be present. Contusions are commoner in the frontal and temporal regions but they can occur anywhere, including the cerebellum and brainstem. Mass effect may be present in contusions; obliteration of pontine, cerebellopontine and perimesencephalic cisterns may result from the mass effect of brainstem contusions. Contusions are frequently observed diagonally opposite foci of increased density and swelling in the scalp because there is often a contrecoup mechanism.Contrecoup contusions are, however, apparently less common in smaller children than in older children and adults [15].

Since there is actual disruption of vessels in cerebral contusion, enhancement following intravenous administration of contrast is to be expected. In fact, some cases of contusion are isodense on noncontrast scans and can be demonstrated only following intravenous contrast as areas of cerebral enhancement [97]. Furthermore, areas of staining with early venous drainage were seen in patients with cerebral contusion; this was when angiography was the standard diagnostic modality in head trauma patients.

In contradistinction to the term contusion, "concussion" is a clinical term which implies no significant degree of structural damage to brain. There is some disagreement with regard to the term concussion [62]. Some authors limit this term to those cases where there is only a brief loss of unconsciousness and no permanent damage to normal neural tissue. Others, on the other hand, interpret the term to include all patients with head injury who do not have objective evidence of cerebral damage regardless of the duration of coma. Coma or loss of contact with the environment of short duration is a characteristic feature of simple concussion.

3.3.8 Cerebral Edema

Edema fluid collects rapidly in the extracellular space once there has been a loss of vascular integrity and extravasation of plasma proteins.

Cerebral edema appears on CT as a low density area measuring around 8–14 EMI units [28, 57]. There may be a mass effect that can result in ventricular compression and displacement (Fig. 3.30). It can appear within a matter of hours (as early as 3–5 h after the insult), it is usually most intense 12–24 h after injury, and it may persist for several weeks as seen at CT.

The reader is reminded that posttraumatic areas of lucency on CT could in actuality represent areas of contusion (Fig. 3.45). This is because tiny collections of blood may be smaller than the resolving capacity of the scanner or may have lost their initial high density. It should also be pointed out that posttraumatic areas of lucency do not always represent edema or contusion. Infarction can also result from trauma and may present at CT as a lucent area involving a vascular distribution of the brain. While mass effect is often lacking, it may be present with infarction.

3.3.9 Acute General Cerebral Swelling

Acute general cerebral swelling is a recently described entity in which there is posttraumatic swelling of the brain [105]. This condition has certain CT and pathologic features that are peculiar to childhood. The cerebral swelling manifests shortly after trauma. CT shows compression or obliteration of the lateral (Fig. 3.46) and third ventricles and the perimesencephalic cisterns, as well as an increase (of about 3

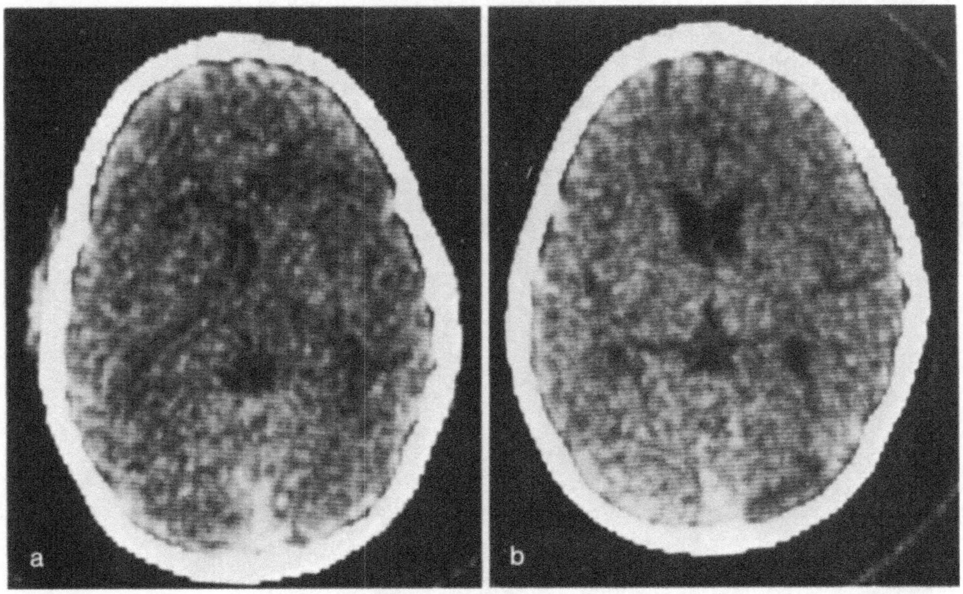

Fig. 3.46 a, b. Acute generalized cerebral swelling. Scans obtained early after trauma (**a**) show very narrow frontal horns due to cerebral swelling. **b** is a scan obtained 3 weeks later in the same patient. Note that the frontal horns have returned to a more normal size following resolution of the cerebral swelling. The interhemispheric fissure (not appreciated on the initial scans) is now evident

Hounsfield units) in average density of the white matter.

The following CT features can be correlated with pathological findings in children dying from head injury: diffuse cerebral swelling, loss of CSF spaces, and venous congestion of the cortex.

Increased density, seen on CT in acute general cerebral swelling, appears to be due to hyperemia and correlates with increased regional blood flow as determined by 133 Xe radionuclide measurements. Higher metabolic rate and greater vasoreactivity in childhood may explain the apparent confinement of these particular features to the pediatric population.

Clinically, almost all the children with acute generalized cerebral swelling have a significant disturbance of consciousness or are comatose. Most will eventually recover and return to a self-supportive state although intellectual deterioration, focal weakness, spastic quadriparesis, or death may supervene.

Edema may develop following hyperemia or may occur secondary to iatrogenic fluid overloading. When edema supervenes, decreased brain densities are recorded in EMI units [105].

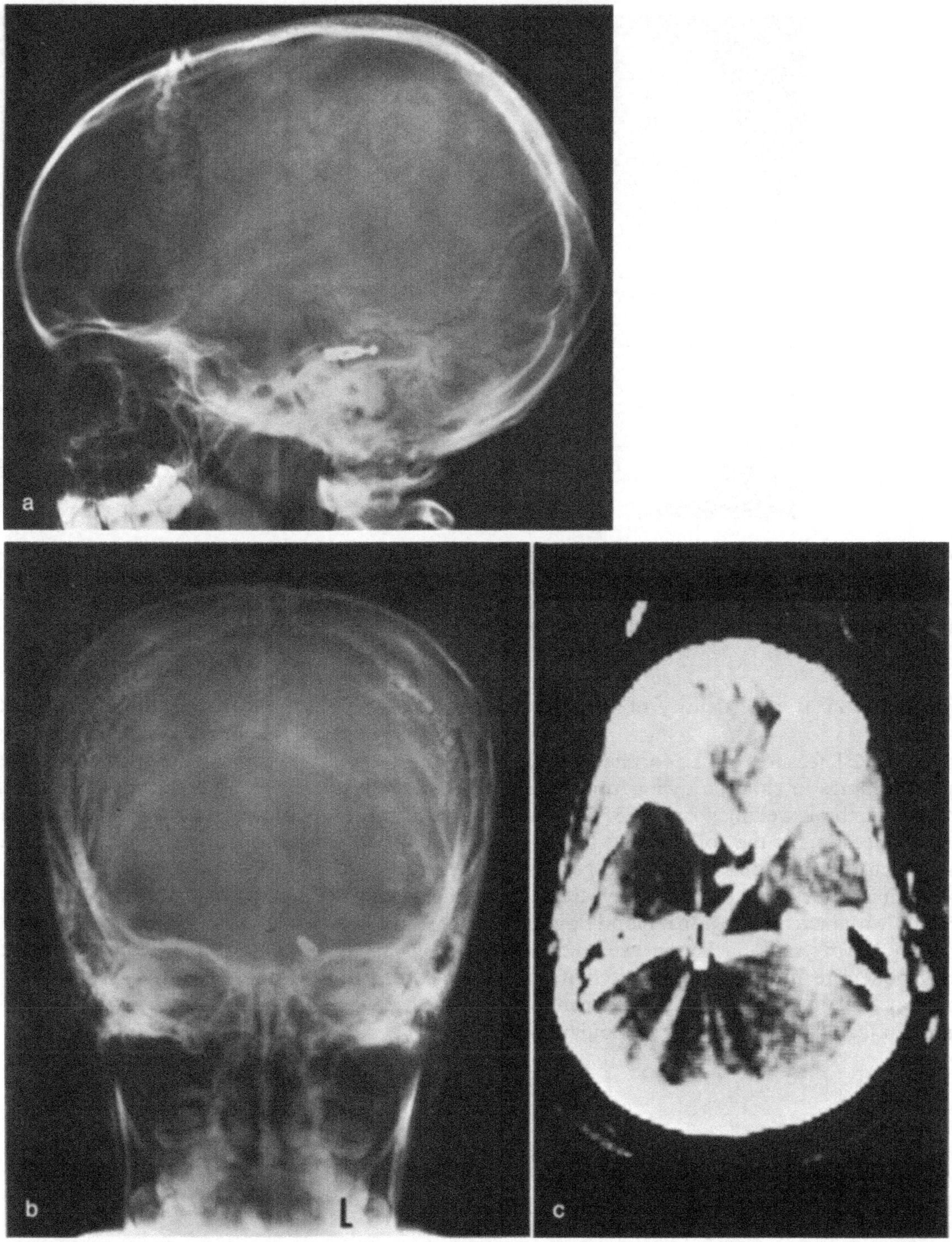

Fig. 3.47 a–c. Metallic umbrella tip in the region of the left cerebellopontine angle cistern. Lateral (**a**) and AP (**b**) skull films show the umbrella tip which was driven intracranially through the superior orbital fissure. No skull fracture or orbital fracture was identified on any one of numerous projections. A CT scan (**c**) shows the metallic foreign body in the region of the left cerebellopontine angle cistern. Note the numerous artifacts associated with the presence of the metallic foreign body. (Case courtesy of Frank M. Anderson, MD)

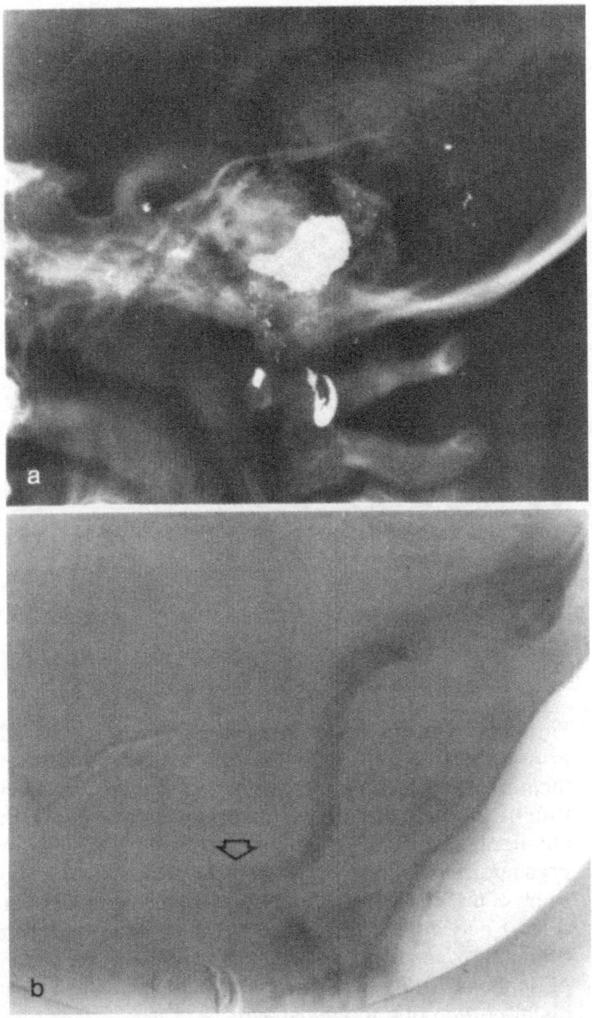

Fig. 3.48 a, b. Metallic intracranial foreign body. A lateral skull film (**a**) shows a metallic bullet involving the posterior part of the petrous bone lodged in the region of the jugular fossa. Note numerous small metallic fragments, as well as the major metallic fragment. A lateral subtraction film (**b**) during the venous phase of cerebral angiography shows that there is occlusion (*arrow*) just distal to the sigmoid sinus

3.4 Traumatic Vascular Lesions

3.4.1 Traumatic Aneurysms

Traumatic aneurysms may involve the cortical vessels (Fig. 3.49), the pericallosal artery, and the vessels at the base of the brain. Traumatic aneurysms may also be situated on extradural vessels such as the middle meningeal artery and the internal carotid artery. They may also occur on scalp vessels.

Traumatic aneurysms are quite uncommon, however, in childhood [4, 8, 23, 60]. Ordinarily, cerebral angiography is necessary for diagnosis, usually showing the lumen of the aneurysm filling with contrast material. Occasionally, however, even angiography may fail to permit the diagnosis of traumatic aneurysm when it is thrombosed. Benoit and Wortzman [8] describe such an aneurysm of traumatic origin. Angiograms in their case were normal, but plain films showed calcification within a suprasellar aneurysm which also displaced the anterior third ventricle at pneumoencephalography. In an occasional case, there may be normal angiography initially following injury with a posttraumatic aneurysm found on a later study. Traumatic aneurysms may also increase in size.

Traumatic cortical aneurysms are not infrequently associated with a nearby skull fracture [83, 84].

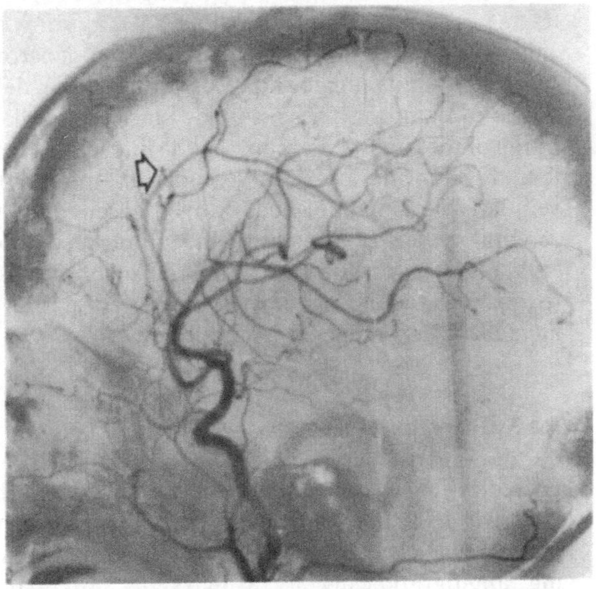

Fig. 3.49. Traumatic cortical aneurysm in an infant. Note the small aneurysm (*arrow*) involving a superficial branch of a middle cerebral artery shown by cerebral angiography. An overlying fracture and small subdural collection were also noted in this infant. Posttraumatic aneurysms are found very infrequently in the pediatric age group

Traumatic anterior cerebral aneurysms, arising from the pericallosal artery are believed to result from the anterior cerebral artery striking the margin of the falx.

3.4.2 Arteriovenous Fistulas

In addition to superficial vessels, such as the superficial temporal artery, occasionally being the site of traumatic aneurysms, traumatic arteriovenous fistulas of the scalp may also occur. These are usually not complicated in their structure and only one or two external carotid arteries branches are involved [72]. In the usual case, the superficial temporal artery wall is weakened by trauma, resulting in aneurysmal dilatation followed by subsequent shunting into the adjacent superficial temporal vein. We have been able to demonstrate the presence of such vascular scalp lesions on CT, but angiography best delineates the abnormalities.

Clinically, posttraumatic arteriovenous fistula of the scalp may present findings after months or years. A thrill may be palpated or a bruit heard and a portion of the affected scalp may be warmer.

Carotid cavernous fistula can occur in the pediatric age group. In this entity, laceration of the intracavernous carotid results from an associated basal skull fracture. Another possible cause is penetrating orbitocranial injury. While CT may show an enlarged superior ophthalmic vein and a generous cavernous sinus, angiography is required for definitive evaluation. These studies show immediate filling of the cavernous sinus, via the internal carotid fistula. Shunting into a large superior ophthalmic vein is typical. Diminished, or even absent flow to cerebral vessels as a result of the shunt may occur [72]. Other types of posttraumatic arteriovenous fistula (such as those involving the vertebral artery) have also been reported in childhood [54].

3.4.3 Dissecting Aneurysm

Dissecting aneurysm has been described in the pediatric age group [47, 87]. The presence of an incomplete vascular occlusion may be seen, appearing angiographically as a markedly attenuated lumen. In some cases of dissecting aneurysm there is a close relationship chronologically to mild or moderate trauma but the proof of a traumatic etiology in many of these cases is far from conclusive [47, 87].

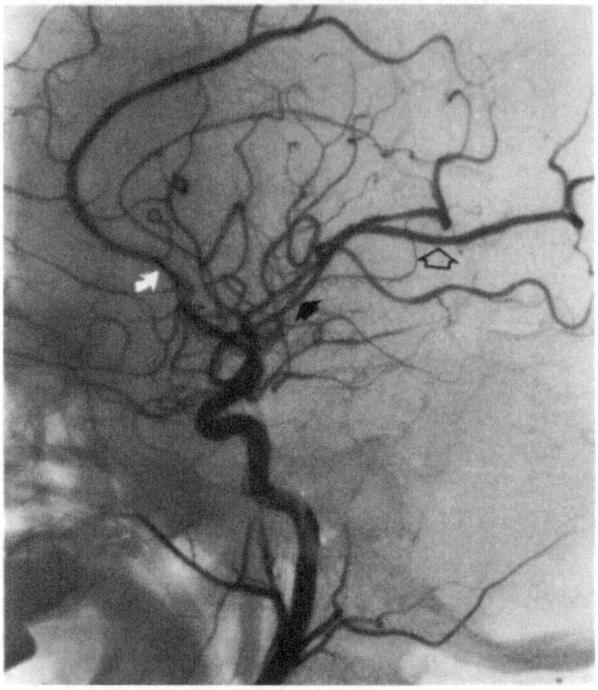

Fig. 3.50. Posttraumatic arterial spasm. Left carotid arteriogram, lateral subtraction film, arterial phase. Note the narrowing of some arteries due to "spasm" following trauma, probably related to the presence of blood in the subarachnoid space. Vessel narrowing is most impressive in the middle cerebral group. Note that the main trunk of the middle cerebral is narrow proximally (*black arrow*) and in fact, it is narrower than one of its distal branches (*open black arrow*). The proximal portion of the pericallosal artery (*white arrow*) is also narrower than its distal portion due to vasospasm

3.4.4 Posttraumatic Spasm

When there is blood in the subarachnoid space following trauma, spasm of cerebral vessels may be noted (Fig. 3.50). Since angiography is now seldom performed for trauma in childhood, angiographic demonstration of spasm will be seen less frequently.

3.4.5 Increased Intracranial Pressure

In children who have sustained head trauma and who are dying with increased intracranial pressure and severe cerebral edema, angiograms prior to death may show absence of flow in the intracerebral arteries, or a markedly prolonged circulation time [75]. The site of obstruction is at the supraclinoid level (Fig. 3.51) where the internal carotid artery pierces the dura and first becomes exposed to elevated intracranial pressure. A common carotid

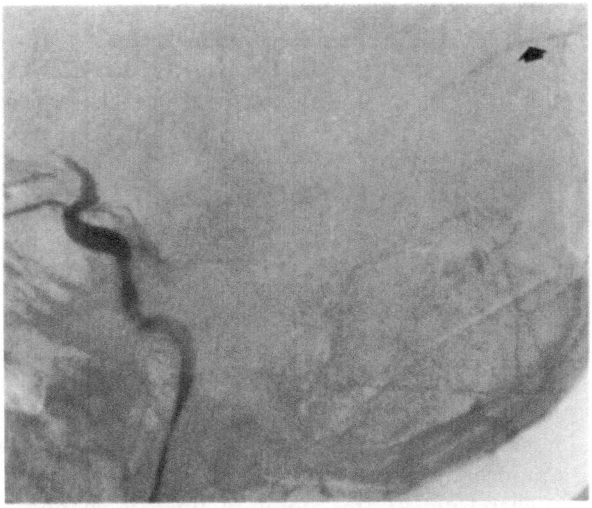

Fig. 3.51. Markedly delayed filling of the intracranial vasculature, secondary to increased inracranial pressure. Note start of filling of the supraclinoid portion of the internal carotid artery (above the level of the ophthalmic artery) 30 s after injection. Note that the distal portion of the posterior branch of the middle meningeal artery has filled (*arrow*). The more proximal portion of the same vessel has already emptied of contrast. Ordinarily, the intracranial branches of the internal carotid artery fill earlier than the middle meningeal artery, related to their larger caliber. In this instance, however, due to increased intracranial pressure, there is not yet filling of the intracranial branches of the internal carotid artery beyond the supraclinoid carotid. The ophthalmic artery and the choroidal-retinal blush are visualized on this subtraction print from a lateral view during carotid arteriography

injection in these patients, on the other hand, may show normal flow in the external carotid artery despite the impediment to intracranial flow (Fig. 3.51).

3.4.6 Posttraumatic Arterial Stenosis and Occlusion

Angiographic changes may be seen following direct trauma to cortical vessels at the time of skull fracture. Occlusions or segments of narrowing adjacent to a fracture line may be seen [83].

The child who falls while running with a Popsicle stick in his mouth may sustain intraoral trauma to the internal carotid artery. Following injury to the cervical portion of the internal carotid artery, stenosis or occlusion due to direct trauma to the vessel may occur [51]. These patients may also embolize, and there may be angiographic demonstration of occlusion of a number of intracranial vessels (Fig. 3.52).

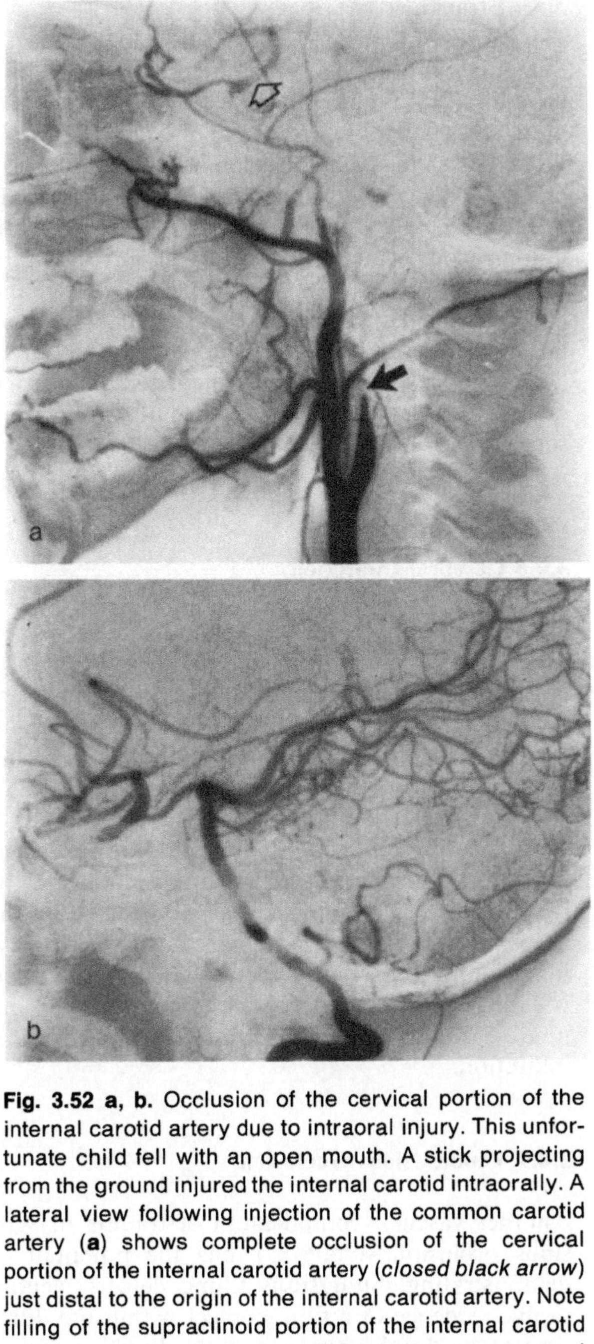

Fig. 3.52 a, b. Occlusion of the cervical portion of the internal carotid artery due to intraoral injury. This unfortunate child fell with an open mouth. A stick projecting from the ground injured the internal carotid intraorally. A lateral view following injection of the common carotid artery (**a**) shows complete occlusion of the cervical portion of the internal carotid artery (*closed black arrow*) just distal to the origin of the internal carotid artery. Note filling of the supraclinoid portion of the internal carotid artery (*open arrow*) due to collaterals between external carotid branches and the ophthalmic artery. Retrograde filling occurs via the ophthalmic artery into the supraclinoid carotid. **b** is from a left vertebral arteriogram, also with subtraction in the same patient. Note that the vertebrobasilar circulation fills readily, The supraclinoid portion of the internal carotid artery above the site of the occlusion fills readily via a posterior communicating artery. Despite good filling of the anterior cerebral branches only a few middle cerebral branches are filled. Embolism from the site of injury in the internal carotid artery has probably resulted in occlusion of several of the middle cerebral branches

3.4.7 Strangling

Someone who survives a strangling attempt may have an asymptomatic interval followed by a progressively evolving neurological disorder. Neuropathological changes have been identified in these cases and CT changes will undoubtedly be delineated in the future. Following strangling, cavitary necrotic lesions have been seen pathologically involving the caudate nucleus, putamen, and part of the globus pallidus [20]. The neuropathological changes simulate those of disease states characterized by severe lactic acidosis; thus it has been theorized that there is not only arterial occlusion involved but also venous stasis associated with lactic acidosis.

3.4.8 Cerebral Infarction

Of course, any of the above-enumerated lesions producing vascular occlusion can result in cerebral infarction. Furthermore, posterior cerebral artery distribution infarction may also result from herniation [91]. Areas of infarction are characteristically low density areas on CT with little mass effect as a rule. Enhancement may occur, particularly in the 1–4 week period following infarction. Atrophic areas involving the brain secondary to infarction may be permanent and recognized by CT long after the occcurrence of infarction. Low density areas involving the brain, as well as ventricular dilatation and widened subarachnoid spaces adjacent to the old infarct, are characteristic CT findings of old areas of infarction.

3.4.9 Venous Sinus Occlusion

Another vascular complication of trauma may be sinus occlusion. While CT has the potential of demonstrating dural sinus filling defects, venographic evidence of a filling defect within the dural sinuses or dural sinus occlusion should be more sensitive. Usually, there is an associated skull fracture, and, perhaps, an extradural hematoma may also be delineated.

3.4.10 Subepicranial Varix

Subepicranial varix may occur under the scalp at the site of a depressed skull fracture. These varices communicate with the diploic veins. Clinically, they are associated with depressed skull fractures and on rare occasions a reducible mass between the scalp may arise at the site of local injury after months or years. Diagnosis may be confirmed either at operation or by direct injection of contrast medium into the swelling [67].

3.5 Conclusion: Neuroradiology in Head Trauma in Perspective

The introduction of CT resulted in a sudden and dramatic change in the neuroradiological investigation of head injury. Without question CT is now the most important imaging modality in evaluating craniocerebral trauma in childhood.

Therefore, at this point in time, a chapter or monograph on head trauma in pediatric patients must reflect the importance of CT especially since existing textbook discussions have largely preceded the era of CT. This chapter provides the forum for the most contemporary consideration of radiology in childhood head trauma to date. To provide a comprehensive update, we have included many different posttraumatic entities. Common as well as uncommon radiological manifestations are described. Pertinent clinical data, physiology and pathology are also presented so as to give greater significance to the radiological material and to catalog some of the interesting information available.

Following injury, what happens to the brain is obviously more important, by and large, than the effect on the skull and scalp. Thus, the material in the Sect. 3.3, "Intracranial Hemorrhage and Cerebral Trauma," is of considerable importance and reflects the vital role of CT. Skull X-rays are obtained without risk and provide some useful information; hence, the habit of obtaining skull films on a nearly routine basis continues in many quarters. Since many skull X-rays in childhood head trauma are seen by radiologists, a fairly substantial section is devoted to skull film findings in pediatric trauma. Nevertheless, in general, skull X-rays are now much less important than CT.

Injury to the intracranial and scalp vessels is obviously of great significance to the patient. The diagnostic considerations are seldom as vital to the neuroradiologist, however, because his neurosurgical colleagues infrequently have the opportunity to justify operation for the sequelae of vascular trauma. Thus, the section devoted to this subject is not extensive.

In some portions of the text, a fair amount of space is devoted to uncommon conditions, since it was our intention to compile an assortment of interesting data rather than to provide merely a primer. Most of the illustrations, however, depict lesions seen with reasonable frequency in a large pediatric institution where trauma patients are treated. On the other hand, a few lesions which are unusual in childhood are depicted; among these are traumatic cortical aneurysm (Fig. 3.49), leptomeningeal cyst (Fig. 3.16), and subdural hematomas which are isodense on CT (Fig. 3.36) or calcify (Fig. 3.39) or thin the calvarium (Fig. 3.40). The angiograms and an air study are shown to demonstrate what has been and can be done with these techniques, but it should be realized that these examinations are now utilized only occasionally in childhood head trauma.

CT has not only given essential diagnostic information of a practical sort in head injury cases but has, in addition, provided new insights into cerebral trauma. For example, acute generalized cerebral swelling was recognized as a clinical-radiological entity only after the emergence of CT [105].

With developments in technology, "fast" scanning is already here. Improvements in resolution continue to be made and ability to reconstruct images in many different planes continues to advance. Thus, CT will show us even more in head trauma and will lessen our need for other imaging modalities to an even greater extent as time passes. Consequently, CT is certainly not a fad, nor will it be just another piece of passing armamentarium in the diagnostic study of pediatric head trauma.

References

1. Alexander E, Davis CH (1969) Intrauterine fracture of the infant's skull. J. Neurosurg 30:446–454
2. Anderson FM (1973) Treatment of subdural hematomas in infants. Bull Los Angeles Neurol Soc 38:103–109
3. Arkins TJ, McLennan JE, Winston KR, Strand RD, Suziki Y (1977) Acute posterior fossa epidural hematomas in children. Am J Dis Child 131:690–692
4. Asari S, Nakamura S, Yamada O, Beck H, Sugatani H, Higashi T (1977) Traumatic aneurysm of peripheral cerebral arteries – Report of two cases. J Neurosurg 46:795–803
5. Azar-Kia B, Sarwar M, Batnitzky S, Schechter MM (1975) Radiology of intracranial gas. AJR 124:315–323
6. Banovetz JD, Duvall AJ (1976) Zygomatic fractures. Otolaryngol Clin North Am 9:499–506
7. Barnes BD, Hoff JT (1976) Radionuclide cisternography after head injury. Arch Neurol 33:21–25
8. Benoit BG, Wortzman G (1973) Traumatic cerebral aneurysms. J Neurol Neurosurg Psychiatry 36:127–138
9. Caffey J (1961) Pediatric X-ray diagnosis, 4th edn. Year Book Medical Publishers, Chicago
10. Carcassonne M, Choux M, Grisoli F (1977) Extradural hematomas in infants. J Pediatr Surg 12:69–73
11. Carter LP, Pittman HW (1971) Posterior fossa subdural hematoma of the newborn – Case report. J Neurosurg 34:423–426
12. Chasler CN (1967) The newborn skull – The diagnosis of fracture. AJR 100:92–99
13. Conway JJ, Vollert JM (1972) The accuracy of radionuclide imaging in detecting pediatric dural fluid collections. Radiology 105:177–183
14. Coppola AR (1976) Acute head injury. Va Med Mon 103:118–121
15. Courville CB (1965) Contrecoupe in injuries of the brain in infancy. Arch Surg 90:157
16. Dandy WE (1926) Pneumocephalus. Arch Surg 12:949
17. Davis KR, Taveras JM, Roberson GH, Ackerman RH, Dreisbach JN (1977) Computed tomography in head trauma. Semin Roentgenol 12:53–62
18. Di Tullio MV (1977) Epidural hematoma with complete third nerve paralysis in an awake patient. Surg Neurol 7:193–194
19. Dolinskas CA, Zimmerman RA, Bilaniuk LT (1978) A sign of subarachnoid bleeding on cranial computed tomograms of pediatric head trauma patients. Radiology 126:409–411
20. Dooling EC, Richardson EP (1976) Delayed encephalopathy after strangling. Arch Neurol 33:196–199
21. Dublin AB, Rennick JM, Sivalingam S (1976) Failure of computerized axial tomography to demonstrate a chronic subdural hematoma. Surg Neurol 6:23–24
22. Dujovny M, Osgood CP, Maroon JC, Jannetta PJ (1975) Penetrating intracranial foreign bodies in children. J Trauma 15:981–986
23. Eichler A, Story JL, Bennett DE, Galo MV (1969) Traumatic aneurysm of a cerebral artery – Case report J. Neurosurg 31:72–76
24. Faber MM (1976) Massive subgaleal hemorrhage: A hazard of playground swings. Clin Pediatr 15:384–385
25. Fein W, Carton CA (1976) Transorbital removal of intracranial foreign body in middle fossa. Ann Ophthalmol 8:89–92
26. Franken EA, Smith JA (1975) Roentgenographic evaluation of infant and childhood trauma. Pediatr Clin North Am 22:301–315
27. Freed TA, Oronzi VR, Frivold WP (1975) Unusual foreign bodies associated with cranial trauma. AJR 125:839–841
28. French BN, Dublin AB (1977) The value of computerized tomography (CT) in the management of 1000 consecutive head injuries. Surg Neurol 7:171–183
29. Front D, Defesche HFHG, Oen TS, Beks JWF, Penning L (1975) Convexity leptomeningeal cysts

diagnosed by scinticisternography. J Neurosurg 43:203–206
30. Genieser NB, Becker MH (1974) Head trauma in children. Radiol Clin North Am 12:333–342
31. Gilles FH Shillito J (1970) Infantile hydrocephalus: Retrocerebellar subdural hematoma. J Pediatr 76:529–537
32. Gresham EL (1975) Birth trauma. Pediatr Clin North Am 22:317–328
33. Gruber FH (1969) Post-traumatic leptomeningeal cysts. AJR 105:305–307
34. Gutierrez FA (1977) Angiographic characteristics of certain subdural collections of fluid. Childs Brain 3:48–61
35. Gutierrez FA, Raimondi AJ (1974) Delayed onset of acute posttraumatic subdural effusion. Am J Dis Child 128:327–331
36. Haar FL (1975) Complication of linear skull fracture in young children. Am J Dis Child 129:1197–1200
37. Hammer B, Gund A (1975) Brain injury due to a blank-shot mortar explosion. Neuroradiol 9:103–106
38. Harbison JW (1974) Neuro-ophthalmology in severe head injury. Q Med Coll Va 10:178–182
39. Harwood-Nash DC (1970) Fractures of the petrous and tympanic parts of the temporal bone in children: A tomographic study of 35 cases. AJR 110:598–607
40. Harwood-Nash DC, Hendrick EB, Hudson AR (1971) The significance of skull fractures in children – A study of 1,187 patients Radiology 101:151–155
41. Harwood-Nash DC Fitz CR (1976) Neuroradiology in infants and children Mosby, St. Louis
42. Hendrick EB, Hoffman HJ, Humpreys RP (1975) Trauma of the central nervous system in children. Pediatr Clin North Am 22:415–424
43. Hillman RSL, Kieffer SA, Ortiz H, Clubb R (1975) Intraosseous leptomeningeal cysts of the posterior cranial fossa. Radiology 116:655–659
44. James HE, Schut L (1974) The neurosurgeon and the battered child. Surg Neurol 2:415–418
45. Jennett B (1976) Assessment of the severity of head injury. J Neurol Neurosurg Psychiatry 39:647–655
46. Jennett B (1976) Some medicolegal aspects of the management of acute head injury. Br Med J 1:1383–1385
47. Johnson AC, Graves VB, Pfaff JP (1977) Dissecting aneurysm of intracr. arteries. Surg Neurol 7:49–52
48. Jonker C, Oosterhuis HJ (1975) Epidural haematoma – A retrospective study of 100 patients. Clin Neurol Neurosurg 78:233–245
49. Kaufman B, Nulsen FE, Weiss MH, Brodkey JS, White RJ, Sykora GF (1977) Acquired spontaneous, nontraumatic normal-pressure cerebrospinal fluid fistulas originating from the middle fossa. Radiology 122:379–387
50. Kogutt MS, Swischuk LE, Fagan CJ (1974) Patterns of injury and significance of uncommon fractures in the battered child syndrome. AJR 121:143–149
51. Koo AH, LaRoque RL (1977) Evaluation of head trauma by computed tomography. Radiology 123:345–350
52. Laster DW, Moody DM, Ball MR (1978) Resolving intracerebral hematoma: Alteration of the "Ring Sign" with steroids. AJR 130:935–939
53. Lende RA (1974) Enlarging skull fractures of childhood. Neuroradiology 7:119–124
54. Linde LM, Fonkalsrud EW, Wilson GH, Batzdorf U (1970) Traumatic vertebral arteriovenous fistula in a child. JAMA 213:1465–1468
55. Lindenberg R (1977) Pathology of craniocerebral injuries. In: Newton TH, Potts DG (eds) Radiology of the skull and brain, vol 3 Mosby, St. Louis
56. Low NL, Correll JW (1966) Head pain due to leptomeningeal cysts. Br J Surg 53:791–793
57. Matson DD (1969) Neurosurgery of infancy and childhood, 2nd edn. Thomas, Springfield
58. McLaurin RL, Tutor FT (1961) Acute subdural hematoma – Review of 90 cases. J Neurosurg 18:61–67
59. Mealey J (1975) Infantile subdural hematomas. Pediatr Clin North Am 22:433–442
60. Menezes AH, Graf CJ (1974) True traumatic aneurysm of anterior cerebral artery – Case report J Neurosurg 40:544–548
61. Merino de Villesante J, Taveras JM (1976) Computerized tomography (CT) in acute head trauma. AJR 126:765–778
62. Merritt HH (1970) A textbook of neurology, 4th edn. Lea & Febiger, Philadelphia
63. Messer HD, Cerza PF (1976) Copper jacketed bullets in the central nervous system. Neuroradiology 12:121–129
64. Messina AV (1976) Computed tomography: Contrast material within subdural hematomas (A preliminary report). Radiology 119:725–726
65. Messina AV, Chermik NL (1976) Computed tomography: The "resolving" intracerebral hemorrhage. Radiology 118:609–613
66. Möller A, Ericson K (1979) Computed tomography of isoattenuating subdural hematomas. Radiology 130:149–152
67. Mori K, Yoneda S, Handa H (1976) Posttraumatic subepicranial varix. Surg Neurol 5:337–339
68. Moseley IF, Zilkha E (1976) The role of computerised tomography (EMI scanning) in the diagnosis and management of cranio-cerebral trauma. J Neuroradiol 3:277–296
69. Moyes PD, Thompson GB, Cluff JW (1965) Subdural peritoneal shunts in the treatment of subdural effusions in infants. J Neurosurg 23:584–587
70. New PFJ, Aronow S (1976) Attenuation measurements of whole blood and blood fractions in computed tomography. Radiology 121:635–640
71. Newton TH Gooding CA (1975) Compression of superior sagittal sinus by neonatal calvarial molding. Radiology 115:635–639
72. Newton TH, Potts DG (1974) Radiology of the skull and brain – Angiography vol 2, book 2. Mosby, St. Louis
73. Norman O (1956) Angiographic differentiation between acute and chronic subdural and extradural

hematomas. Acta Radiol [Diagn] (Stockh) 46:371–378
74. Osborn AG, Heaston DK, Wing SD (1978) Diagnosis of ascending transtentorial herniation by cranial computed tomography. AJR 130:755–760
75. Parvey LS, Gerald B (1976) Arteriographic diagnosis of brain death in children. Pediatr Radiol 4:79–82
76. Pollak K, Payne EE (1976) Fractures of the frontal sinus. Otolaryngol Clin North Am 9:517–522
77. Rabe EF (1967) Subdural effusion in infants. Pediatr Clin North Am 14:831–850
78. Ramsden RT, Block J (1976) Traumatic pneumocephalus. J Laryngol Otol 90:345–355
79. Raynor R, Parsa M (1968) Nonsurgical elevation of depressed skull fracture in an infant. J Pediatr 72:262–264
80. Roberts F, Shopfner CE (1972) Plain skull roentgenograms in children with head trauma. AJR 114:230–240
81. Ross G (1975) Spontaneous elevation of a depressed skull fracture in an infant – Case report. J Neurosurg 42:726–727
82. Rothman L, Rose JS, Laster DW, Quencer R, Tenner M (1976) The spectrum of growing skull fracture in children. Pediatrics 57:26–31
83. Rumbaugh CL, Bergeron RT, Kurze T (1972) Intracranial vascular damage associated with skull fractures – radiographic aspects. Radiology 104:81–87
84. Rumbaugh CL, Bergeron RT, Talalla A, Kurze T (1970) Traumatic aneurysms of the cortical cerebral arteries – radiographic aspects. Radiology 96:49–54
85. Sarsfield JK (1974) The neurological sequelae of non-accidental injury. Dev Med Child Neurol 16:826–827
86. Sato O, Tsugane R, Kageyama N (1975) Growing skull fractures of childhood: Possible mechanism of its focal ventricular dilatation. Childs Brain 1:148–157
87. Sato O, Bascom JF, Logothetis J (1971) Intracranial dissecting aneurysm – Case report. J Neurosurg 35:483–487
88. Scotti G, Terbrugge K, Melançon D, Bélanger G (1977) Evaluation of the age of subdural hematomas by computerized tomography. J Neurosurg 47:311–315
89. Silverman FN (1972) Unrecognized trauma in infants, the battered child syndrome, and the syndrome of Abroise Tardieu – Rigler Lecture. Radiology 104:337–353
90. Slepyan DH (1976) A case of orbital floor eruption. J Trauma 16:320–322
91. Stovring J (1977) Descending transtentorial herniation: Findings on computed tomography. Neuroradiology 14:101–105
92. Svendsen P (1976) Computer tomography of traumatic extracerebral lesions. Br J Radiol 49:1004–1012
93. Taveras JM, Wood EH (1964) Diagnostic neuroradiology. Williams and Wilkins, Baltimore
94. Teal JS, Huprich JE, Eto R, Tsai FY, Segall HD (1978) Computed tomography in the evaluation of apparent delayed post-traumatic intracerebral hemorrhage. 1978 Annual meeting of the Western Neuroradiological Society, Newport Beach, California, October 15, 1978
95. Teasdale G (1976) Assessment of head injuries. Br J Anaesth 48:761–766
96. Tenner MS, Stein BM (1970) Cerebral herniation in the growing fracture of the skull. Radiology 94:351–355
97. Tsai FY, Huprich JE, Gardner FC, Segall HD, Teal JS (1978) Diagnostic and prognostic implications of computed tomography of head trauma. J Comput Assisted Tomogr 2:323–331
98. Watts C (1976) The management of intracranial calcified subdural hematomas. Surg Neurol 6:247–250
99. Webber RL, Folio J (1976) Radiographic detectability of occipital and temporal-parietal fractures induced in cadaver heads. J Trauma 16:115–124
100. Weber SC, Cohn AM (1977) Fracture of the frontal sinus in children. Arch Otolaryngol 103:241–244
101. Williams JP, Fowler GW, Pribram HF, Delaney CA, Fish CH (1972) Roentgenographic changes in head bangers. Acta Radiol [Diagn] (Stockh) 13:37–42
102. Wolter JR, Leenhouts JA, Coulthard SW (1976) Clinical picture and management of subperiosteal hematoma of the orbit. J Pediatr Ophthalmol 13:136–138
103. Zilkha A, Irwin GAL (1976) The rim sign in epidural hematoma: Case report. J Nucl Med 17:977–979
104. Zelson C, Lee SJ, Pearl M (1974) The incidence of skull fractures underlying cephalhematomas in newborn infants. J Pediatr 85:371–373
105. Zimmerman RA, Bilaniuk LT, Bruce D, Dolinskas C, Obrist W, Kuhl D (1978) Computed tomography of pediatric head trauma: Acute general cerebral swelling. Radiology 126:403–408
106. Zimmerman RD, Leeds NE, Naidich TP (1977) Ring blush associated with intracerebral hematoma. Radiology 122:707–711

4 Injuries to the Spine

Philip Stanley

Spinal injuries are uncommon in children, particularly with major neurological complications [13, 59]. Some spinal injuries are associated with certain activities. Breech deliveries are a significant cause in neonates, but in later life sporting injuries and motor vehicular accidents predominate. It is very important to recognize the possibility of spinal cord damage in a traumatized child so that he may be protected against further damage and transported safely to the X-ray department where studies may be performed to determine whether the fracture/dislocation is stable or unstable.

It is important to realize that patients with one spinal level of injury may also have injuries at other levels [14]. If not recognized and treated early, these other injuries may prove very significant.

Several mechanisms are responsible for cord damage following trauma. The damage may be purely mechanical, due to compression by bone/ligaments or hematoma, or due to severe traction [7], or may have been due to a compromised blood supply [2, 75] arising sometimes, from a more distant injury [37]. In some dislocations and usually with traction and vascular injuries, the radiographs may be normal in a patient who has severe neurological deficit.

On account of the anatomical and functional differences, the spine can be conveniently divided into cervical, thoracolumbar, and sacral regions.

4.1 Cervical Spine

Because the atlas and axis are structurally and functionally distinct from the other five cervical vertebrae, and consequently suffer different types of injuries, the two regions will be considered separately.

4.1.1 Occipital-atlantoaxial Region

Before describing the traumatic events that may affect this region, it is important to describe the embryology, function, and special anatomy of the region because these are highly relevant to the injuries sustained and for accurate recognition of important congenital variants.

Embryologically, the rim of the foramen magnum, including occipital condyles and the apical segment of the dens, are formed from the fourth occipital sclerotome. The base of the odontoid is derived from the body of the atlas which comes primarily from the first cervical sclerotome. The axis, apart from the odontoid, is derived from the second cervical sclerotome. Secondary centers and anomalous ossification centers should not be confused with fractures. The atlas normally has three primary ossification centers, one for the body and one for each neural arch. The body may arise from two centers which ultimately fuse. The vertical cleft between the two centers should not be mistaken as fracture [67] nor should the cleft between the two lateral centers before they unite in the 7th year [5]. The axis has four primary ossification centers; one each for the body and for the odontoid, and two for the neural arches. The dens can arise from two centers which may not unite; the vertical cleft between them could be misinterpreted as a fracture, as could the synchondrosis separating the primary centers.

Many anomalies may be associated with maldevelopment of the odontoid. In the condition "ossic-

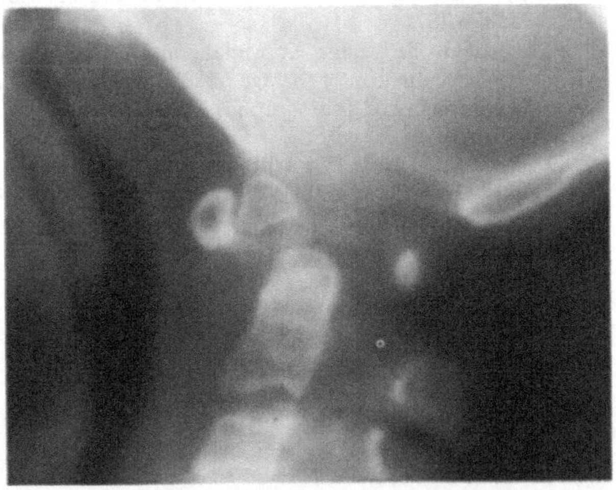

Fig. 4.1. A lateral tomogram of a 16-year-old with intermittent cord compression. There is an ossiculum terminale with forward slip of the ossiculum and atlas on the axis

ulum terminale" there is failure of fusion at the apical segment of the dens to the base which is normally fused with the body of the axis. The ossiculum may ride forward with the atlas with the potential danger of cord compression (Fig. 4.1). If the base of the dens has failed to develop completely and there is an ossified apical segment, then the condition is "agenesis of the odontoid base." This is rare [31]. There may be agenesis of the apical segment or agenesis of both the base and the apical segment. There is, of course, potential subluxation with the latter. The most controversial anomaly is the os odontoideum. Greenberg [30] believes that the dens has developed normally but not fused with the body of the axis, but Shapiro [82] is of the opinion that the os odontoideum is a hypertrophic remnant of the proatlas.

Function. The occipito-atlantoaxial joints function together as a unit, providing a complex range of mobility at the expense of some stability. Flexion and extension take place mainly at the occipito-atlantoid joint, and rotation and some lateral flexion at the atlantoaxial joint. These functions are reflected in the anatomy peculiar to the region.

Anatomy. Only the important bony structures and ligaments will be described. The occipital condyles articulate with the superior articular facets of the atlas. The odontoid process lies within the anterior ring of the atlas, being held forward by the transverse atlantal ligament which arises from a tubercle on the inner aspect of each atlantal mass (Fig. 4.2). The axis is connected to the occiput by the thick alar ligaments each running from the dorsolateral aspect of the dens to the medial surface of the condyles. The tectorial membrane, which is an extension of the posterior longitudinal ligament, is another important ligament. The apical ligament running from the odontoid peg tip to the anterior lip of the foramen magnum is of limited strength. These are the anterior ligaments, and posteriorly there is a strong posterior atlanto-occipital ligament and the ligamentum nuchae.

Radiology. The routine projections of the occipito-atlantoaxial region consist of a lateral, an antero-posterior film, and an anteroposterior film with an open mouth. If needed, tomograms, oblique views, and lateral flexion and extension projections are helpful. The last should not be performed except under strict supervision if there is a question of atlantoaxial instability. Certain radiographic appearances in this region are open to misinterpretation. In the open-mouth view, the biting surface of the upper incisor teeth and the posterior occiput or posterior arch of the atlas can give the spurious appearance of a fracture. Likewise, Mach bands may resemble a fracture of the base of the odontoid [19]. On forward flexion of the neck there can be considerable apparent subluxation of the atlas on the axis with increase in the distance between the posterior surface of the anterior arch of the atlas and the anterior odontoid process. Greenberg [30] gives a formula for normal limits, while 3 mm is quoted by Shapiro [82] and 5 mm by Martel [57] as the upper limit of normal. However, if there is any doubt, then a line joining the most anterior part of the posterior arches of the cervical spine should be a continuous smooth curve in normals. With hyperextension in children, there may be overriding of the anterior arch of the atlas over the odontoid process [15].

Rotary subluxation of C1 on C2 is a controversial subject. A child presents with a wry neck, and on the open-mouth views there may be unilateral offset of one of the articular masses of the atlas on the axis; if there is bilateral lateral displacement this could indicate a Jefferson fracture [48]. Jacobson and

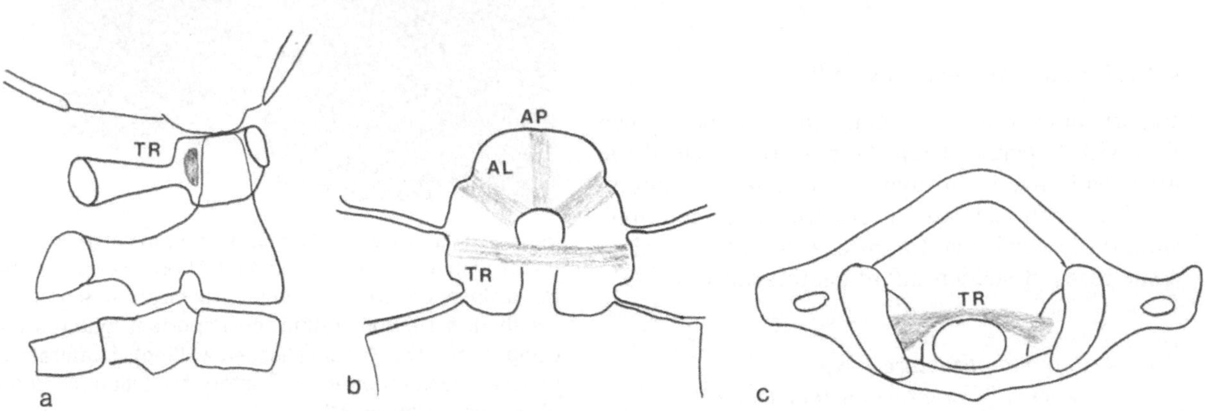

Fig. 4.2. The relationship of the import ligaments to the occiput, atlas and axis; lateral (**a**), frontal (**b**), and axial diagrams (**c**). *TR*, transverse atlantal ligament; *AL*, alar ligament; *AP*, apical ligament

Adler [44] believe that medial offset of a single articular mass is indicative of rotary subluxation of C1 on C2. However, this is most probably a normal finding [20, 64] and only if, in addition, there is an increased distance between the dens and the anterior arch of the atlas will Shapiro [82] accept that rotary subluxation is present.

4.1.1.1 Pseudosubluxation of Axis

Up to about the age of 10 years, maximum anteroposterior movement of the cervical spine takes place at C2/C3. In flexion, "excessive" angulation is apparent in some children at C2/C3 with some forward slip. This movement comes about because of the lax posterior ligaments and the horizontal alignment of the articular facets at this level. The line formed by the posterior arches of the vertebrae in the lateral projection is continuous and smooth. These appearances of pseudosubluxation of C2 on C3 are normal and the child should not be treated as a genuine dislocation. Jacobson [45] found that these children may have up to 5 mm slip on the lateral projection when comparing flexion and extension views.

4.1.1.2 Atlanto-occipital Dislocation

Considerable force is required for this rare injury. The occipital condyles are dislocated anteriorly. This lesion is usually fatal with compression of the medulla oblongata. A lateral view will show the dislocation with extensive prevertebral soft tissue swelling [82] (Fig. 4.3). There was increase in the distance between the occipital condyles and the superior articulating facets of the atlas in Gabrielsen's case [27], in whom rupture of the spinal meninges and anterior atlanto-occipital membrane was demonstrated on myelography.

4.1.1.3 Atlanto-occipital Instability

Experimental work with infant cadavers has shown that with hyperextension the posterior arch of the atlas will invert through the foramen magnum, causing potential bilateral vertebral artery compression. It is possible that this mechanism could explain some cases of sudden infant death syndrome [29].

4.1.1.4. Jefferson Fracture [48]
(Vertical Compression Injury of C1)

This is a fracture of the atlas due to vertical compression forces. Because of the oblique inward

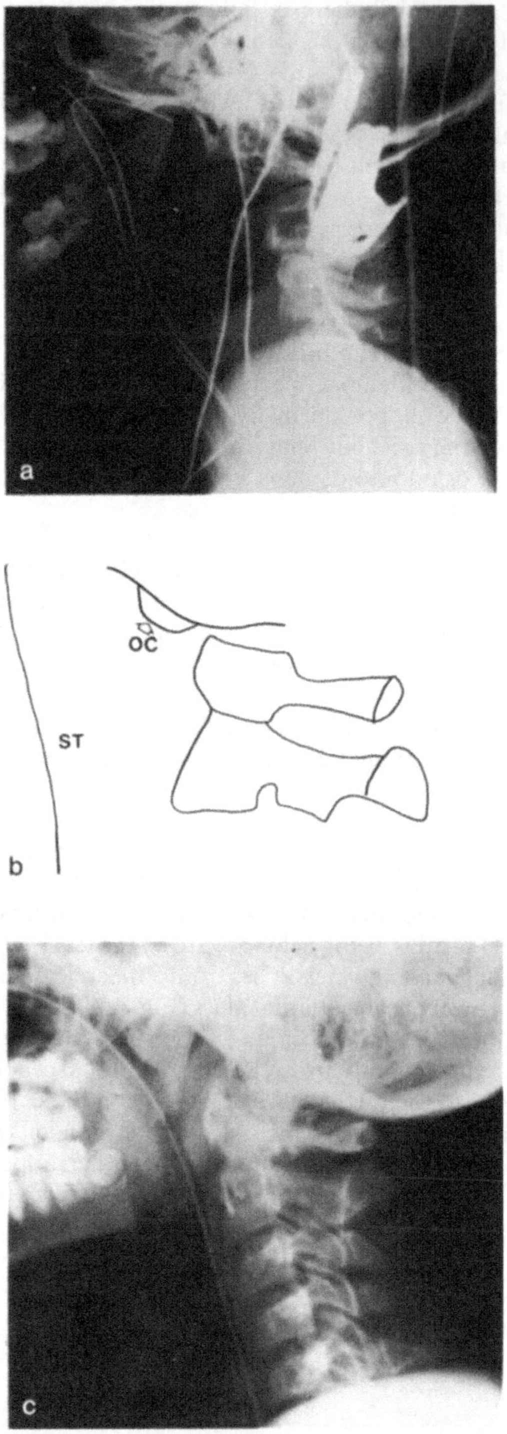

Fig. 4.3. a Lateral view of the cervical spine of a 6-year-old involved in a road traffic accident. There is occipitoatlantal dislocation with massive prevertebral soft tissue swelling. **b** Demonstrating the important features (*OC*, occipital condyle; *ST*, soft tissue swelling). **c** Lateral view showing position after satisfactory reduction. (Courtesy of Richard Graviss. MD)

orientation of the occipital condyles, a downward force wedges apart the articular surfaces of the lateral masses of the atlas. There are usually two anterior and two posterior fractures of the ring of C1 [82]. This fracture is unstable but spinal cord damage is rare. A lateral view of the cervical spine will demonstrate the posterior arch fracture, and an open-mouth anteroposterior view will demonstrate lateral displacement of both articular masses. Tomograms are often helpful and the role of computerized tomography has recently been discussed [50]. It has been shown not only that can the fracture be demonstrated, but also that intraspinal fragments can be located.

4.1.1.5 Extension Fracture of Atlas

With excessive extension, the posterior arch of the atlas is compressed between the occiput and the posterior elements of the axis. The fracture, which involves the posterior arch of the atlas, is usually single but may be multiple. Horizontal fractures of the anterior arch of the atlas are associated with other hyperextension fractures of the cervical spine, particularly through the base of the dens. This is easily overlooked on routine projections but if diagnosed can usually be better demonstrated by tomography [88].

4.1.1.6 Isolated Atlanto-axial Dislocation

Atlantoaxial dislocation without a fracture of the dens occurs as a result of incompetence of the transverse atlantal ligament [30]. This may be congenital, seen in mongolism [22, 30, 57] and in various skeletal dysplasias or occurs for no known reason. It is unusual for acute trauma to rupture the transverse atlantal ligament as the weaker odontoid peg usually fractures first, although there have been isolated case reports of such ruptures [8, 30]. However, if there are defects of segmentation, with either atlanto-occipital assimilation [58] or a block vertebra between C2 and C3, then increased stress is applied to the ligament and a chronic fatique fracture may occur [30]. Incompetence of the transverse atlantal ligament secondary to pharyngeal infections has been well documented and there have been reports of fatal cord compression secondary to "hyperemic" ligamentous rupture [30].

Apart from infection, there is another group of conditions in which there is a laxity of the transverse atlantal ligament, and dislocation of the atlas on the axis may then occur. These conditions are found in the rheumatoid group, which includes rheumatoid arthritis and ankylosing spondylitis (Fig. 4.4). Atlantoaxial dislocations have been found in a moderate percentage of patients with these conditions [83, 85]. Although not causing spinal cord compromise initially, the laxity of the atlantal ligament may be of critical importance even with minor trauma or during endotracheal intubation.

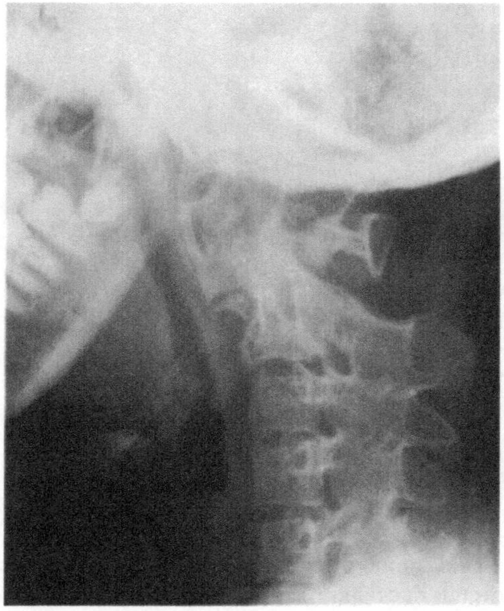

Fig. 4.4. Fifteen-year-old with long-standing rheumatoid arthritis showing atlantoaxial subluxation due to weakness of the transverse atlantal ligament. Fusion of the posterior elements of the cervical spine is present, another manifestation of rheumatoid arthrithis

4.1.1.7 Fractures of the Odontoid

Odontoid fractures form about 13% of fractures affecting the cervical spine [3]. Anderson [4] describes three main types of odontoid process fracture. In type I, there is an oblique avulsion fracture of the odontoid tip, most probably due to sudden tension on the alar ligaments. Types II and III are fractures at the odontoid base. Type II is at the junction of the odontoid with the second cervical vertebra (Fig. 4.5) whereas type III is a true fracture through the body of the axis. Type II fractures may not unite but occur less frequently in children [74]. The odontoid is usually, but not invariably, angled forward and there is usually forward slip of the atlas on the axis [43]. Backward displacement and angulation occur with extension injuries. Lateral tomograms are helpful. There can be acute neurological compromise or delayed myelopathy [60]. Because of the similarity clinically and radiologically it can be difficult at times to distinguish between a fracture of the base of the odontoid and a congenitally separate odontoid even if a history of injury is available [25,

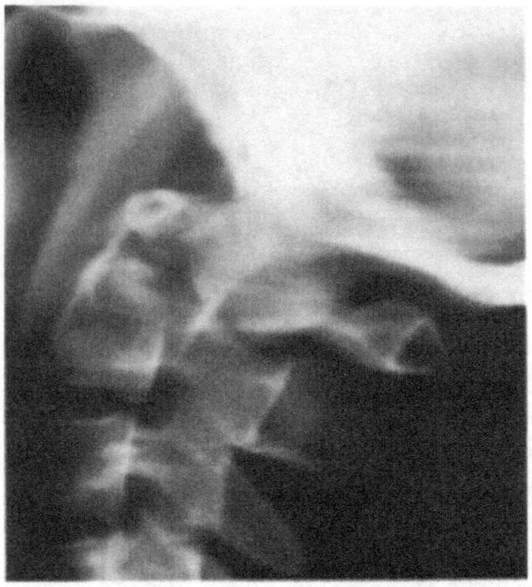

Fig. 4.5. Lateral tomogram of a 16-year-old boy involved in a hang-glider accident. There is a fracture through the base of the dens with backward dislocation

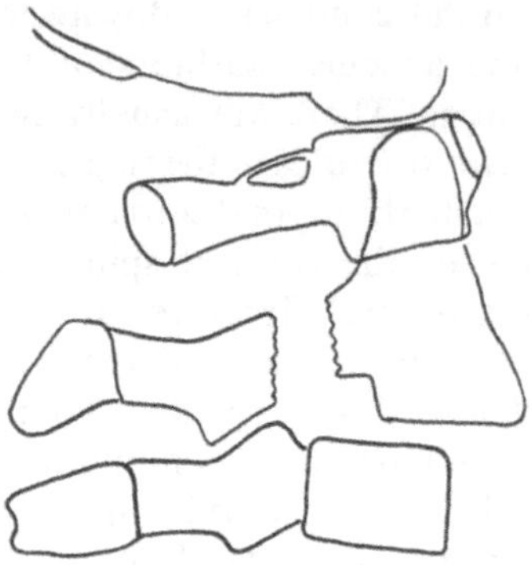

Fig. 4.6. Diagram of the fracture lines and displacement associated with a hangman's fracture

27, 30, 77, 82]. Greenberg offers several differentiating features of congenital separation of the odontoid versus trauma. These include the site of separation which is usually between the base and the apical segment of the dens in congenital abnormalities. This suprafacet separation is in contradistinction to the fractured odontoid where the separation line is usually below the superior articular facet. The line of separation is usually irregular in a fracture, and smooth and corticated in a congenital separation [34, 69].

4.1.1.8 Hangman's Fracture

This title is a misnomer as the injury occurs to the person who is hanged and not to the hangman. However, a specific fracture of the axis has been associated with hanging, with submental placement of the knot and a moderately long drop [79]. An identical injury is seen in hyperextension injuries caused by chin or forehead striking the dashboard of a car during an accident. The basic injury is a bilateral fracture of the neural arch of the axis with an intact odontoid peg [24, 79]. In fatal cases, usually judicial hanging, death is caused by the body of the axis, odontoid peg, and atlas remaining mutually united and moving forward with the skull, the detached neural arch of the axis remaining attached to the third cervical vertebra (Fig. 4.6). The odontoid peg remains intact and does not directly contribute to the cord injury. It should be noted that the majority of these injuries are not fatal, probably because the causative force is not continuous and the canal/cord ratio in this region is favorable [24]. Usually, cord compression is not seen, although a high incidence has been reported in one series [56].

The fracture line usually passes through the interarticular segment of the pedicles which is the weakest part of the arch. The fracture line occurs anterior to the inferior articular facet on both sides but is often slightly asymmetric. The intra-articular segment of the pedicles is the weakest part of the arch, which is pierced by the foramen transversarium containing the vertebral artery. (It is of interest that the vertebral artery is rarely affected.) The superior articular process of the axis bears the weight of the skull and contents transmitted via the occipital condyles and lateral masses of the atlas. The force is then transmitted caudally in three distinct vectors: anteriorly through the vertebral bodies and bilaterally posteriorly through the pedicles onto the articular facets [24, 79]. This distribution of force combined with an inherent weakness in the arch of the axis explains the consistency of the fracture lines in a hangman's fracture.

Radiographically, it is usually difficult to see the fracture line in the anteroposterior view. On the lateral view, bilateral fractures through the neural arch anterior to the inferior facet can be seen. The occipito-atlantal and the atlantoaxial joint are normal and the odontoid is intact. (The transverse atlantal ligament is intact.) Forward dislocation of C2 on C3 nearly always occurs although there have been isolated reports of a hangman's fracture without subluxation [79]. Other bony injuries have been described in association with this fracture. An avulsion chip fracture of the anteroinferior margin of the axis or anterior-superior margin of C3 may be present reflecting damage to the anterior longitudinal ligament. Fractures of the posterior arch of C1 and disruption of the pedicles of C3 have been reported [79]. Although unusual, fractures of the odontoid have been described in a pedicle fracture of the axis but in these cases the axis fracture is usually unilateral which probably accounts for the associated odontoid damage [21] (Fig. 4.7).

With classical hangman's fracture, extensive prevertebral soft tissue swelling is invariably present, sometimes sufficient to require a tracheostomy [79].

4.1.2 Injuries Below the Axis

Injuries to this region are due mainly to hyperextension or excessive flexion. With the latter, there may be some rotary component and the flexion can be accompanied by vertical compression. Because of the almost horizontal alignment of the zygapophyseal joints, excessive flexion, usually with an element of rotation, can cause subluxation of one cervical vertebra on another, causing or contributing to the neurological deficit.

In any person suspected of having a severe neck injury, a lateral view of the cervical spine with a horizontal ray, with the patient supine, is the first projection. If there are neurological signs, then traction should be applied to the head, and if the patient is moved, then traction should be applied to the head and feet, and the trunk supported [37]. If the lateral view is normal or the fracture seen appears to be stable, then other views are taken.

Because of the association of cervical spine trauma with head injuries [84] it is important in patients with head trauma to radiograph the cervical spine. If the patient is unconscious, attention may otherwise not be directed to the cervical spine.

Patients who have congenital anomalies of the cervical spine (e. g., Klippel-Feil-syndrome) appear to be more susceptible to trauma [37].

In the cervical region it is possible to apply considerable distraction to the vertebrae without apparent bony injury and yet cause tearing of the dura with subdural and extradural hematomas and laceration of the cord [37]. This is best demonstrated radiographically by myelography. There has been considerable controversy about the role of myelography and the type of contrast medium to use in acute cervical cord injury [73]. The difference of opinion regarding the choice of contrast medium

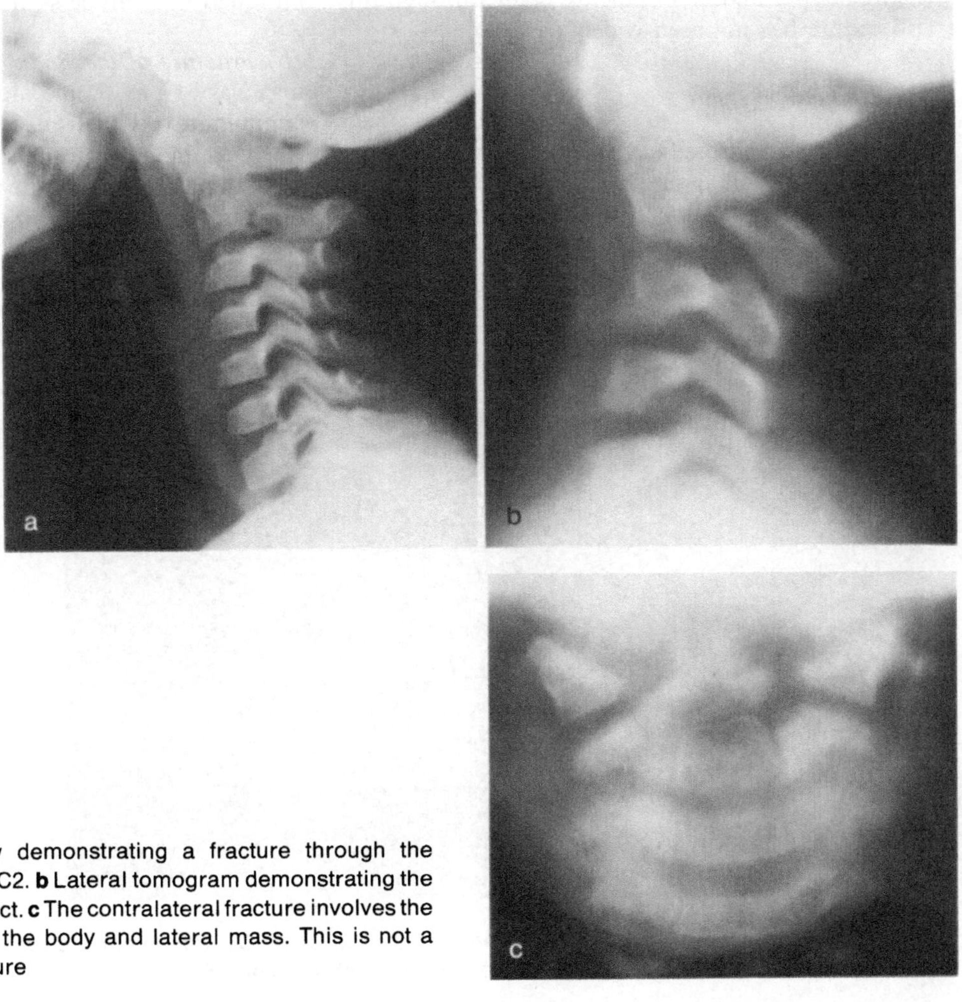

Fig. 4.7. a Lateral view demonstrating a fracture through the interarticular isthmus of C2. **b** Lateral tomogram demonstrating the fracture line to better effect. **c** The contralateral fracture involves the synchondrosis between the body and lateral mass. This is not a typical hangman's fracture

Pantopaque *vs* air has been partly resolved by the introduction of a suitable water-soluble contrast agent – Amipaque (Metrizamide). In a patient with cervical cord compromise following trauma, myelography is performed in the supine position with a lateral C1/C2 approach which usually requires an image intensifier with a C arm [89]. A moderately high concentration of Amipaque (270 mg/ml) is required for satisfactory visualization in both the anteroposterior and lateral projections [65]. In a patient with an unstable fracture or dislocation, continuous traction should be applied.

Myelography in the acute phase will demonstrate compressing bone fragments, extruded intervertebral discs, torn membranes, hematomas and cord swelling. In the chronic phase, cord atrophy and arachnoid pouches may be shown.

If there has been severe trauma to the neck and spine producing neurological deficit, then arteriography may demonstrate main vessel occlusion or narrowing which may be primarily responsible for the deficit.

There have been reports of spinal arteriography being helfpul in deciding therapy [90] although this procedure has not been widely accepted.

4.1.2.1 Flexion Injuries

These may be classified as to whether there is primarily (a) soft tissue injury, (b) fracture of the body and/or neural arch, (c) facet dislocations, or (d) avulsion fractures. There may, in some patients, be a combination of these injuries. Although flexion is usually the primary movement causing these injuries, it may be combined with vertical compression and rotation.

(a) Soft Tissue Injuries. If there is tearing of the ligamentum nuchae along with the ligamentum flavum and interosseous spinous ligaments, then there may be excessive forward movement of one cervical vertebra upon another. This is not usually associated with cord injury as the anterior and posterior longitudinal ligaments are intact, preventing gross subluxation. It may be regarded as a stable injury. On neutral or flexion view, there is widening of the interspinous space at the level of the injury. There will be excessive angulation of the body of one cervical vertebra upon another with some narrowing of the disc space anteriorly and widening posteriorly [32]. Extension views may well be normal. During healing, calcification may be seen within the interspinous ligaments. With minor soft tissue damage there may just be loss of the normal cervical lordosis, although this can be seen in normals [15].

(b) Fracture of the Body and/or Neural Arch. This may vary from simple anterior wedging to severe comminution with displacement of fragments posteriorly to impinge on the spinal cord.

A simple wedge fracture is stable without subluxation and is not usually associated with neurological

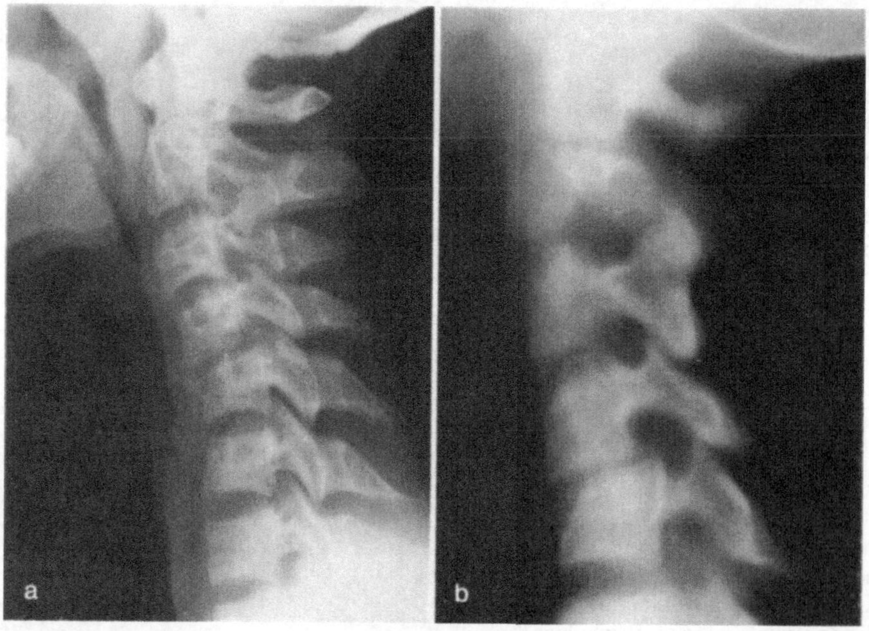

Fig. 4.8. a Lateral view showing a fracture/dislocation of C4 on C5 with anterior teardrop fracture of C5. **b** Lateral tomogram demonstrates "perching" of the inferior facèt of C4 on C5

damage [6, 32] although neurological sequelae following diving injuries have been described with this injury [51].

If the fracture of the body is comminuted with posterior extrusion of a fragment (so-called flexion teardrop fracture [32, 78], then neurological damage is likely. The fracture tends to be unstable. This fracture can be associated with posterior element damage [32], and if the zygapophyseal joints and their ligaments are affected then dislocation may occur (Fig. 4.8).

If a more vertical force has been applied to the cervical vertebrae then a bursting-type fracture may occur. In the atlas, this was first described by Jefferson (see earlier) In the lower cervical spine there is often comminution of the vertebral body sometimes with a vertical cleft [32]. There may be some impingement upon the cord but usually the posterior element remains intact.

With a severe flexion injury with marked disruption of the posterior ligaments and capsules of the zygapophyseal joints then bilateral facet dislocations may occur. Usually an element of rotation contributes to the injury. The inferior facets of the superior vertebrae are "locked" anteriorly over the superior articular facets of the vertebrae below. On the anteroposterior view, there is usually an increase in the distance between the spinous processes immediately above and below the dislocated segment [11]. The lateral and oblique views are characteristic. This lesion is often seen in football injuries [76] and with difficult breech deliveries (Fig. 4.9).

If there has been an element of rotation as well as flexion, then unilateral facet dislocations can occur [10]. The radiographic findings are subtle on the anteroposterior and lateral views; oblique views are most helpful. On the anteroposterior projection, the spinous process is displaced towards the side of the subluxation. On the lateral radiographs, there is a "step" in the line of zygapophyseal joints on one side. Oblique views will show the inferior facet projected in the intervertebral foramen. Usually, unilateral facet locking occurs in the lower cervical spine.

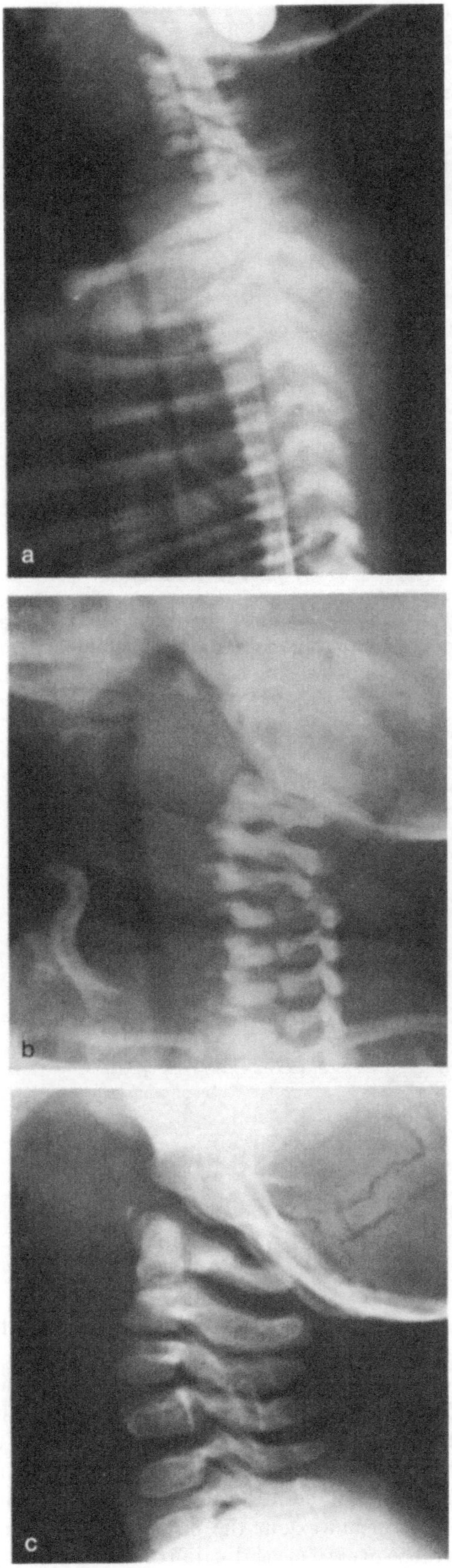

▷

Fig. 4.9. a Lateral view showing forward dislocation of C3 on C4. **b** Oblique view demonstrating locking of the inferior facet of C3 under the superior facet of C4, a child weighing 10,25 lb, had a difficult breech delivery. **c** Lateral radiograph 1 year later showing almost complete realignment with posttraumatic overgrowth of the body of C4

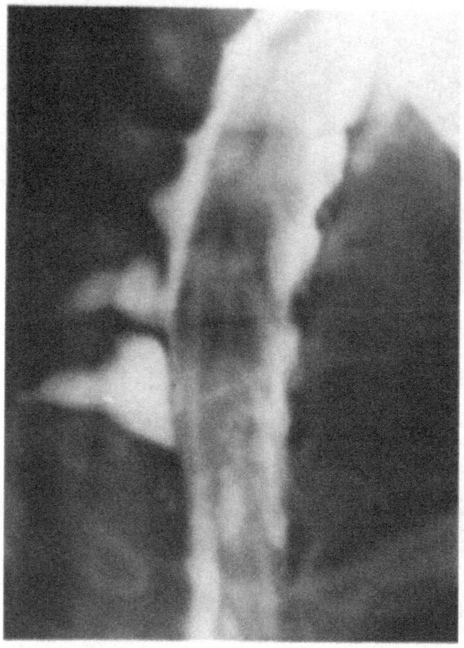

Fig. 4.10. Myelogram demonstrating posttraumatic diverticula formation. The nerve roots are not visualized at this level; indicative of avulsion

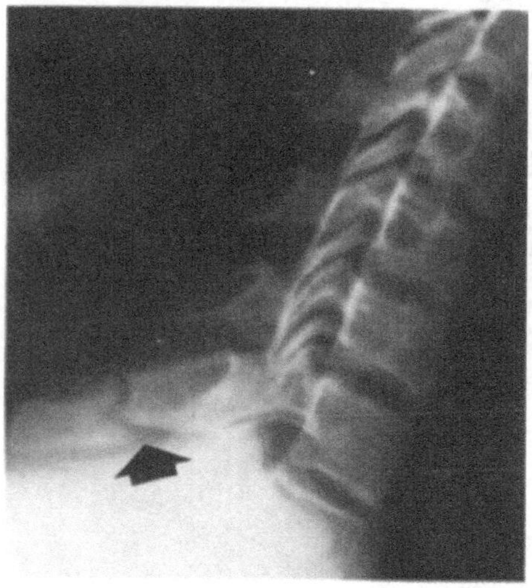

Fig. 4.11. Fracture through the spinous process of C7 (a clay shoveler's fracture)

(c) Lateral Flexion Injuries. Some injuries of the cervical spine may be due purely to lateral flexion. It is important to recognize the injury so that treatment does not cause further lateral separation of the vertebrae [72]. In severe cases there is often injury to the brachial plexus, due to stretching or avulsion of the nerve roots, in addition to a spinal cord injury [72]. To a certain extent the position of the arm, whether it be in extreme abduction or adduction, will determine which roots are affected [94]. Characteristic myelographic findings of lateral meningocele formation have been described with brachial plexus nerve root avulsion [61, 94] (Fig. 4.10) but the myelogram may be normal if the meningoceles have been sealed off by adhesions [80]. Prognosis regarding recovery is poor although a recent report showed good functional restitution in a patient with typical myelographic findings [54].

Routine radiographs usually show vertebral crush injuries on the concave side with some separation of the lateral masses and bodies on the convex side.

(d) Avulsion Injury. A fracture through the posterior spinous process of C7 can be due to indirect trauma, avulsion occurring as the result of sudden severe muscular forces (clay shoveler's fracture) (Fig. 4.11), or as a result of direct trauma. In this situation there is no spinal cord injury and the fracture is stable.

4.1.2.2 Hyperextension Injuries

Hyperextension may be the only abnormal movement causing damage to the cord meninges and vertebral column or it may be associated with a secondary hyperflexion of the spine that contributes to, or may be the dominant factor in, the injury (extension/flexion injury [47]).

It is hyperextension that is responsible for the majority of spinal cord injuries that occur during birth. The most potentially damaging position appears to be hyperextension of the neck in a breech presentation, particularly with forcible extraction [1, 12]. Although there may be severe neurological damage, plain films of the cervical spine can be normal although a complete block on myelography may be demonstrated [1]. The dura can be scarred and the cord will show extensive demyelination or transection [12]. With a breech presentation, the most common site of the spinal cord lesion is between the fifth cervical vertebra and the first thoracic vertebra [12]. In investigative work, performing myelography with hyperextension of the neck in a full-term infant who had died of heart disease, it was shown that maximum angulation occurred at the cervico-thoracic junction where the subarachnoid space was most narrow [1]. In addition, sudden flexion of the neck as the fetus descends into the birth canal probably also contributes. Cesarean section for a breech or transverse presentation with a hyperextended head is promoted as being the best way to protect the baby [1, 12, 36] although, even with cesarean section, this does not do so consistently [12] since the lesion may occur before the onset of labor [12].

In the older child, a hyperextension injury to the cervical spine is usually the result of a deceleration injury. In most healthy people, forward and lateral flexion of the spine in a deceleration injury is within physiological limits. However, with hyperextension, the head can be thrown backward until it strikes a solid object which acts as a fulcrum (e. g., car seat without head support) or the posterior chest wall. The injuries may vary from minor soft tissue damage to severe fracture/dislocation, causing tetraplegia.

Experimental data have shown soft tissue changes which have parallels in humans [55]. Muscle injuries included tears in the sternocleidomastoid area and avulsion of the longus colli. The latter was associated with the development of a retropharyngeal hematoma and damage to the sympathetic nerves. In addition, hemorrhages were present in the muscle layer of the esophagus. Perhaps more significantly there was tearing of the anterior longitudinal ligament and separation of the disc from the adjacent vertebrae. The disc damage can be demonstrated radiologically by discography, although this is rarely performed in children.

If the hyperextension injury is severe and there has been extensive damage to the anterior longitudinal ligament and intervertebral discs, then there may be a dislocation, with cord trauma. Spontaneous reduction often occurs. However, a small avulsed fragment pulled off the anterior/inferior edge of the vertebral body at the point of ligamentous tear may sometimes be seen [26].

As Forsyth [26] has pointed out, in many hyperextension injuries the force is not simply backward and downward but through a rotational arch with the main force to the cervical spine traveling forward and being counteracted by the relatively rigid bony cage and thoracic spine. The resultant injury depends to a certain degree on the strength of the anterior longitudinal ligament. If the ligament remains intact, then the force is transmitted directly to the articular facets, the spinous processes, and then to the laminae and pedicles. With continuous force and with fracture of the articular processes there will be anterior displacement of the vertebral body. Radiographs if not carefully scrutinized will give the spurious appearance of a flexion injury with forward displacement of one vertebra on another [26]. However, further observation will disclose that there are, in addition, fractures and compressions of the posterior bony elements and a chip fracture from trauma to the anterior longitudinal ligament. Usually, the damage is to the inferior articular facet of the vertebra above the site of maximum trauma rather than a fracture of the superior articular facet of the vertebra below, the latter usually being seen with flexion injuries [26].

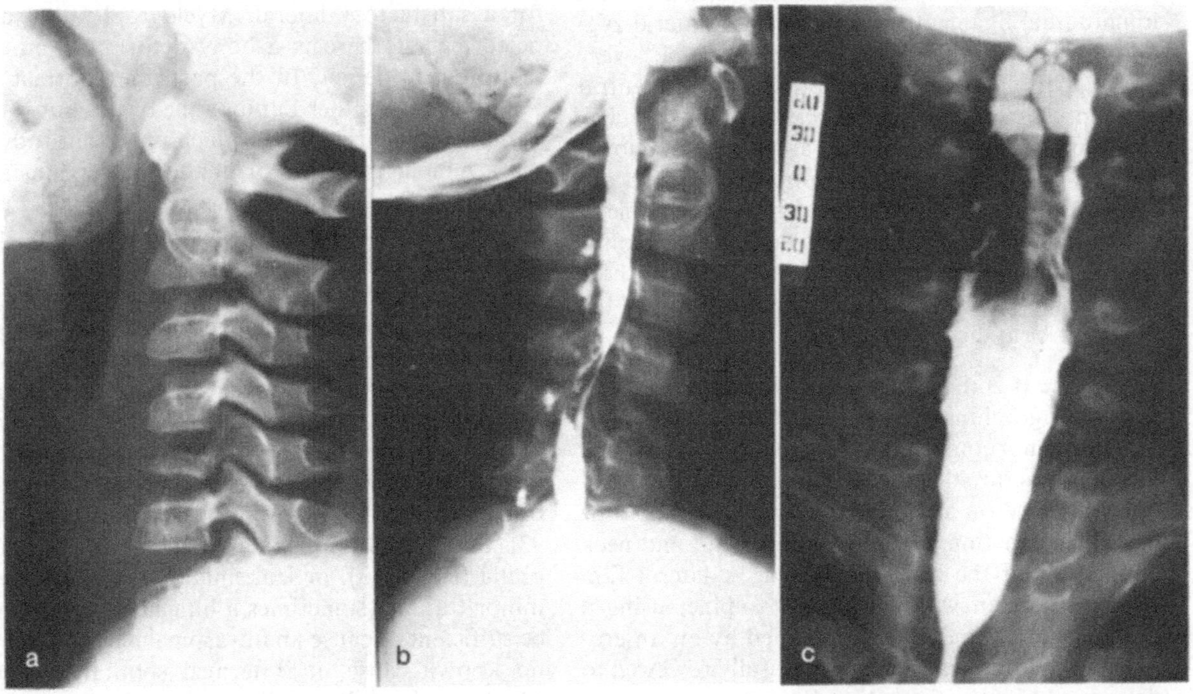

Fig. 4.12. a Symmetric loss of height of the body of C5 with preservation of the disc space. These are the appearances of histiocytosis X. **b** Lateral and **c** frontal views of a cervical myelogram demonstrating an anterior extradural mass compressing the subarachnoid space

If there has been frank rupture of the anterior longitudinal ligament, then there will be severe trauma angulation between the vertebral bodies, with misalignment and "opening up" of the disc space [26].

4.1.2.3 Pathological Fractures

It is uncommon in children for a fracture to occur in an area of preexisting disease in the cervical spine. However, occasionally histiocytosis X will present with a wedge fracture of the cervical spine. If there is a history of trauma, it is often minimal and out of all proportion to the vertebral compression. The lateral view of the cervical spine will demonstrate a wedge fracture of the body, sometimes with posterior extension that involves the subarachnoid space and cord, as shown on myelography (Fig. 4.12). Healing may result in reconstitution of the vertebral body or it may remain collapsed. There are often associated skeletal lesions to support the diagnosis of histiocytosis X.

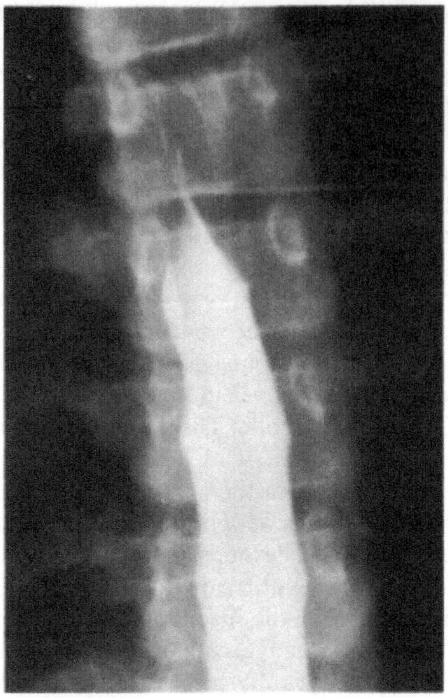

Fig. 4.13. AP view of a myelogram demonstrating a complete block at T6 due to a left-sided extradural mass which was a chronic hematoma in a 13-year-old hemophiliac. (Courtesy of Gordon McComb, MD)

4.2 Thoracolumbar Spine

Anatomy. All the thoracic and lumbar vertebrae articulate the same way. There is a central intervertebral disc with accompanying anterior and posterior longitudinal ligaments and two posterolateral zygapophyseal joints. The intervertebral disc has a very strong peripheral annulus fibrosis and a central incompressible fluid-filled nucleus pulposus. The two components of the disc act as a single functional unit of great strength. The apophyseal joints are supported by the "posterior ligament complex" consisting of the intraspinous and supraspinous ligaments and the ligamentum flavum [39]. For there to be dislocation, there must be interruption of the posterior bony ligamentous complex.

Radiology. It is most important when transporting and radiographing the patient that neurological function is not compromised in a patient who has an unstable fracture/dislocation. The patient is transported supine on a firm board, and if he has to be lifted then traction is applied to the head and neck and feet, and the back supported. A lateral film should be taken with the patient supine, using a horizontal ray, and be accompanied by an anteroposterior film. These films are carefully reviewed to determine whether the patient has an unstable spine before oblique views and/or tomography are performed. Special attention has to be applied to the lower cervical and upper thoracic region. Swimmers views and traction on the arms are often necessary for a satisfactory lateral. Myelography is usually performed if there is a bony deformity and/or a neurological deficit. In the past, the contrast medium has been either Pantopaque or air, but is now Amipaque (metrizamide), which may be introduced via a lumbar puncture or, if the spine is unstable, through a C1/C2 approach. Cord swelling due to edema and extradural compression by bony fragments and hematomas can be demonstrated.

Epidural and subdural hematomas may be difficult to diagnose accurately on clinical findings alone. They may mimic cord edema if following acute trauma, vascular accidents to the cord, and other extramedullary causes of cord compression, particularly metastasis. These hematomas may follow severe injuries or occur after minor trauma, often when the initial event has been forgotten [23, 93]. Sometimes anticoagulant therapy [81], hemophilia (Fig. 4.13), or leukemia [23] combined with minor trauma (sometimes a lumbar puncture) may be sufficient to cause an intraspinal bleed. If there is no known cause, it is termed spontaneous [68]. Myelography will usually localize the level of the block and demonstrate its extent.

Recently, computerized axial tomography has been used in demonstrating narrowing of the spinal canal with fractures of the dorsolumbar spine [17]. Computerized axial tomography has the advantage of demonstrating soft tissue deformities not seen with regular transverse axial tomography of the spine [46].

The thoracolumbar spine can be subjected to five main types of force which may act singularly or in combination. These are flexion (which may be forward or lateral), compression, rotation, extension, and shearing [40].

4.2.1 Flexion Injuries

In children, forward flexion injuries usually result from a fall or traffic accident [35, 41]. Although rare, tetanus can cause these injuries (Fig. 4.14). The injury is more common in boys [41]. With pure forward flexion, it is extremely rare for the posterior ligaments to be ruptured or a fracture to occur through the posterior bony elements [71], although it can happen [62] and has been seen in abused children [18, 52], although in these cases there may be an element of shearing. Knowledge of the mechanics involved with forward flexion will explain the infrequency of posterior bony/ligamentous damage. The centrum of the forward flexion is through the nucleus pulposus of the intervertebral disc and, therefore, the anterior body is subjected to about four times the disruptive forces affecting the posterior bony ligamentous complex and takes the brunt of the force [71]. In addition, the posterior bony ligamenous complex is resistant to pure forward flexional forces. The posterior ligament complex being intact, the fracture is stable. In the thoracic region the ribs add to the stability.

On a lateral radiograph there will be loss of height anteriorly (anterior wedging) and a normal adjacent intervertebral disc [71], although disc damage has been reported in child abuse [52]. The most common site for the fracture is between T4 and L2 and specifically at the thoracolumbar junction [35]. There are often multiple vertebral body fractures [35]. Occasionally, there may be some increased density within the vertebral body caused by bone compaction and sometimes anterior beaking of the vertebra may be demonstrated, particularly at the thoracolumbar junction [38]. This can come about as a result of chronic flexion in conditions in which there is chronic flexion stress at the thoracolumbar junction (e. g., cretinism and mongolism). If many fragments are involved, then a gibbus may result. Loss of height with some lateral bulging may be seen on the anteroposterior film. A paravertebral hematoma may also be demonstrated in the acute phase (Fig. 4.15).

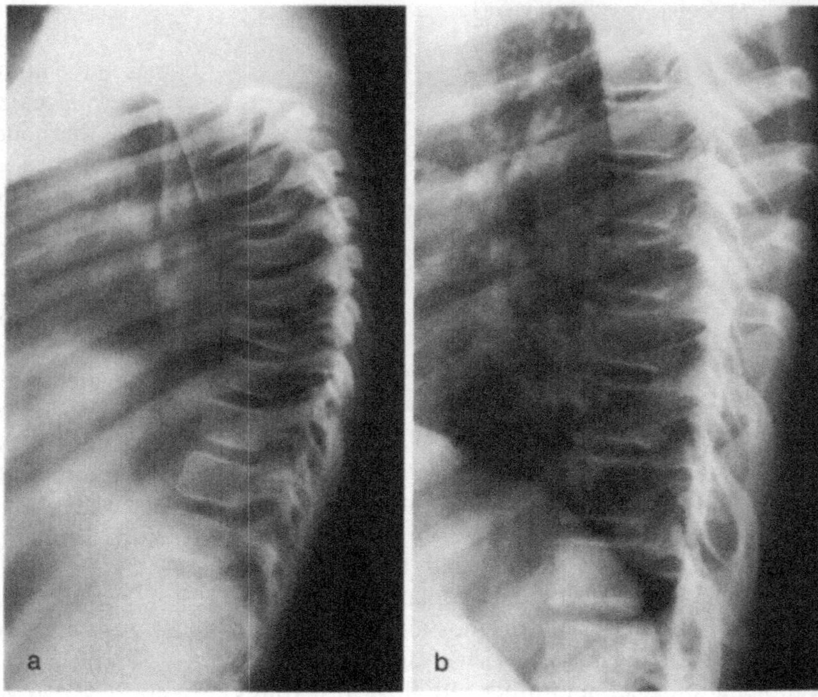

Fig. 4.14. a Multiple anterior wedge fractures in a 5-year-old boy with tetanus. **b** Lateral view 5 years later shows complete restitution of the shape and height of the vertebral bodies

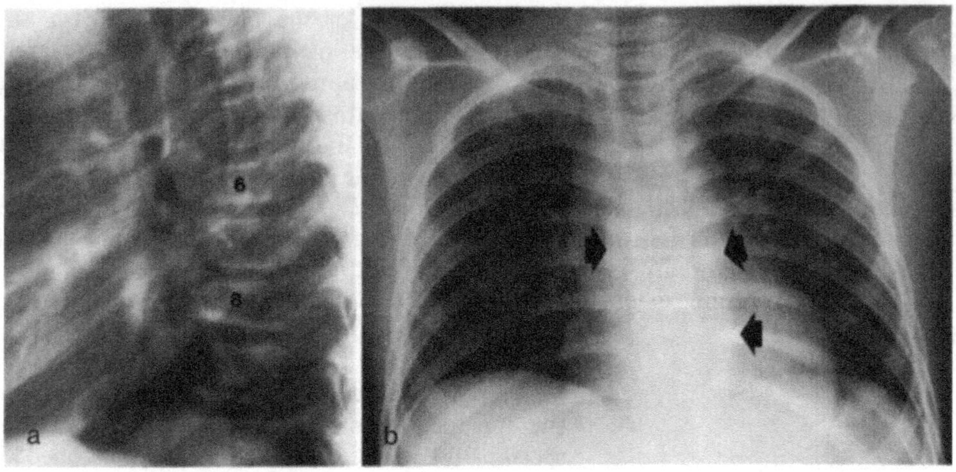

Fig. 4.15. a Fractures of the bodies of T6 and T8 with an associated paravertebral hematoma (**b**)

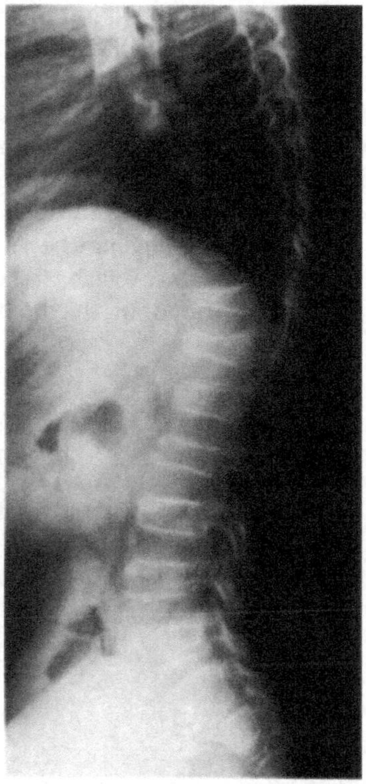

Fig. 4.16. Osteopenic vertebrae with wedging of several of the bodies due to leukemia

The differential diagnosis of anterior wedging includes Scheuermann's disease in which there is irregularity of end plates not usually seen in trauma. Osteogenesis imperfecta and neoplastic infiltration (Fig. 4.16) are important diagnostic considerations along with histiocytosis X. Usually, there are clinical, hematological, and other radiological features to help distinguish these conditions. It should be noted that slight anterior wedging of vertebral bodies in the midthoracic region may be physiological. Lack of pain and no history of injury should separate this condition from trauma, and if there is any doubt then a bone scan will be helpful as it is usually positive in acute trauma.

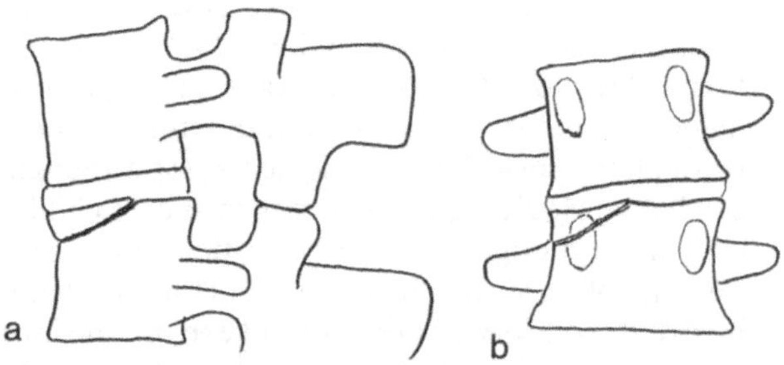

Fig. 4.17. Frontal (**a**) and lateral (**b**) diagrams demonstrating a marginal plateau fracture of a lumbar vertebra

Traumatically induced wedge vertebrae usually reconstitute themselves, often taking over a year before returning to normal [35] (Fig. 4.14). Scheuermann's disease does not appear to be an end result of acute vertebral trauma.

With lateral flexion, particularly with an element of compression, a marginal plateau fracture may result (Fig. 4.17) which should not be confused with a slice fracture, the latter often being unstable (see later). With a marginal fracture there is an oblique fracture through the end plate.

4.2.2 Seat-belt Hyperflexion Injury

In crashes involving cars traveling usually in excess of 80 km/h there is a characteristic lumbar spine injury associated with lap seat belts. It is rare in

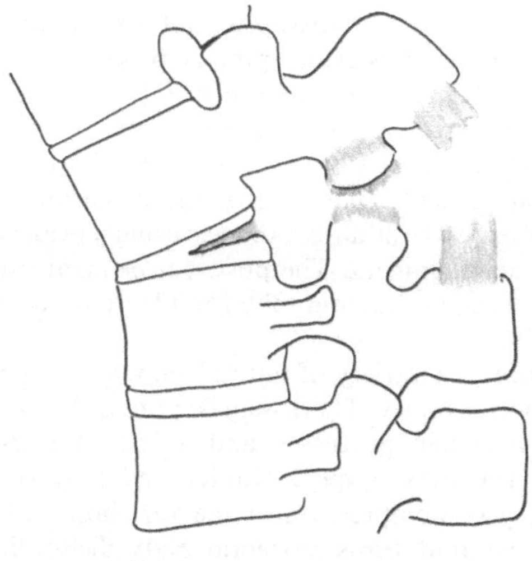

Fig. 4.18. Typical lap seat belt injury with rupture of the posterior ligaments

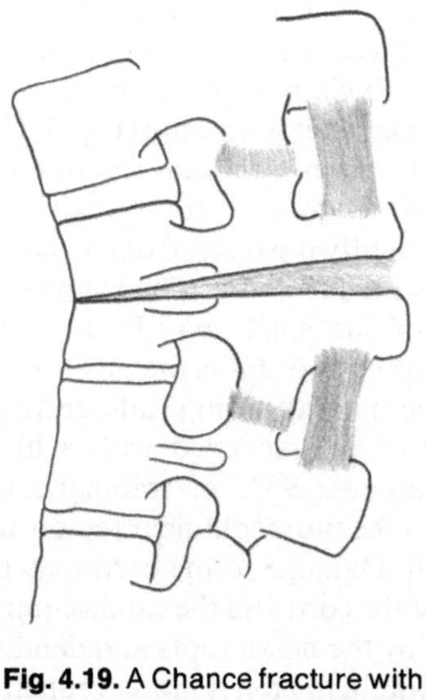

Fig. 4.19. A Chance fracture with horizontal splitting of the body, transverse processes and spinous processes. The posterior ligaments are intact

drivers because hyperflexion is prevented by the steering wheel. With a restraining lap seat belt, during sudden deceleration there is acute hyperflexion as well as compression of the abdominal contents. Unlike "ordinary" flexion injuries, the fulcrum of rotation is the seat belt, which is immediately anterior to the vertebral bodies. Hence, tremendous vertical disruptive forces are applied to the posterior bony ligamentous complex which tends to "open up" the posterior joints. Usually, the first to the third lumbar vertebrae are affected, there are seat-belt contusion marks on the skin, and sometimes associated abdominal visceral injuries. Radiographs usually show widening of the interspinous distance and increase in the height of the intervertebral foramina [86] (Fig. 4.18). There may be avulsion of the superior articular facets and avulsion fractures of the vertebral bodies. There is no or minimal forward or lateral subluxation and usually no or little, vertebral body compression. Usually, this particular pattern of injury is not associated with neurological damage unless rotational forces have been applied. Occasionally, this particular seat-belt injury will result in a Chance fracture [16] with horizontal splitting of the body, pedicles, transverse processes, and spinous process (Fig. 4.19). In this situation, the interspinous ligaments are intact. With modern combination lap and seat belts and head supports this type of injury should be seen less frequently. It should also be noted that other injuries to the lumbar spine may occur in belt wearers in car crashes. Such injuries are not directly linked to wearing a lap seat belt [42].

4.2.3 Compression

With a pure vertical compression force, the vertebral end plates take the brunt of the force. The end plate at first bulges inward, with consequent squeezing of blood out of the cancellous bone of the vertebral body [71]. There is very little change in the intervertebral disc until the end plate cracks and allows nuclear material to intrude into the body of the vertebra. If sufficient vertical compression is applied, then not only will the end plate "give" but there will also be a vertical fracture of the body, which can be comminuted with some backward displacement of fragments into the canal, the so-called burst fracture (Fig. 4.20). Cord damage may be present. The posterior elements are intact and the fracture is stable. Vertical compressive forces are

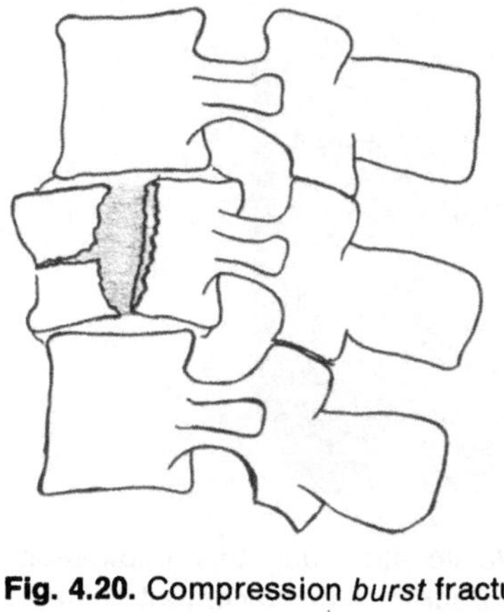

Fig. 4.20. Compression *burst* fracture with backward extrusion of the posterior elements

often associated with forward flexion, to cause vertebral body injuries (e. g., fall from a height).

4.2.4 Rotation

This force is often combined with forward flexion and sometimes with vertical compression. The intervertebral discs, capsules of the zygapophyseal joints, and posterior ligaments are resistant to forward flexion, extension and compressive forces but vulnerable to rotation [71]. In rotation combined with flexion there is tearing of the posterior ligamentous complex and the capsule of the zygapophyseal joints, occasionally causing damage to the posterior bony elements. As a result of the posterior disruption, dislocation can occur and the condition is unstable (Fig. 4.21). The zygapophyseal joints may simply be opened up or there may be perching of the facets or forward dislocation with fracture of the posterior bony elements and facet locking [49]. It should be noted that it is possible to have forward slip of one vertebra upon another and bilateral fractures through the pars interarticularis, there being forward displacement of the superior facet, and the inferior facet remaining behind, similar to classical spondylolisthesis [49, 62]. In this situation, the posterior ligaments are intact (Type V Kaufer and Hays). This is an extremely rare type of injury. Forward slip is rare above L4 [62] but does occur.

Often, the posterior ligaments rupture without associated bony posterior element fracture, but if the injury is severe then disruption of the laminae, articular facets, posterior spinous processes, and fracture of the pedicles will be seen [87]. On a lateral view of the vertebra, the damage to the posterior ligamentous complex may be inferred if there is abnormal vertical separation of the posterior spinous processes. In addition, there is usually evidence of facet malalignment. The posterior element fractures may require tomography for adequate visualization [87].

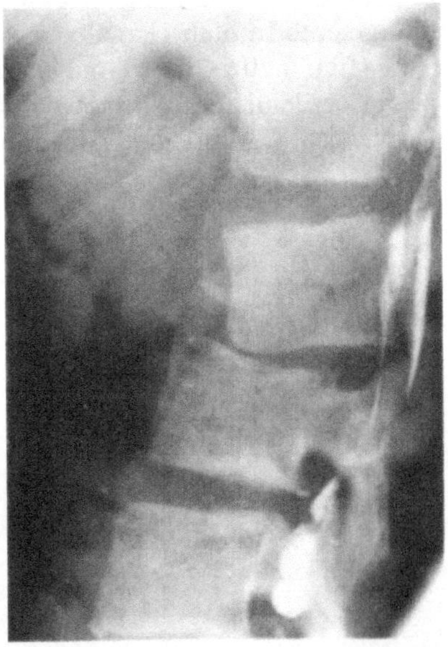

Fig. 4.21. Fracture/dislocation due to combination of flexion and rotation. Backward displacement of the cord has been demonstrated by myelography

Anteriorly, a variety of injuries may accompany this posterior injury. There may be pure dislocation of the articular processes and vertebral bodies without fractures (Type I Kaufer and Hayes) or there may be compression of the vertebral bodies with or without frank vertebral body dislocation (Types II and III respectively) (Figs. 4.22, 4.23). A more complex injury is seen in Type IV which is also referred to as the rotational or slice fracture [39, 62, 71]. Anteriorly, there is a rotational tear through the disc and a slice fracture through the superior surface of the body which may be comminuted, usually with a transverse process fracture (Fig. 4.24). Comminution and a transverse process fracture on the convex side help separate a rotational slice fracture, which is inherently unstable, from a marginal plateau fracture which is stable. The rotational fracture/dislocation of the spine may be reduced when the patient is supine and this is the position in which to maintain the patient during radiography. This particular fracture is associated with a high incidence of cord damage: 95% of traumatically induced paraplegias in the thoracolumbar region are due to this injury [39]. Damage to the cord may be related to the fact that the cord and the cauda equina are tethered laterally by the nerve roots and dentate ligament so that the lateral flexion is more traumatic to the cord than pure forward flexion.

Dislocation of the lumbar spine occurs more frequently with anomalies of segmentation. Presumably as a result of limited movement at the anomalous sites a disproportionate amount of stress is placed upon the normal segments during trauma [49].

4.2.5 Extension

With hyperextension, the posterior ligamentous complex remains intact but there are "compressive" fractures of the laminae and pedicles. The anterior ligament is often ruptured with opening up of the disc space. However, it should be noted that this is an extremely rare injury in the thoracolumbar spine.

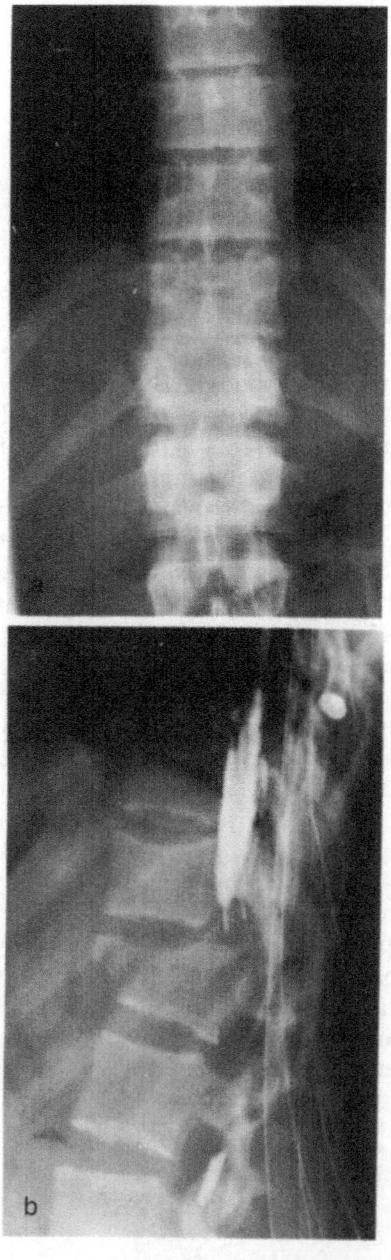

Fig. 4.22. a Frontal projection showing narrowing of the T11–12 disc space with slight frontal misalignment. **b** Lateral projection with cisternally introduced Pantopaque showing almost complete obstruction. There is forward subluxation of T11 on T12 with a fracture of the body of T12. This injury was due to a combination of flexion and shearing

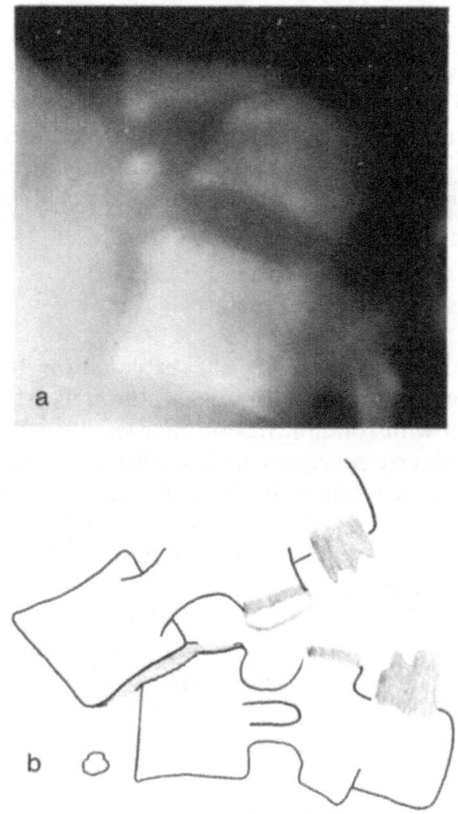

Fig. 4.23. a Tomogram demonstrating forward slip of L1 on L2 with fracture of the superior surface of L2 and displacement of chip fracture. **b** Fracture and associated ligamentous injury. This is equivalent to Kaufer and Hayes, Type II

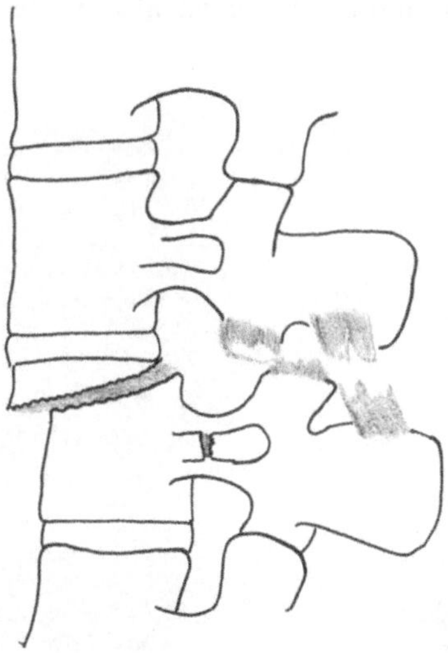

Fig. 4.24. Rotational slice fracture with a fracture through the body and transverse process associated with ligamentous rupture. This is equivalent to Kaufer and Hayes, Type IV

4.2.6 Shearing

This occurs when a violent force is applied directly to the back. The upper part of the spine is sheared off, the vertebral body being displaced forward, resulting in fracture of the articular processes and/or pedicles and rupture of all of the posterior ligaments [40].

4.2.7 Transverse Process Fractures

Direct violence is probably the explanation for fractures of the transverse processes although these can be seen with rotation/flexion injuries. Usually, several transverse processes are involved with some separation at the fracture site due to the action of the quadratus lumborum (Fig. 4.25). Because of the site of insertion of quadratus lumborum into the tips of the transverse processes, this muscle is no longer effective and the contralateral quadratus lumborum, now unopposed, causes a scoliosis which is convex to the side of the fracture [Gilsanz, personal communication 1979].

4.2.8 Posttraumatic Deformity

Due to a combination of alteration of the bony contour and alignment, in association with damage to the growing end plate, progressive spine deformity (scoliosis/lordosis/kyphosis) is sometimes seen in the thoracolumbar spine. As a rule, the younger the child and the higher the lesion the greater is the chance of deformity, and the curve will also be more severe.

Deformity may result from extensive laminectomy for neurosurgical procedures.

4.3 Lumbosacral Spine

4.3.1 Fatigue or Stress Changes

In the past, there has been considerable controversy regarding the etiology of "defects" in the pars interarticularis. If there is a defect and no slip, then the condition is termed "spondylolysis" and if there is forward slip "spondylolisthesis." It is most probable that the defect represents a fatique fracture resulting from a repeated minor trauma, although it can occur following one acute episode [70, 92] (Fig. 4.26). However, as Wilste [92] points out, there are certain differences between this particular fatigue fracture and other stress fractures. In fatigue fractures of the pars interarticularis, the fractures occur at an earlier age, exuberant callus is rarely seen, and healing is rare. There appears to be a very strong hereditary factor, the pars and laminae being hypoplastic and prone to fracture [92]. Boys are affected more than girls probably because boys undergo more violent exercise. There is considerable experimental data [54] to support the fatigue fracture hypothesis demonstrated clinically and by serial radiography. Not only will congenitally hypoplastic posterior arch be more prone to fracture but, if excessive stresses are applied following spinal fusion to the adjacent vertebrae, a fatigue fracture may occur [33]. There may be an associated disc protrusion which can only be demonstrated by myelography (Fig. 4.27).

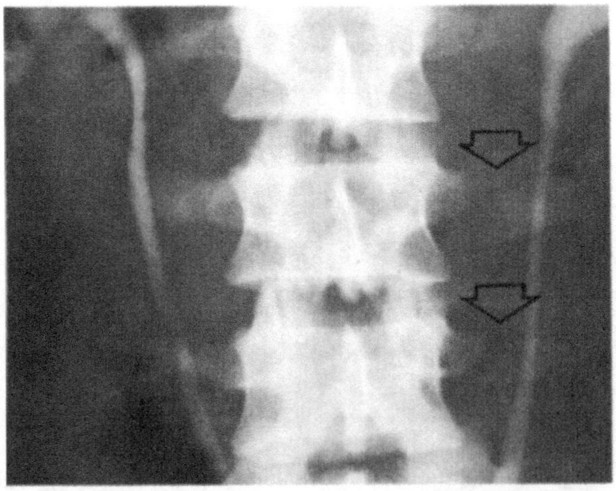

Fig. 4.25. Fracture of left transverse processes of L2 and L3

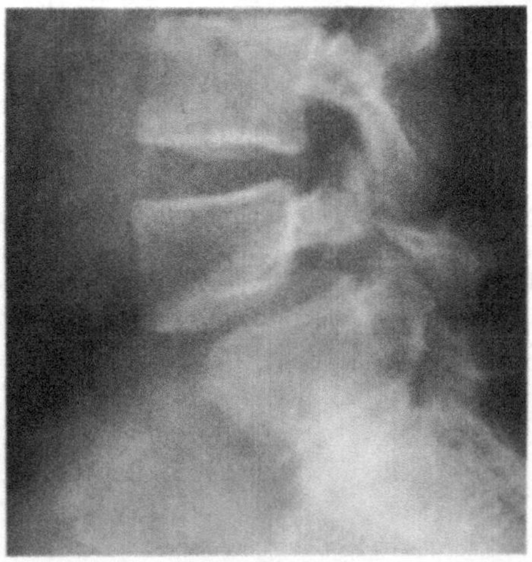

Fig. 4.26. Spondylolisthesis of L5 on S1 with a break in the pars interarticularis following acute trauma

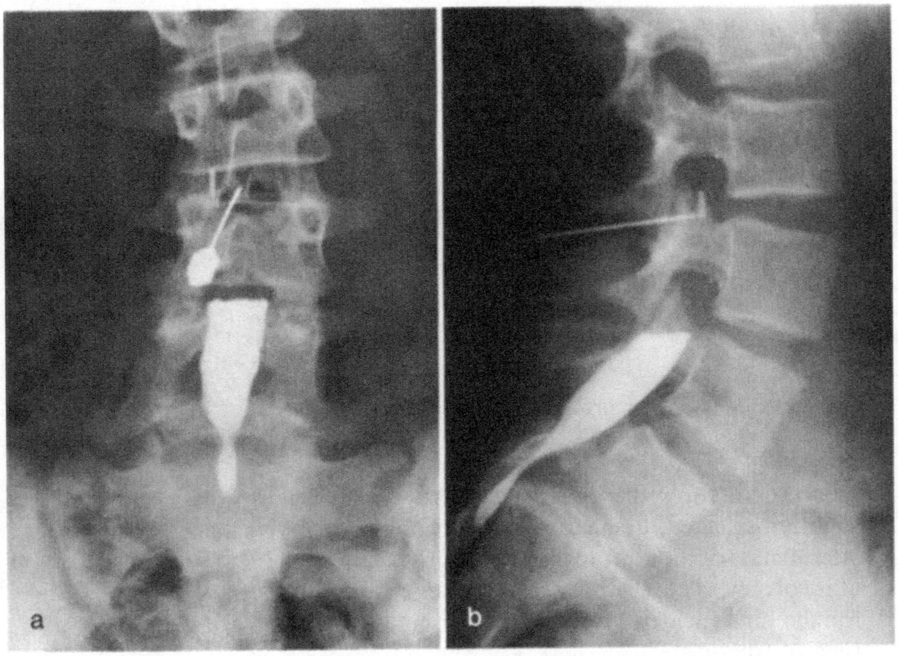

Fig. 4.27. Myelograms showing protrusion at L5/S1 at site of a spondylolisthesis; frontal (a) and lateral (b) projection

Wilkinson [91] has drawn attention to the presence of bony hypertrophy of the pars interarticularis and pedicles opposite a unilateral break in the pars interarticularis. This sclerosis represents a compensation for instability of the posterior arch complex and should not be confused with a neoplasm or infection.

4.3.2 Fractures of the Sacrum and Coccyx

The sacrum forms the posterior element of the pelvic ring, and because of this fractures of the sacrum are frequently associated with innominate bone fractures [66]. A brief review of the anatomy will explain the types of fracture seen, occurring as they do through the weaker bony elements.

The sacrum articulates with the innominate bone through the sacroiliac articulation which extends from the upper margin of the first sacral foramen to the upper margin of the third. The first and second anterior and posterior sacral foramina which join the lateral mass with the body are areas of weakness through which fracture lines often start and spread. The sacrum is most often involved due to indirect violence transmitted through the innominate bone although it can also be subjected to direct violence and avulsion strain.

The sacrum appears to be very resistant to compression and is usually fractured by tension and by shearing. Bonnin [9] has described the three main forces causing indirect violence to the sacrum: rotation, leverage, and shearing. In rotation, there is disruption of the anterior part of the pelvic ring (separation of the symphysis pubis or fractures of the ischiopubic rami). There is hyperextension, with rotation of the innominate bone around the horizontal axis of the sacroiliac joint. Rotational force is therefore applied to the upper sacral foramina with consequent fracture. With a leverage fracture, the symphysis pubis is opened up, and, with further abduction after distracting the sacroiliac joint, the sacrum is further wedged with a fracture through the first and second sacral foramina (Fig. 4.28). In

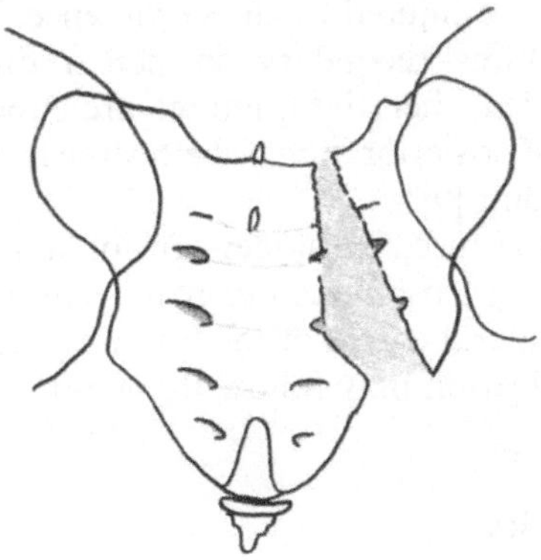

Fig. 4.28. Common site of fracture through the sacral foramen

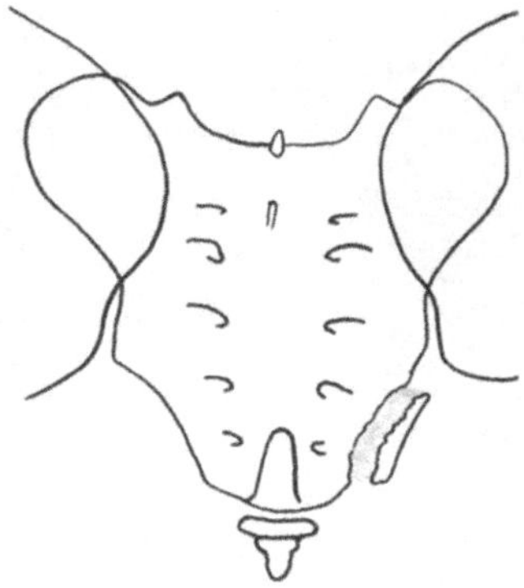

Fig. 4.29. Avulsion fracture through body of the sacrum

shearing fractures, the leg is driven backward and, if slightly abducted, a shearing fracture through the lateral mass of the sacrum may result. The frequency of involvement of the upper sacral foramen accounts for the high incidence of nerve involvement in this type of fracture.

Demonstrating the vertical fracture line through the sacral foramen due to indirect violence can be difficult. The sacrum is not perpendicular to a central anterior-posterior ray and the innominate bones obscure the sacrum in the lateral projection. Often, feces obscure the fine detail of the pelvis in the frontal projection and it is all too easy to overlook important sacral fractures in the presence of extensive innominate bone injuries. The anterior-superior sacral line as noted by Bonnin [9] and Northrup [63] is a useful landmark in diagnosing vertical sacral fractures. The anterior-superior sacral lines form the superior boundaries to the anterior exit foramen of the first, second, and third sacral nerves. They are visualized in the anteroposterior view. Disruption of the continuity of the line is seen with vertical fractures involving the anterior sacral foramen. If necessary, this can be confirmed by frontal tomography.

The sacrum can be injured by direct violence. If comminuted fractures secondary to penetrating wounds are excluded, then the fractures are either compression of the posterior arch or below the level of the sacroiliac joint [9].

Avulsion injuries caused by sudden tension in the sacrotuberous and sacrospinous ligaments cause a slice through the lateral cortex of the lower sacrum (Fig. 4.29). Calcification may follow this injury.

4.3.3 Coccyx Injuries

Fracture of the coccyx and forward dislocation at the sacrococcygeal junction may occur due to direct violence, the patient suddenly falling and landing on their "bottom" (Fig. 4.30). This injury may be painful but be of little consequence except it could interfere with childbirth later.

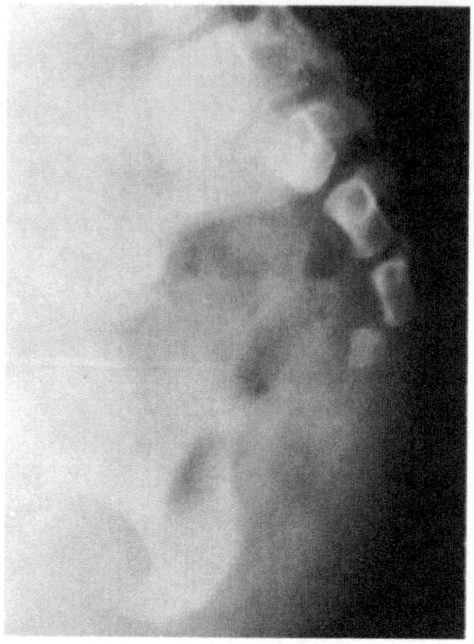

Fig. 4.30. Fracture/dislocation of last sacral segment with forward displacement

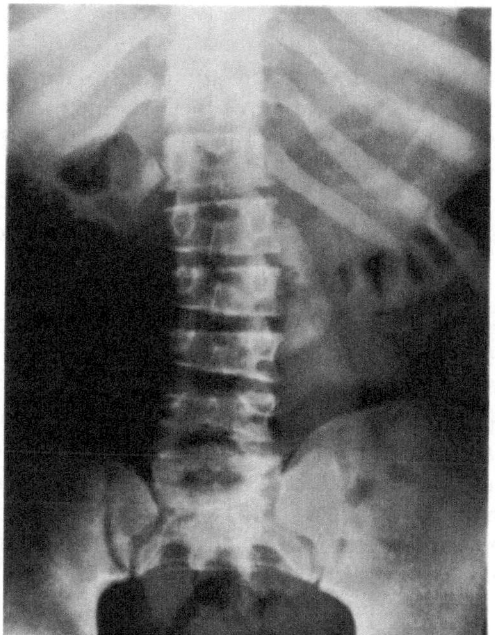

Fig. 4.31. Lateral wedging and scoliosis in the lumbar region secondary to irradiation of a right Wilms' tumor

4.3.4 Radiation Injury to the Lumbar Spine

Depending on the surgical and pathological staging, radiation may be given to the renal fossa following nephrectomy for Wilms' tumor. In the past, this was given with an orthovoltage machine whose isodose curve characteristics are such that the ipsilateral half of the spine is often irradiated along with the planned field. The growth of the spine is adversely affected, there is lateral wedging of the vertebra, and consequent scoliosis, which in part is also due to postirradiation soft tissue contracture (Fig. 4.31). With more modern sources of irradiation there is less "scatter" and the bone absorption at higher voltage is less.

References

1. Abroms IF, Bresnan MJ, Zuckerman JE, Fischer EG, Strand R (1973) Cervical cord injuries secondary to hypertension of the head in breech presentation. Obstet Gynecol 41:369–378
2. Ahmann PA, Smith SA, Schwartz JF, Clark DB (1975) Spinal cord infarction due to minor trauma in children. Neurology (Minneap) 25:301–307
3. Amyes EW, Anderson FM (1956) Fracture of the odontoid process (report of 63 cases). Arch Surg 72:377–393
4. Anderson LD, D'Alonzo RT (1974) Fractures of the odontoid process of the axis. J Bone Joint Surg [Am] 56a:1663–1674
5. Bailey DK (1952) The normal cervical spine in infants and children. Radiology 59:712–719
6. Barnes R (1948) Paraplegia in cervical spine injuries. J Bone Joint Surg [Br] 30b:239–244
7. Bedbrook GM (1966) Pathological principals in the management of spinal cord trauma. Paraplegia 4:43–56
8. Bell C (1830) The nervous system of the human body. Longman, Rees, Orme, Brown and Green, London
9. Bonnin JG (1945) Sacral fractures and injuries to the cauda equina. J Bone Joint Surg [Br] 27:113–127
10. Braakman R, Vinken PJ (1967) Unilateral facet interlocking in the lower cervical spine. J Bone Joint Surg [Br] 49b:249–257
11. Braakman R, Vinken PJ (1968) Old luxations of the lower cervical spine. J Bone Joint Surg [Br] 50b:52–60
12. Brans YW, Cassady G (1975) Neonatal spinal cord injuries. Am J Obstet Gynecol 123:918–919
13. Burke DC (1974) Traumatic spinal paralysis in children. Paraplegia 11:268–276
14. Calenoff L, Chessaare JW, Rogers LF, Toerge J, Rosen JS (1978) Multiple level spinal injuries: importance of early recognition. AJR 130:665–669
15. Cattell HS, Filtzer DL (1965) Pseudosubluxation and other normal variations in the cervical spine in children. J Bone Joint Surg [Am] 47a:1295–1309
16. Chance GQ (1948) Note on a type of flexion fracture of the spine. Br J Radiol 21:452–453
17. Coolley DP, Dunsker SB (1978) Traumatic narrowing of the dorsolumbar spinal canal demonstrated by computer tomography. Radiology 129:95–98
18. Cullen JC (1975) Spinal lesions in battered babies. J Bone Joint Surg [Br] 57b:364–366
19. Daffner RH (1977) Pseudofracture of the dens: mach bands. AJR 128:607–612
20. Dankmeijer J, Rethmeier BJ (1943) Lateral movement in the atlanto-axial joints and its clinical significance. Acta Radiol [Diagn] (Stockh) 24:55–66
21. Daum W, Archer CR (1977) Fracture of the odontoid associated with pedicle fracture of the axis: a previously undescribed entity. J Trauma 17:381–386
22. Dzenitis AJ (1966) Spontaneous atlanto-axial dislocation in a mongoloid child with spinal cord compression. J Neurosurg 25:458–460
23. Edelson RN, Chernik NL, Posner JB (1974) Spinal subdural hematomas complicating lumbar puncture. Arch Neurol 31:134–137
24. Elliott JM, Rogers LF, Wissinger JP, Lee JF (1972) The hangmans fracture. Radiology 104:303–307
25. Fielding JW (1965) Disappearance of the central portion of the odontoid process. J Bone Joint Surg [Br] 47:1128–1230
26. Forsyth HF (1964) Extension injuries of the cervical spine. J Bone Joint Surg [Am] 46a:1792–1797
27. Freiberger RH, Wilson PD, Nicholas JA (1965) Acquired absence of the odontoid process. A case report. J Bone Joint Surg [Am] 47a:1231–1236
28. Gabrielsen TO, Maxwell JA (1966) Traumatic atlanto-occipital dislocation. AJR 97:624–629
29. Gilles FH, Binna M, Sotrel A (1979) Infantile atlanto-occipital instability. Am J Dis Child 133:30–37
30. Greenberg AD (1968) Atlanto-axial dislocations. Brain 91:655–684
31. Gwinn JL, Smith JL (1962) Acquired and congenital absence of the odontoid process. AJR 88:424–431
32. Harris JH, Edeiken J (1976) Acute cervical spine trauma. Weekly Radiology Science Update, Number 17
33. Harris RI, Wiley JJ (1963) Acquired spondylolysis as a sequel to spinal fusion. J Bone Joint Surg [Am] 45a:1159–1170
34. Hawkins RJ, Fielding JW, Thompson WJ (1976) Os odontoideum: congenital or acquired. J Bone Joint Surg [Am] 58a:413–414
35. Hegenbarth R, Ebel KD (1976) Roentgen findings in fractures of the vertebral column in childhood. Pediatr Radiol 5:34–39
36. Hellstrom B, Sallmander U (1968) Prevention of spinal cord injury in hyperextension of the fetal head. JAMA 204:107–110
37. Hoffman HJ, Hendrick EB, Humphrics RP (1975) Spinal cord injuries in care for the injured child. Williams & Wilkins, Baltimore
38. Hohl M, Baker HR (1964) The atlantoaxial joint. J Bone Joint Surg [Am] 46a:1739–1752

39. Holdsworth FW (1963) Fractures, dislocations and fracture-dislocation of the spine. J Bone Joint Surg [Br] 45b:6–20
40. Holdsworth F (1970) Fractures, dislocations, and fracture-dislocations of the spine. J Bone Joint Surg [Am] 52a:1534–1539
41. Horal J, Nachemson A, Scheller S (1972) Clinical and radiological long term follow up of vertebral fractures in children. Acta Orthop Scand 43:491–503
42. Huelke DF, Kaufer H (1975) Vertebral column injuries and seat belts. J Trauma 15:304–318
43. Husby J, Srensen KH (1974) Fracture of the odontoid process of the axis. Acta Orthop Scand 45:182–192
44. Jacobson G, Adler DC (1956) An evaluation of lateral atlanto-axial displacement in injuries of the cervical spine. Radiology 61:355–362
45. Jacobson G, Bleeker HH (1959) Pseudosubluxation of the axis in children. AJR 82:472–481
46. Jacobson RE, Gargano FP, Rosomoff HL (1975) Transverse axial tomography of the spine. J Neurosurg 42:406–419
47. Janes JM, Hooshmand H (1965) Severe extension-flexion injuries of the cervical spine. Mayo Clin Proc 40:353–369
48. Jefferson G (1920) Fracture of the atlas vertebra. report of four cases and a review of those previously recorded. Br J Surg 7:407–422
49. Kaufer H, Hayes JT (1966) Lumbar fracture-dislocation. J Bone Joint Surg [Am] 48a:712–730
50. Kershner MS, Goodman GA, Perlmutter GS (1977) Computed tomography in the diagnosis of an atlas fracture. AJR 128:688–689
51. Kewalraman LS, Kraus JF (1977) Acute spinal-cord lesions from diving – epidemiological and clinical features. West J Med 126:353–361
52. Kogutt MS, Swischuk LE, Fagan CJ (1974) Patterns of injury and significance of uncommon fractures in the battered child syndrome. AJR 121:143–149
53. Jelasic F, Piepgras U (1974) Functional restitution after cervical avulsion injury with "typical" myelographic finding. Eur Neurol 11:158–163
54. Lafferty JF, Winter WG, Gambaro SA (1977) Fatigue characteristics of posterior elements of vertebrae. J Bone Joint Surg [Am] 59a:154–158
55. Macnab I (1964) Acceleration injuries of the cervical spine. J Bone Joint Surg [Am] 46a:1797–1799
56. Marar BC (1975) Fracture of the axis arch. Clin Orthop 106:155–165
57. Martel W, Tishler JM (1966) Observations on the spine in mongoloidism. AJR 97:630–637
58. McRae DL (1953) Bony abnormalities in region of foramen magnum: correlation of anatomic and neurologic findings. Acta Radiol [Diagn] (Stockh) 40:335–355
59. Melzak J (1969) Paraplegia among children. Lancet II:45–48
60. Miyakawa G (1952) Congenital absence of odontoid process. J Bone Joint Surg [Am] 34a:676–677
61. Murphy F, Hartung W, Kirklin JW (1947) Myelographic demonstration of avulsing injury of the brachial plexus. AJR 58:102–105
62. Nicoll EA (1949) Fractures of the dorsolumbar spine. J Bone Joint Surg [Br] 31b:376–394
63. Northrop CH, Eto RT, Loop JW (1975) Vertical fracture of the sacral ala. AJR 124:102–106
64. Paul LW, Moir WW (1949) Non-pathologic variations in relationship of the upper cervical vertebrae. AJR 62:519–524
65. Pay NT, George AE, Benjamin MV, Bergeron T, Lin JP, Kricheff II (1977) Positive and negative contrast myelography in spinal trauma. Radiol. 123:103–111
66. Peltier LF (1965) Complications associated with fractures of the pelvis. J Bone Joint Surg [Am] 47a:1060–1069
67. Polga JP, Cramer GG (1974) Cleft anterior arch of atlas simulating odontoid fracture. Radiology 113:341
68. Posnikoff J (1968) Spontaneous spinal epidural hematoma of childhood. J Pediatr 73:178–183
69. Ricciardi JE, Kaufer H, Louis DS (1976) Acquired os odontoideum following acute ligament injury. J Bone Joint Surg [Am] 58a:410–412
70. Roche MB (1948) Bilateral fracture of the pars interarticularis of the lumbar neural arch. J Bone Joint Surg [Am] 30a:1005–1008
71. Roaf R (1960) A study of the mechanics of spinal injuries. J Bone Joint Surg [Br] 42b:810–823
72. Roaf R (1963) Lateral flexion injuries of the cervical spine. J Bone Joint Surg [Br] 45b:36–38
73. Rossier AB, Berney J, Rosenbaum AE, Hachen J (1975) Value of gas myelography in early management of acute cervical spine cord injuries. J Neurosurg 42:330–337
74. Schatzker J, Rorabeck CH, Waddell JP (1971) Fractures of the dens (odontoid process). J Bone Joint Surg [Br] 53b:392–405
75. Scher AT (1976) Trauma of the spinal cord in children. S Afr Med J 50:2023–2025
76. Scher AT (1977) Rugby injuries to the cervical spinal cord. S Afr Med J 51:473–475
77. Schlesinger EB, Taveras JM (1958) Lesions of the odontoid and their management. Am J Surg 95:641–650
78. Schneider RC, Kahn EA (1956) Chronic neurological sequelae of acute trauma to the spine and spinal cord. J Bone Joint Surg [Am] 38a:985–997
79. Schneider RC, Livingston KE, Cave AJE, Hamilton G (1965) "Hangmans fracture" of the cervical spine. J Neurosurg 22:141–154
80. Seddon, H (1972) Surgical disorders of the peripheral nerves. Williams & Wilkins, Baltimore, pp 183–196
81. Senelick RC, Norwood CW, Cohen GH (1976) "Painless" spinal epidural hematoma during anticoagulant therapy. Neurology 26:213–215
82. Shapiro R, Youngberg AS, Roth SLG (1973) The differential diagnosis of traumatic lesions of the occipito-atlanto-axial segment. Radiol Clin North Am 11:505–526

83. Sharp J, Purser DW (1961) Spontaneous atlanto-axial dislocation in ankylosing spondylitis and rheumatoid arthritis. Ann Rheum Dis 20:47–76
84. Shrago GG (1973) Cervical spine injuries: association with head trauma. AJR 118:670–673
85. Skok P, Kapp J, Troland CE (1964) Spontaneous dislocation of the atlas. Report of a case simulating syringomyelia with a discussion of etiology and methods of treatment. J Neurosurg 21:219–222
86. Smith WS, Kaufer H (1969) Patterns and mechanisms of lumbar injuries associated with lap seat belts. J Bone Joint Surg [Am] 51a:239–254
87. Smith GR, Northrup CH, Loop JW (1977) Jumpers' fractures: patterns of thoracolumbar spine injuries associated with vertical plunges. Radiology 122:657–663
88. Stewart GC, Gehweller JA, Laib RH, Martinez S (1977) Horizontal fracture of the anterior arch of the atlas. Radiology 122:349–352
89. Sypert GW, Mozingo JR (1976) A technique for early pantopaque myelography in cervical cord injuries. Surg Neurol 6:221–222
90. Wener L, Dichiro G, Gargour GW (1974) Angiography of cervical cord injuries. Radiology 112:597–604
91. Wilkinson RH, Hall JE (1974) The sclerotic pedicle: tumor or pseudotumor. Radiology 111:683–688
92. Wiltse LL, Widell EH, Jackson DW (1975) Fatigue fracture, the basic lesion in isthmic spondylolisthesis. J Bone Joint Surg [Am] 57a:17–22
93. Zilkha A, Nicoletti JM (1974) Acute spinal subdural hematoma. Case report. J Neurosurg 41:627–630
94. Zorub DS, Nashold BS, Cook WA (1974) Avulsion of the brachial plexus. Surg Neurol 2:347–353

5 Facial and Temporal Bone Trauma

John H. Miller and Charles J. Schatz

5.1 Facial Trauma

Facial bone fractures are less frequent in children than adults; however, they present unique problems and considerations in terms of diagnosis and treatment. Vehicular trauma accounts for approximately 45%, and falls approximately 30% of facial injuries in children. There is almost a 60% incidence of associated multiple injuries [33]. As the child matures and approaches adulthood, inflicted trauma due to assault takes becomes second place to vehicular (e. g., bicycle, skateboard, moped) injury.

Pediatric facial injury differs from the adult in that a child is more difficult to examine both clinically and radiographically; anesthesia may even be required. The lack of development and pneumatization reduces radiographic contrast between the facial bones and soft tissues. In addition, the bones are thin and incompletely mineralized. Hence false negative roentgen examinations are not uncommon. However, clinical examination may be even less rewarding. The maxilla and mandible of a child are usually full of unerupted teeth or mixed dentition which can obscure fracture lines. The structures of the developing face may lend to greater facial elasticity and stability in a child than in an adult. Rapid healing necessitates early definitive diagnosis and treatment [37]. Generally, the younger the child at the time of injury the greater the likelihood of residual deformity. Parents must be warned that, irrespective of the treatment, there is a likelihood of facial or dental deformity [17]. Surgical intervention must be carefully planned to avoid damage to growth centers and to avoid compounding the chances of eventual deformity. Repeated facial trauma could suggest the possibility of a battered child.

5.1.1 Roentgenographic Evaluation

Roentgenographic evaluation by plain film examination (Table 5.1) should be tailored to the individual. The radiologist should review the examination before the patient leaves the department and not hesitate to obtain supplemental views (Table 5.1) to evaluate the patient completely. Frequently, it will be necessary to obtain complex motion tomography (Table 5.1) to complete this evaluation.

Table 5.1 Examinations in Facial Trauma

Routine plain film	Supplemental views	Complex motion tomography
Nasal bones		
Waters'	Occlusal view	
Lateral		
Facial bones		
Posteroanterior	Jughandle	Anteroposterior coronal section
Waters'		
Lateral	Stereo	Submentovertex axial section Lateral sagittal section
Mandible		
Posteroanterior	Panoramic	Lateral
Oblique lateral		
Temporomandibular joint		
Oblique lateral with open and closed mouth		Lateral Anteroposterior
Towne		

In any case of facial injury that has been severe enough to produce a loss of consciousness a full skull series is mandatory. "Dashboard" facial injury calls for a cervical spine series [21]. A Waters' view is used to evaluate the orbital floor. For suspected zygomatic arch injury a submentovertex (SMV) view will be helpful. Also slight lateral rotation of the head from this projection will produce the so-called "jughandle" view which gives an excellent evaluation of the zygomatic arch (Fig. 5.1)

A radiograph with a horizontal X-ray beam may reveal an air-fluid level in any of the sinuses and should be part of the examination in facial trauma. Plain or panoramic views of the mandible with the teeth in occlusion may show malocclusion caused by condylar fracture or displacement. When available, a stereo view of facial bones gives an added dimension to the examination [25].

Complex motion tomography may demonstrate fractures not seen on plain films (Fig. 5.8). To obtain a satisfactory examination in an apprehensive child sedation or general anesthesia may be necessary. Anteroposterior (AP) complex motion tomography is used routinely with supplemental SMV tomography and lateral tomography when necessary. Good quality tomography requires excellent radiographic positioning. The usual anatomic landmarks may be unreliable since there may be retrodisplacement of the bony structures of the face. Therefore, the sphenoid bone, particularly the pterygoid plates, may serve as radiographic landmarks since they are rarely displaced. For the SMV tomographic examination, a foam pad 15 cm thick, in the method of Harwood-Nash, is utilized in such a manner as to allow the patient's head to hang over the top edge and rest on the table top [13]. In general 2-mm interval sections are used in the very young child and 5-mm intervals in older children.

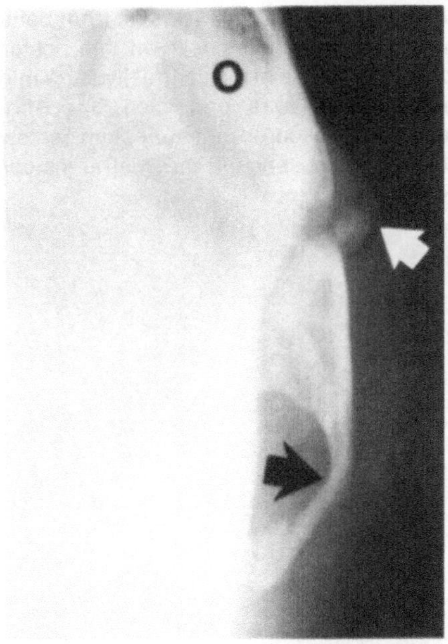

Fig. 5.1. A "jughandle" radiographic view is obtained by slight lateral rotation of the head from the submentovertex projection. Sharp angulation (*dark arrow*) indicates a fracture site associated with a fracture of the frontal process of the zygoma (*white arrow*) (*0*, orbit)

To localize the site of protracted cerebrospinal fluid (CSF) rhinorrhea, radionuclide studies may be useful (cf. Chap. 6). Rarely will contrast medium studies be performed because of the high risk and low yield [16, 30].

5.1.2 Patterns of Facial Injury

5.1.2.1 Soft Tissues

Soft tissue swelling is nonspecific radiographically but may direct the radiologist's attention to areas of injury.

5.1.2.2 Nasal Bones

Radiological examination of the nasal bones has historically been unrewarding. Figures range from only 45%–50% positive roentgenographic examination in cases of clinically documented nasal fracture [19]. Some authors have felt that the radiological examination is of sufficiently low yield actually to discourage its use in the evaluation of nasal trauma [5], yet it has been reported that approximately one-half of nasal fractures occur in children [10]. Significant deformity can also arise, in children, from small displacements of the nasal bone [19]. Because of edema and the special problems entailed in examining children, many clinicians feel more comfortable having obtained a radiographic examination.

The displaced fracture is easy to diagnose radiographically; however, the nondisplaced fracture presents difficulty to radiologists. Any sharply defined line reaching the anterior border of the nasal bone should be regarded as a fracture [5] (Fig. 5.2). However, fractures must be distinguished from the groove for the nasal branch of the nasocillary nerve and the nasomaxillary sutures [6].

The nasal spine of this maxilla must be included on the film examination of the nasal bones (Fig. 5.3). A fracture of the nasal spine can alert one to the possibility of a nasal septal hematoma. This complication of a blow to the nose is secondary to the lack of ossified support. Left untreated, a nasal septal hematoma may cause avascular necrosis of the

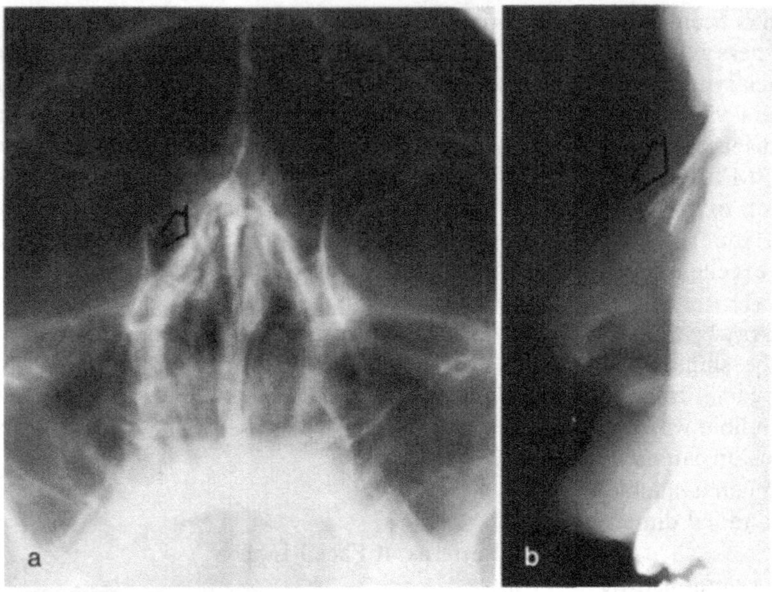

Fig. 5.2 a, b. A 13-year-old girl was struck on the nose during a basketball game. **a** Posteroanterior radiograph of the nasal bones reveals slight depression at the site of the fracture with displacement (*open arrow*). **b** Lateral radiograph of the nasal bones demonstrates a step-off (*open arrow*) at the site of the fracture

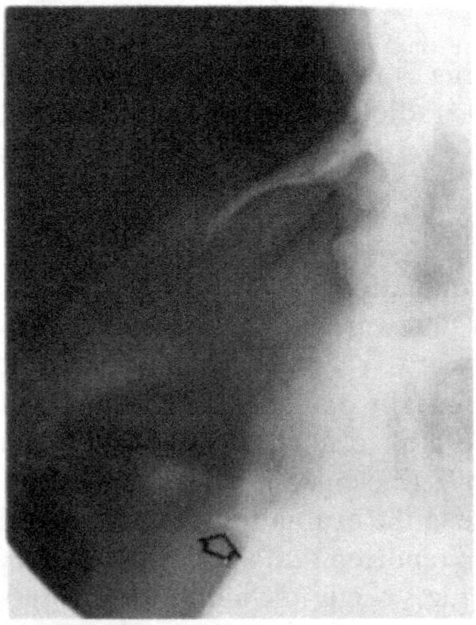

◁ **Fig. 5.3.** Fourteen-year-old boy with a "bloody nose" following an altercation at school. Lateral radiograph reveals a fracture of the nasal spine of the maxilla (*open arrow*)

▽ **Fig. 5.4 a, b.** Nine-year-old boy who was hit from behind while drinking at a water fountain. **a** On this posteroanterior radiograph absence of the central incisors might be overlooked, but the Waters' projection (**b**) confirms their absence. The unobscured nasal septum (*arrows*) should alert one to the absence of the central insicors

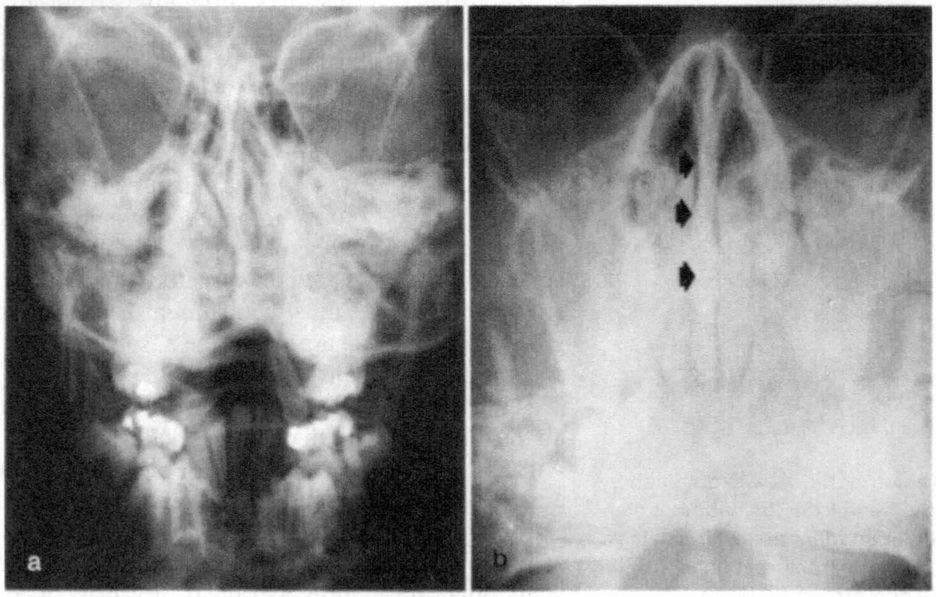

septal cartilage and a septal abscess [19]. This may lead to erosion and absorption of the septal cartilage with sagging of the cartilaginous dorsum. This can give rise, eventually, to the saddle deformity of obstruction to the nasal passages [7].

5.1.2.3 Teeth

The radiologist must discipline himself to evaluate the teeth on the film examination (Fig. 5.4). One must account for a missing tooth, since it may be in the hypopharynx or tracheobronchial tree. An unusual dental injury is the "water fountain accident" where an incisor can be driven into the alveolar ridge with the root acting as a wedge. This tooth can become devitalized or abnormal growth of the maxillary region can result [15].

5.1.2.4 Mid Face

Maxillofacial injuries manifest differently in children than adults. In our experience it is unusual for a child to sustain a classic Le Fort's fracture. More frequently the fracture tends to follow Campbell's lines. These are vertical lines which divide the face through the midorbit into lateral and medial aspects, and horizontal lines which divide the face above and below the orbit, along the maxilla, into thirds [30].

The trimalar or "tripod" fracture is a common facial injury in children. This fracture can be difficult to diagnose on a plain film examination. There are several signs that can alert the observer to the possibility of this complex fracture: zygomatic arch fracture, zygomaticofrontal suture diastasis, lateral maxillary wall fracture, inferior orbital rim fracture, opacification of maxillary antrum, rotation of the zygoma, or decreased motion of the temporomandibular joint (TMJ). For example, with decreased range of motion of the TMJ following trauma, the retrodisplaced temporal process of the zygoma may be seen impinging on the coronoid process, markedly reducing motion of the mandible [9] (Fig. 5.5). One should obtain a facial bone series following an accident, if the TMJ has a decreased range of motion (Figs. 5.6, 5.7).

In infants and young children the plain film examination may reveal clouding of the maxillary antrum (Fig. 5.8). In such circumstances complex motion tomography should be obtained in order to establish that the facial structures show no evidence of a fracture.

5.1.2.5 Orbital

Most frequently, disruption of the orbital floor is part of the trimalar fracture [1] (Fig. 5.6). However, blunt trauma to the orbit may cause an orbital blowout fracture, which may be associated with entrapment of the inferior rectus muscle. This can produce loss of upward gaze and diplopia [29]. The orbital floor was fractured in 46% of a series of 363 trimalar fractures [4]. Typically, there is a fracture of the

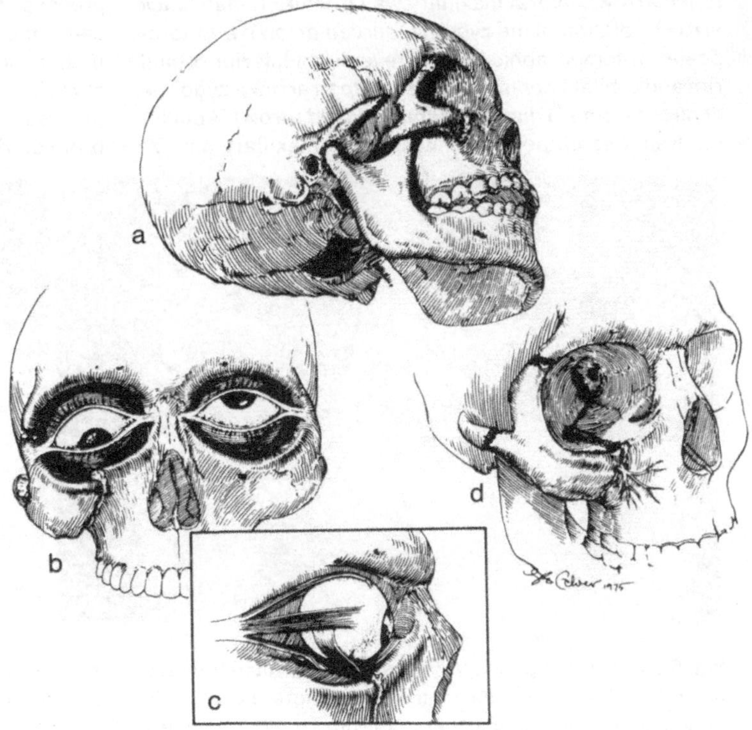

Fig. 5.5 a–d. The trimilar fracture. **a** Rotation of the fracture segment compromises the motion of the mandible by pressure on the coronoid process. **b** Depression of the fracture producing visual changes without entrapment. **c** Entrapment of the inferior oblique and inferior rectus muscles of the eye by the fracture. **d** Compromise of the infraoribtal nerve which frequently produces hypesthesia of the cheek below the eye. (Reproduced with permission from Gerlock and Sinn [9])

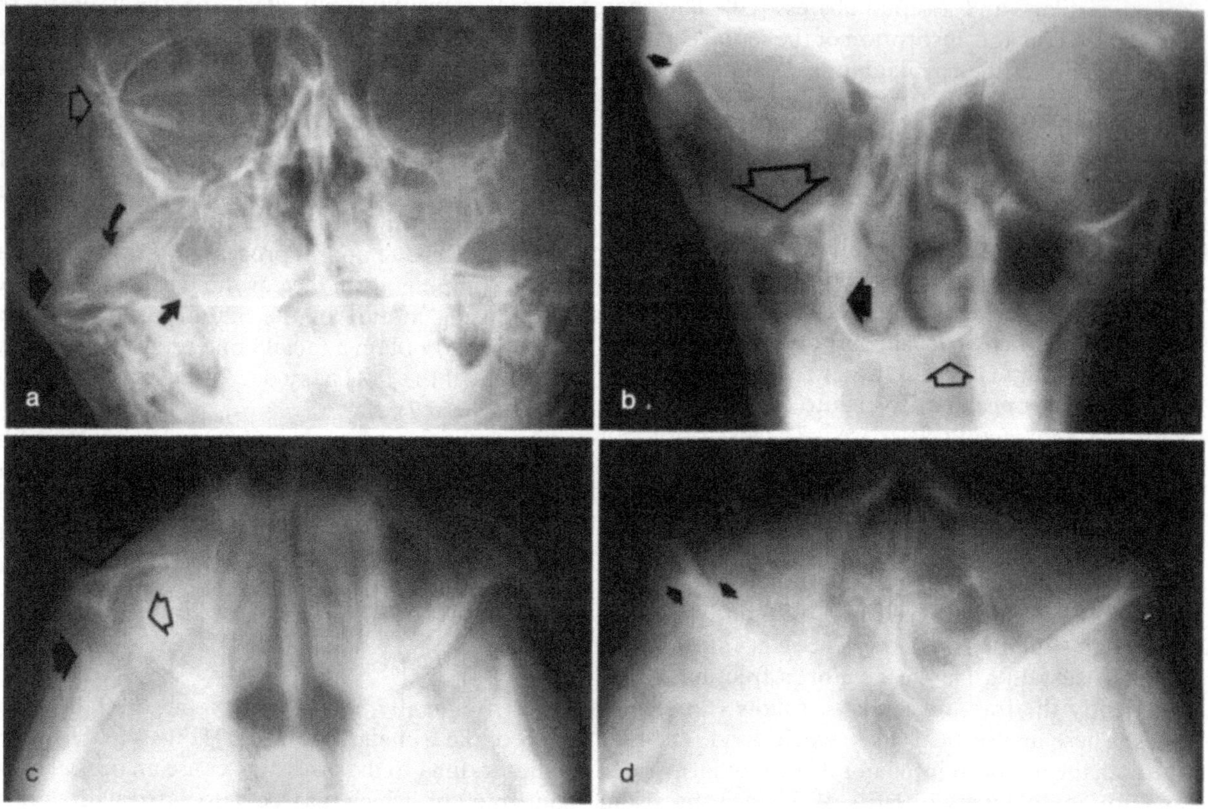

Fig. 5.6 a–d. Seventeen-year-old girl who struck her face on a tree while riding a bicycle and sustained a trimalar fracture. **a** Waters' view demonstrates the major components of a trimalar fracture: zygomatic arch fracture (*large black arrow*), zygomaticofrontal suture diastasis (*open arrow*), lateral maxillary wall fracture (*small black arrow*), rotation of the zygoma (*curved arrow*). **b** Anteroposterior tomographic section reveals an inferior orbital rim and orbital floor fracture (*large open arrow*), zygomaticofrontal suture diastasis (*small closed arrow*). Additional fractures of the medial wall of the maxillary antrum (*large closed arrow*) and anterior alveolar ridge fracture (*small open arrow*) are noted. **c** Submentovertex tomogram reveals retrodisplacement of the zygoma (*large open arrow*) and a fracture of lateral wall of the maxilla (*small open arrow*). Note the proximity of the coronoid process of the mandible (*closed arrow*) to the retrodisplaced and rotated zygoma. This can compromise motion of the mandible. **d** Submentovertex tomogram reveals a fracture through the lateral wall of the orbit (*arrows*). This can entrap the lateral rectus muscle and produce diplopia

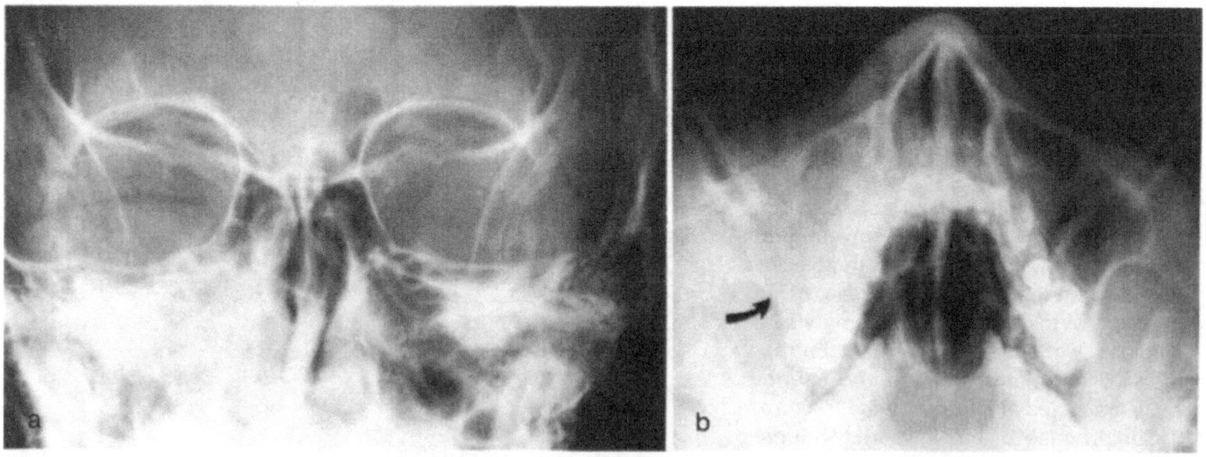

Fig. 5.7 a–e. Boy aged $15^1/_2$ years who was hit in the face by a baseball. **a** Posteroanterior radiography reveals opacification of the maxillary antrum. **b** Waters' view reveals a fracture of the lateral wall of the maxillary antrum (*arrow*).

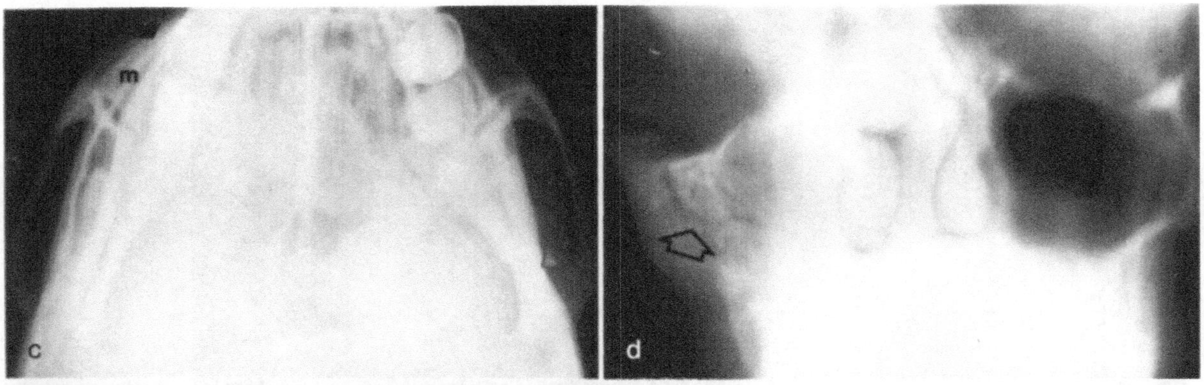

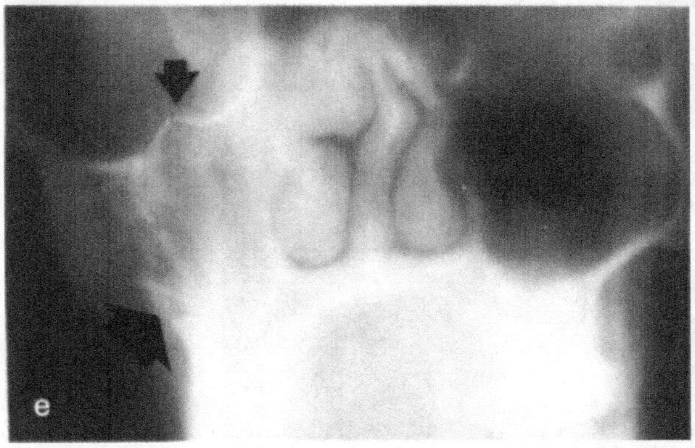

Fig. 5.7. **c** Submentovertex view reveals flattening and posterior displacement of the malar eminence (*arrow*) and cloudiness of the maxillary antrum (*m*). **d** Anteroposterior complex motion tomographic section reveals the extensive fracture with considerable displacement of the lateral wall of the maxillary antrum (*arrow*). In comparison with the opposite normal side, one can appreciate the retrodisplacement of the malar eminence. **e** A further posterior section reveals superior displacement of the orbital floor: "blow-in" orbital floor fracture (*small closed arrow*). A fracture of the lateral wall of the maxillary antrum is seen (*large arrow*)

orbital floor adjacent to the infraorbital nerve. However, the fracture occurs posterior and medial to the infraorbital nerve canal in the majority of cases [11]. "Blow-out" encompasses a wide spectrum of fractures from a simple fracture with no displacement to a large fracture with herniation of orbital contents into the maxillary antrum [4, 24]. Roentgenographically the fracture may be manifest by a "hanging drop" on the roof of the maxillary antrum (Fig. 5.9). This appearance may represent herniated muscle, orbital fat, or a hematoma beneath the mucoperiosteum of the maxillary sinus. The entire maxillary sinus may be opacified and the plain film examination will not adequately evaluate the floor of the orbit (Fig. 5.10). Complex motion tomography should be used to evaluate adequately the orbital floor. Any irregularity of the floor or any discontinuity of the walls of the infraorbital canal should be considered evidence of an orbital floor fracture. It should be kept in mind that, during the injury, the fracture could entrap structures such as the inferior rectus and oblique muscles as well as the fascia of these muscles. Any of these can produce gaze disturbance.

Orbital emphysema (Fig. 5.11) usually occurs with medial wall blow-out fractures, but it rarely occurs with inferior blow-out fractures [16]. The medial wall of the orbit and the lamina papyracea can be as thin as 0.2–0.4 mm and be easily fractured [11]. Both the superior oblique and medial rectus muscles are related anatomically to this bone: hence, entrapment of these muscles can occur following fracture, with concomitant gaze disturbance. Following trauma, partial or complete opacification of the ethmoid air cells, or orbital emphysema, must be considered evidence of a medial orbital wall blow out fracture. Complex motion tomography in the AP and SMV projections adequately evaluates the medial wall of the orbit.

Both the orbital roof (Fig. 5.12) and lateral wall (Fig. 5.6d) can be fractured and similar entrapment syndromes occur. Most frequently they are part of a complex facial fracture and almost never happen as isolated events. The roof fractures occur as a part of frontal bone fractures, whereas lateral wall fractures are part of the trimalar or zygoma injury (Fig. 5.7).

An orbital "blow-in" fracture is a rare injury which accompanies a zygomatic or maxillary fracture with the orbital floor pushed upward into the orbit. There is a high risk of injury to the globe secondary to manipulation of the fracture segments or "blind" orbital floor repair [28, 3] (Fig. 5.7d).

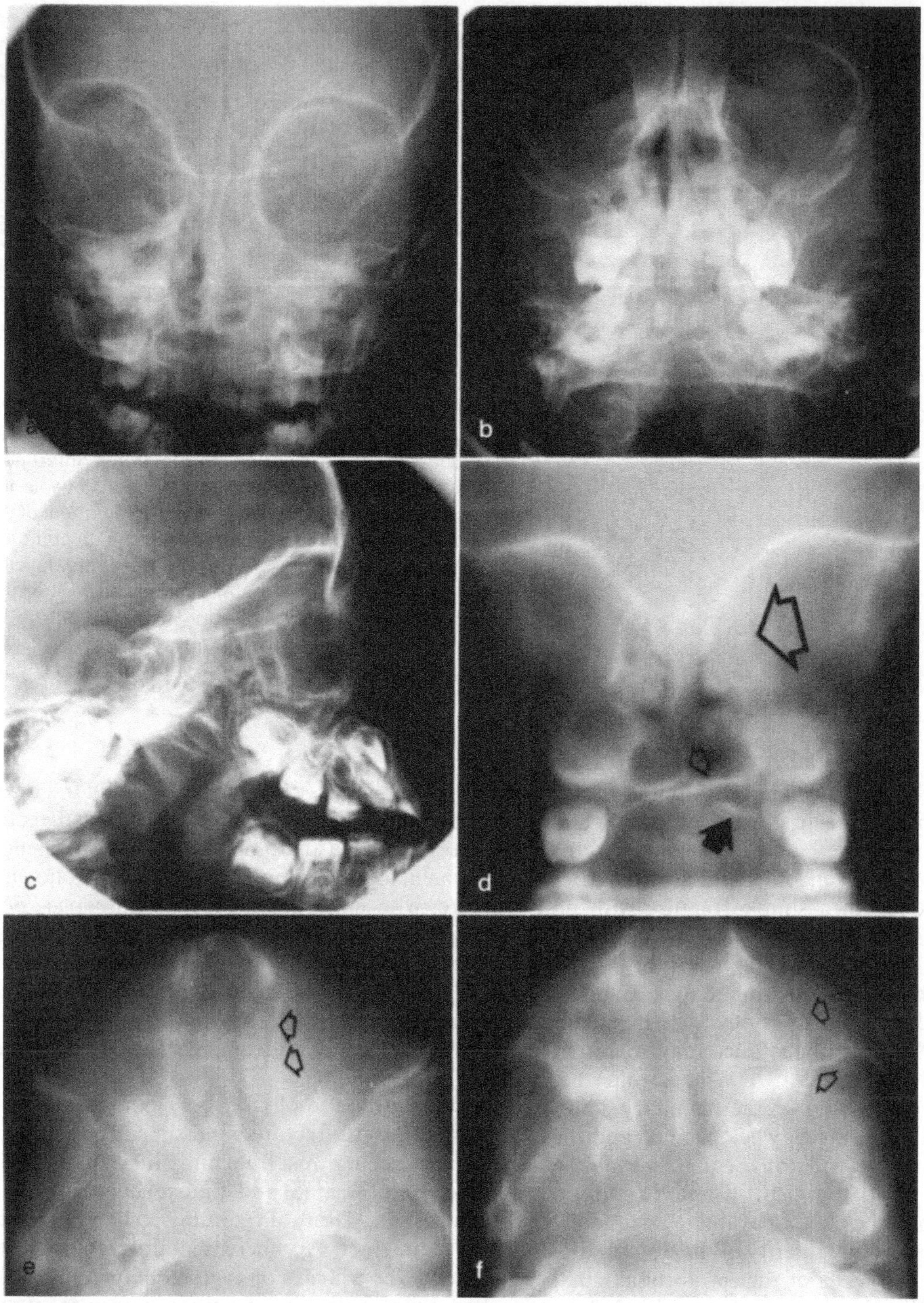

Fig. 5.8 a–f. Two-year-old boy hit the dashboard during a collision. Anteroposterior (*a*), Waters' (*b*), and lateral views (*c*) reveal opacification of the left maxillary antrum and ethmoid air cells. **d** Anteroposterior tomogram reveals a fracture of the medial wall of the orbit (*large open arrow*) and a complex fracture of the palate (*small open and closed arrows*). **e** Submentovertex tomogram confirms the medial displacement (*arrows*) of the medial orbital wall (lamina papyracea). **f** Additional SMV section reveals a fracture through the zygomatic process of the maxilla

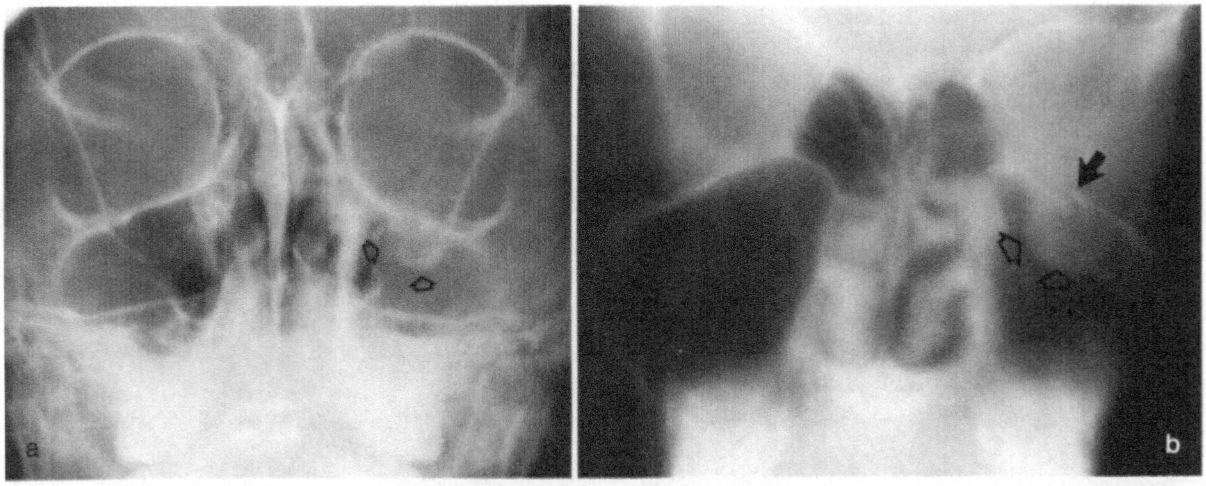

Fig. 5.9 a, b. Fourteen-year-old girl who had been kicked in the face by a horse. She had diplopia on upward gaze following this accident. **a** Waters' view demonstrates "hanging drop" in the roof of the maxillary antrum **b** Anteroposterior tomogram confirms the mass (*open arrows*) and a disruption of the orbital floor ar the level of the intraorbital nerve canal (*closed arrow*)

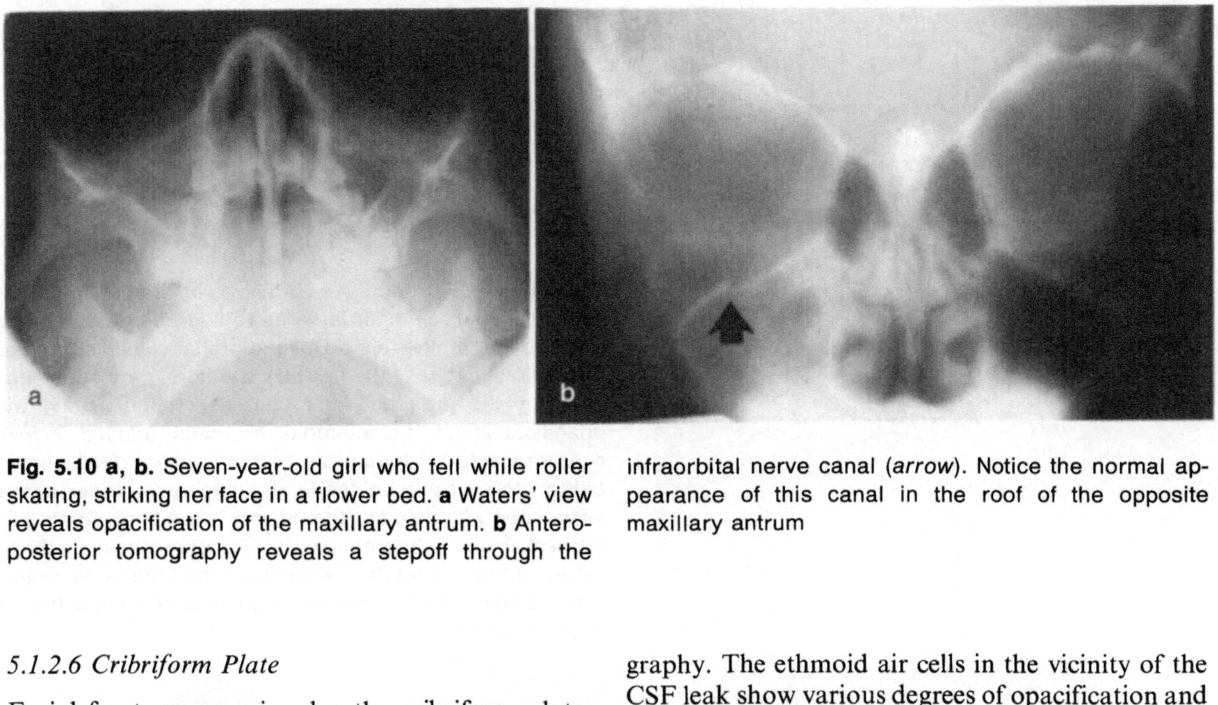

Fig. 5.10 a, b. Seven-year-old girl who fell while roller skating, striking her face in a flower bed. **a** Waters' view reveals opacification of the maxillary antrum. **b** Anteroposterior tomography reveals a stepoff through the infraorbital nerve canal (*arrow*). Notice the normal appearance of this canal in the roof of the opposite maxillary antrum

5.1.2.6 Cribriform Plate

Facial fractures may involve the cribriform plate, sometimes causing CSF rhinorrhea. Recurrent bouts of meningitis may follow this serious fracture. Although, in the majority, CSF rhinorrhea will spontaneously stop, in a few patients it will continue and require surgical treatment. A vexing problem is the facial fracture patient who has persistent serous discharge from his nose. To determine if there is a CSF leak a radionuclide cisternogram can be performed. Once CSF rhinorrhea is established further evaluation should include complex motion tomography. The ethmoid air cells in the vicinity of the CSF leak show various degrees of opacification and give the radiologist a clue to the site of the leakage (Fig. 5.13). Good quality complex motion tomograms in the AP projection will generally prove the most useful. Lateral tomograms occasionally demonstrate the fracture sites.

5.1.2.7 Temporomandibular Joint

We have found that evaluation of the TMJ by plain film examination (Fig. 5.14) is not as useful as evaluation by complex motion tomography. A frac-

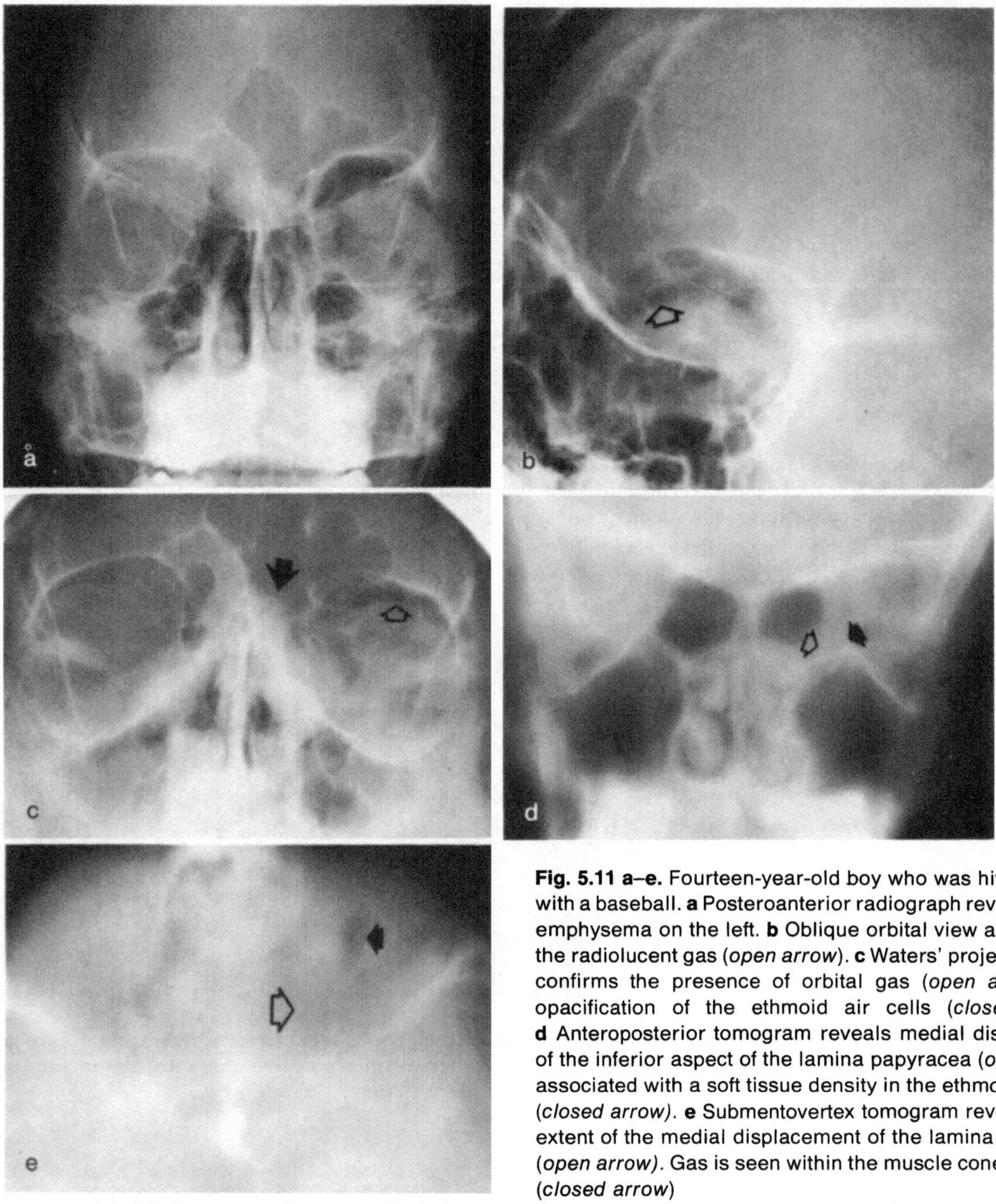

Fig. 5.11 a–e. Fourteen-year-old boy who was hit in the eye with a baseball. **a** Posteroanterior radiograph reveals orbital emphysema on the left. **b** Oblique orbital view also reveals the radiolucent gas (*open arrow*). **c** Waters' projection again confirms the presence of orbital gas (*open arrow*) with opacification of the ethmoid air cells (*closed arrow*). **d** Anteroposterior tomogram reveals medial displacement of the inferior aspect of the lamina papyracea (*open arrow*) associated with a soft tissue density in the ethmoid air cells (*closed arrow*). **e** Submentovertex tomogram reveals the full extent of the medial displacement of the lamina papyracea (*open arrow*). Gas is seen within the muscle cone of the eye (*closed arrow*)

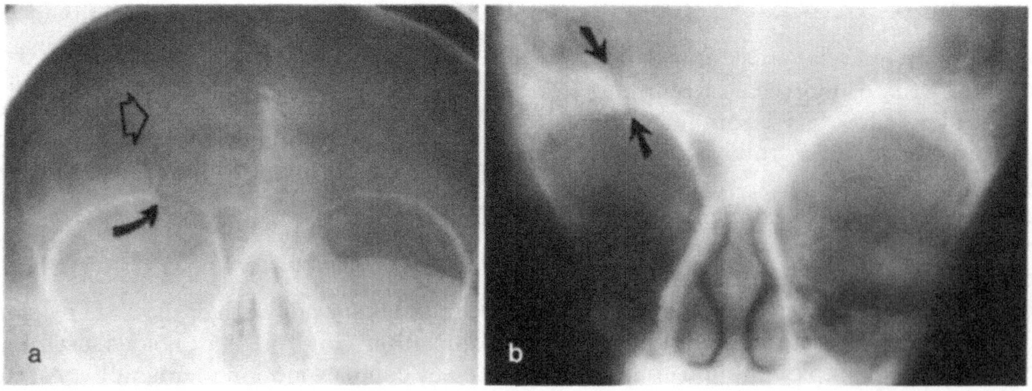

Fig. 5.12 a, b

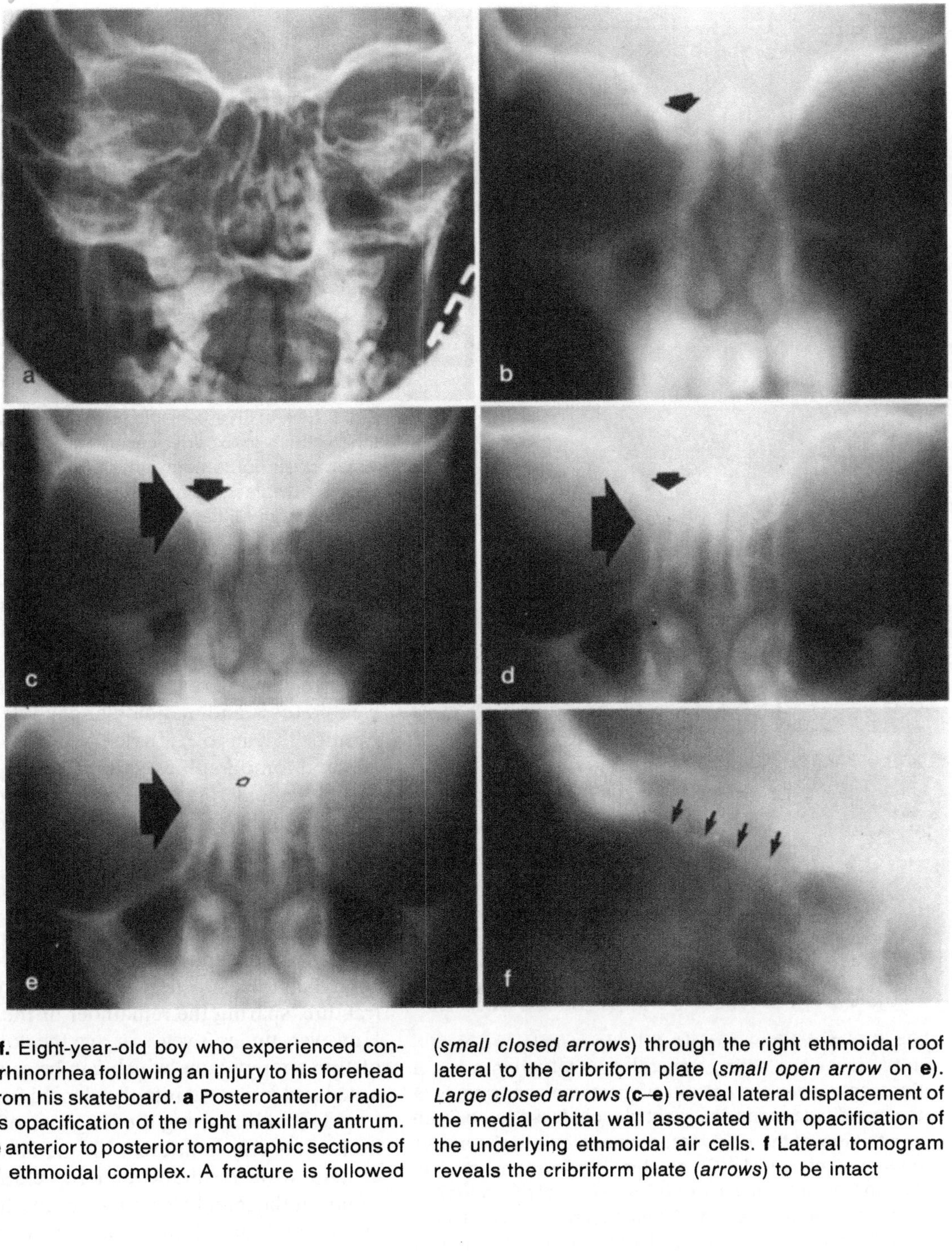

Fig. 5.13 a–f. Eight-year-old boy who experienced continuing CSF rhinorrhea following an injury to his forehead after a fall from his skateboard. **a** Posteroanterior radiograph shows opacification of the right maxillary antrum. **b–e** Multiple anterior to posterior tomographic sections of the anterior ethmoidal complex. A fracture is followed (*small closed arrows*) through the right ethmoidal roof lateral to the cribriform plate (*small open arrow* on **e**). *Large closed arrows* (**c–e**) reveal lateral displacement of the medial orbital wall associated with opacification of the underlying ethmoidal air cells. **f** Lateral tomogram reveals the cribriform plate (*arrows*) to be intact

◁ **Fig. 5.12 a, b.** Four-year-old boy who hit his forehead on the dashboard during an accident, following which he experienced a gaze disturbance. **a** Waters' projection reveals a frontal bone fracture (*open arrow*) entering the orbital roof (*curved arrow*). **b** Anteroposterior tomography reveals the extent and displacement of the fracture which had entrapped the superior rectus muscle

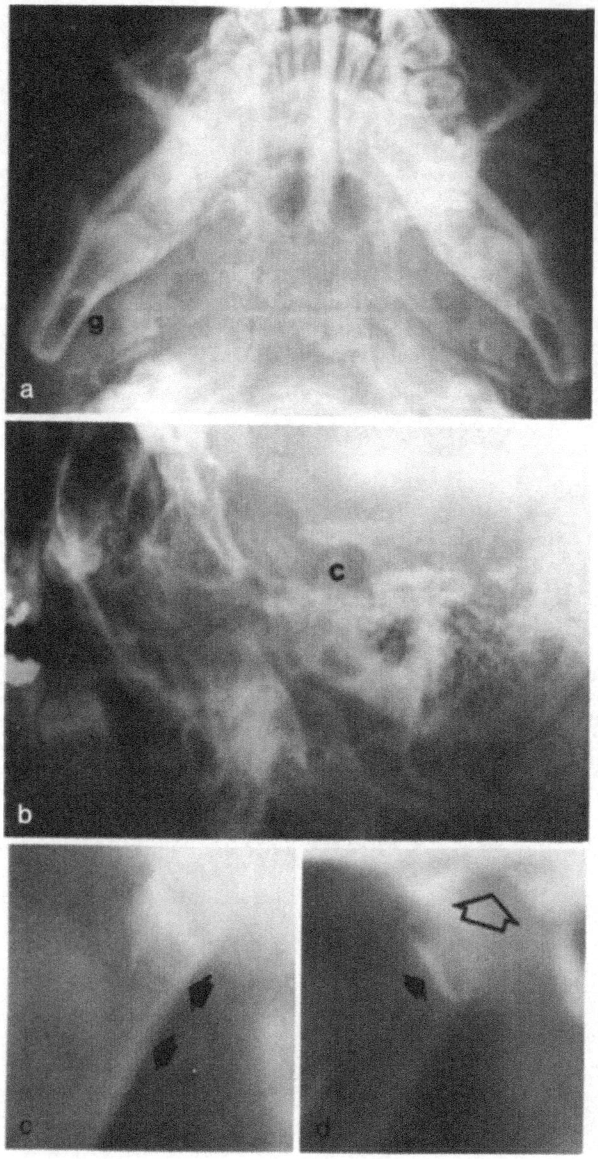

Fig. 5.14 a–d. Nine-year-old girl who complained of pain in the jaw while eating, several days following a fall. **a** Submentovertex radiograph suggests no abnormality of the mandibular condyles; right glenoid fossa (*g*). **b** Open mouth view of the right temporomandibular joint shows no motion of condyle (*C*). **c** Lateral tomography, section 11 mm from table top, reveals the ramus of the mandible (*arrow*) to be in focus. **d** 17-mm section: the condyle is identified (*closed arrow*) dislocated from the glenoid fossa (*open arrow*) because of a fracture at the base of the condyle

ture in the vicinity of the TMJ may be present with a plain film examination being within normal limits. The need for further evaluation by complex motion tomography includes: decreased range of motion of the mandibular condyle on open- and closed-mouth films, dental malocclusion, slight lateral deviation of

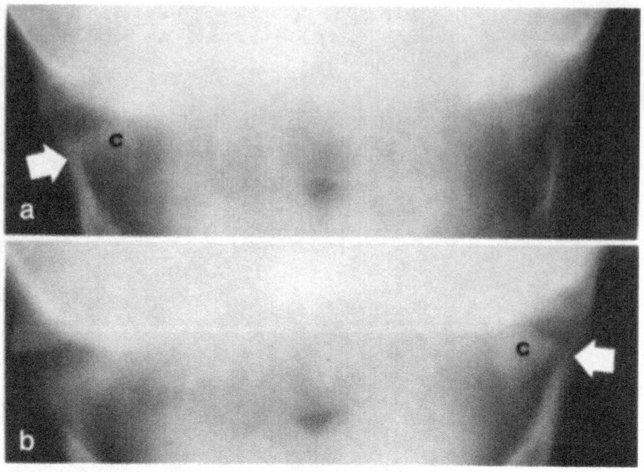

Fig. 5.15 a, b. Five-year-old boy who fell, striking his chin the midline. He experienced trismus following this injury. Anteroposterior tomography at (**a**) 8.6-cm and (**b**) 9.0-cm levels reveals medial subluxation of the mandibular condyle from bilateral condylar neck fractures

the central lower incisors as compared to the upper central incisors, or a clinical evaluation suggesting a fracture. Complex motion tomographic examination is usually limited to the lateral projection in order to demonstrate completely the anatomy of the glenoid fossa and mandibular condyle in the resting position. Then, to evaluate the function of the joint, a lateral tomographic section through the midplane of the glenoid fossa is obtained in the open- and closed-mouth positions (Fig. 14c, d). Only rarely will AP complex motion tomography be needed to evaluate medial subluxation or displacement of fracture segments (Fig. 5.15).

The mandibular condyle is unique in children. The elasticity of the bone and joint structures protect the condylar process. Therefore the condylar neck will fracture, sparing the remainder of the condyle [33]. However, under 3 years of age the condyle consists of thin spongy bone which can be severely comminuted and impacted into the glenoid fossa secondary to a direct blow along the long axis of the condylar neck. This can interfere with the condylar growth centers with resultant underdevelopment of the ramus of the mandible and micrognathism as well as abnormal biomechanics of the joint leading to malocclusion problems in later life. There is almost never an indication for open reduction of fractures of the condylar ramus or neck because of the risk of injury to the subcondylar growth center of the ramus of the mandible [33, 37].

5.1.2.8 Mandible

The TMJs allow some dissipation of forces applied to the body of the mandible, for this reason the bipartite "closed ring" fracture is less frequent than the single fracture [22]. However, one must carefully evaluate the possibility of a second fracture or TMJ dislocation when faced with a fracture of the mandible. Remember that the developing dental structures in a child's mandible may mask a fracture.

5.1.2.9 Complications

Complications of facial bone fractures include: pneumocephalus [34], extracranial CSF loculation [18], intracranial abscesses [14], diabetes insipidus [12] hypertelorism, and multiple visual problems [2] The long-term facial cosmetic deformity is difficult to predict in a given case. Generally the younger the child the greater the likelihood of residual deformity from serious injury. When possible, reconstructive procedures should be delayed until most of the growth period is over to avoid damaging growth centers [33].

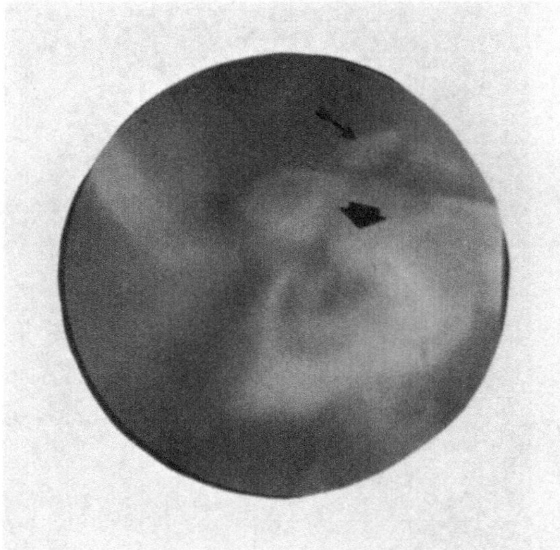

Fig. 5.16. Three-year-old child injured as a passenger in an automobile. Lateral tomogram at the level of the ossicles (*arrowhead*) reveals depressed fragments of bone from the tegmen tympani into the middle fossa (*arrow*)

5.2 Temporal Bone Trauma

Trauma to the temporal bone is a rare but serious consequence of severe blunt trauma to the head. Most temporal bone fractures result from high-speed automobile or motorcycle accidents. Because children are frequently unrestrained passengers in automobiles they can become projectiles, striking the windshield or dashboard during rapid decelaration of the vehicle. In older children, motorcycle accidents can result in severe head trauma with consequent temporal bone fractures. Other causes of temporal bone fractures in children include gunshot injuries and any other traumatic episode which results in a severe blow to the head.

This author (CJS) has examined over 200 patients with temporal bone fractures and their consequences. Of these patients over 50% have been in the pediatric age group and the majority were involved in automobile or motorcycle accidents.

Fractures of early childhood may differ from those of teenagers and adults. The inner ear structures are fully developed at birth [20]. However, the mastoid process does not start developing until 2 years of age; it continues to develop through early childhood and is complete by adolescence. In addition, the external auditory canal is short in infancy and early childhood because of the absence of its osseous portion [27] and so fractures in these areas are rare in infancy. Although longitudinal and transverse fractures do occur in infancy and early childhood, atypical fractures are also seen (Fig. 5.16). Fractures in teenagers do not differ significantly from fractures in adults (i. e., longitudinal and transverse type).

Classification. Traditionally, linear temporal bone fractures have been described as "longitudinal" and "transverse." Longitudinal fractures usually parallel the long axis of the petrous pyramid and are frequently related to a conductive hearing loss. These fractures usually extend from the temporal squamosa inferiorly through the long axis of the external auditory canal. This canal is a ring. When the ring is fractured, two fracture lines are usually visualized. One of the fractures approximates the glenoid fossa. The other fracture line usually extends superiorly or posteriorly through the tegmen tympani or mastoid (Fig. 5.17).

Transverse fractures are perpendicular to the long axis of the petrous pyramid and are frequently related to fractures of the skull base. They can cause neurosensory hearing loss by fracturing through the internal auditory canal, cochlea, semicircular canal, or vestibule (Figs. 5.18–5.20).

Technique of Evaluation. In evaluating patients with temporal bone injury, conventional radiography with plain films may reveal a fracture or mastoid clouding but may have a considerably lower yield than complex motion tomography [8] (Fig. 5.17). Since a negative plain film examination does not rule out a fracture or ossicular dislocation, the authors usually proceed to complex motion tomography in

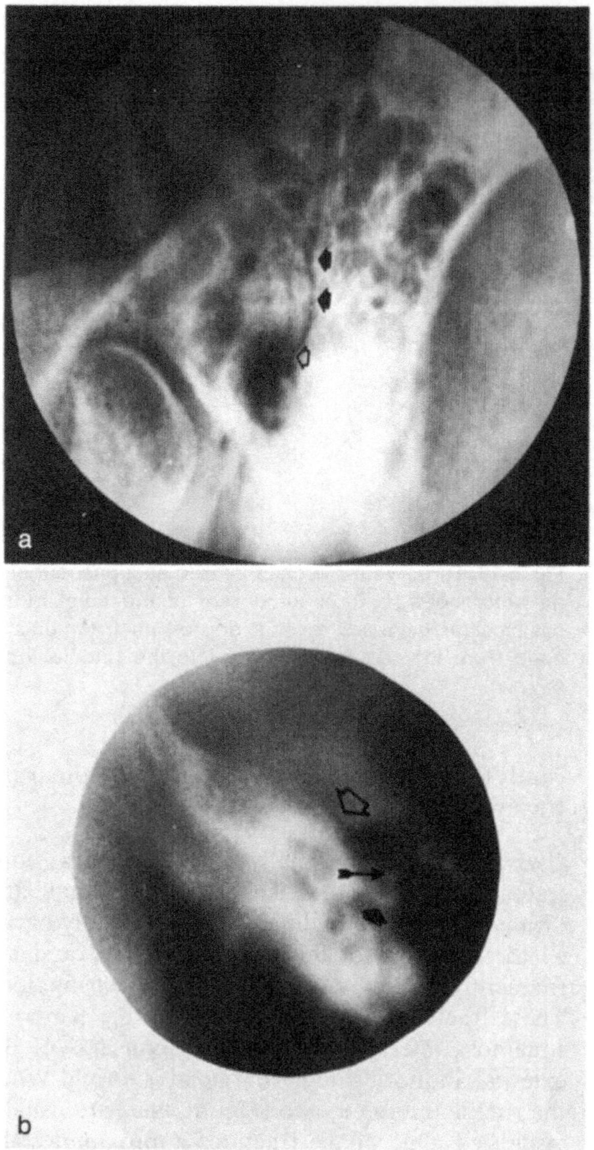

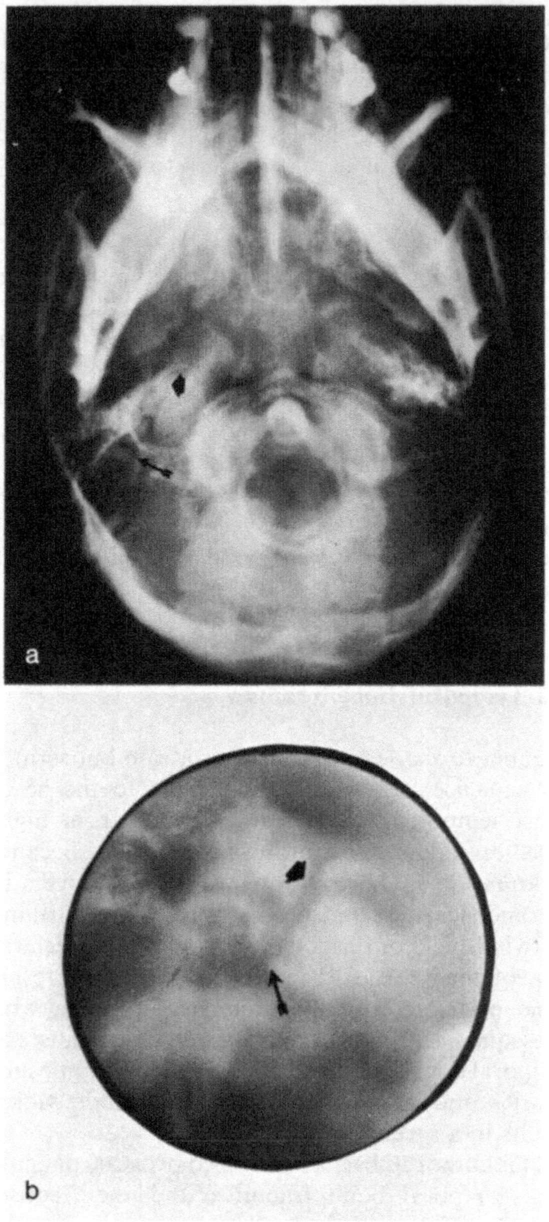

Fig. 5.17 a, b. Sixteen-year-old male presented with a conductive hearing loss after head trauma from a motorcycle accident. **a** Owens projection showing linear fracture (*closed arrowheads*) entering external auditory canal (*open arrowhead*). **b** Submentovertex tomogram revealing a longitudinal fracture (*open arrowhead*) and ossicular dislocation: malleus head (*arrow*) in normal location, incus body rotated (*closed arrowhead*)

Fig. 5.18 a, b. Male patient who fell 15 ft onto his head. He had an immediate facial nerve palsy and complete neurosensory hearing loss on the right. **a** Submentovertex view of the skull showing an occipital fracture (*arrow*) extending transversely across petrous bone (*arrowhead*). **b** Anteroposterior tomogram of the right temporal bone showing fracture extending through lateral end of internal auditory canal (*arrowhead*) and basal turn of the cochlea (*arrow*)

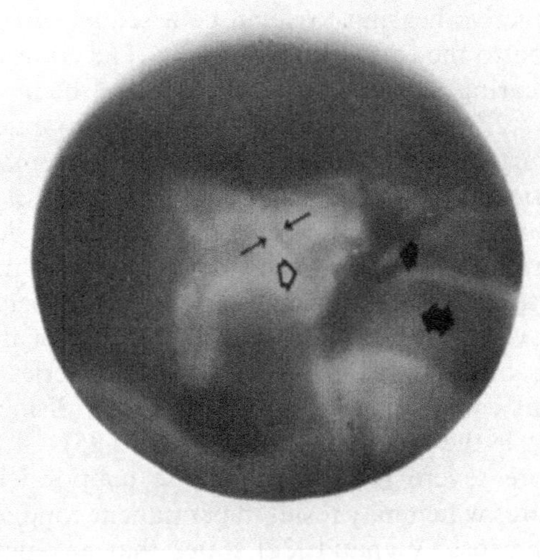

Fig. 5.19. Fourteen-year-old male entered hospital with a left facial nerve palsy and complete neurosensory hearing loss after blunt trauma to head (same patient as in Fig. 5.26). Left semiaxial tomogram demonstrates a transverse fracture (*arrows*) entering the vestibule (*open arrow*); external auditory canal (*double- headed arrow*), incus (*closed arrowhead*)

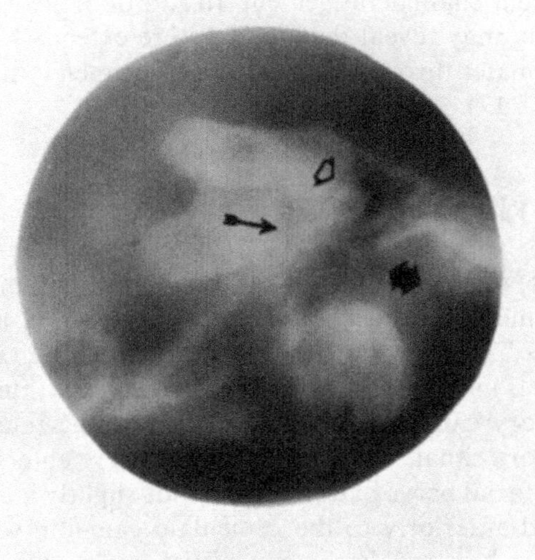

Fig. 5.20. Teenage male involved in motorcycle accident suffered an immediate neurosensory hearing loss on the left. Left semiaxial tomogram through the posterior portion of the vestibule (*arrow*). External auditory canal (*double-headed arrow*); transverse fracture (*open arrowhead*) extends through the horizontal semicircular canal

the evaluation of posttraumatic hearing loss, facial nerve palsy or CSF otorrhea. Other conventional films may be helpful in identifying additional skull fractures or cervical spine fractures. The radiographic positioning after trauma depends entirely on clinical and audiometry examinations [23, 26, 31]:

Neuro-hearing sensory loss
1. Anteroposterior tomography
2. Lateral tomography
3. Routine skull series with base view to evaluate additional fractures

Conductive hearing loss
1. 15–20 degree semiaxial to the pyramid tomography (Guillen projection)
2. Lateral or inclined lateral tomography
3. Submentovertex tomography for further evaluation of the malleus and incus in a patient with suspect ossicular dislocation if not demonstrated in above projections

Facial nerve palsy
1. 15–20 degree semiaxial to the pyramid tomography (Guillen projection)
2. Lateral tomography
3. Stenver's projection tomography (when the seventh cranial nerve canal is not seen on the lateral projection)

Sedation. Below the age of 5 years, sedation is usually required for tomographic studies. In order to obtain the proper tomographic level, centering, and technique, the patient must not be allowed to move during the examination.

It is beyond the scope of this chapter to discuss medications for sedation, but there are times when general anesthesia may be required.

5.2.1 Neurosensory Hearing Loss

Transverse fractures can cause neurosensory hearing loss. The fracture can involve the cochlea (Fig. 5.18), internal auditory canal, vestibule (Fig. 5.19), or semicircular canals (Fig. 5.20). When the internal auditory canal is fractured there is frequently involvement of the facial nerve. In our series, under 10% of documented temporal bone fractures had involvement of the bony labyrinth. These fractures are commonly related to basilar skull fractures in which either the occipital bone posteriorly or the sphenoid bone anteriorly are involved. We have also seen a fracture of the sphenosquamosal suture extend posteriorly to the petrous portion of the temporal bone, causing a transverse fracture (Fig. 5.21).

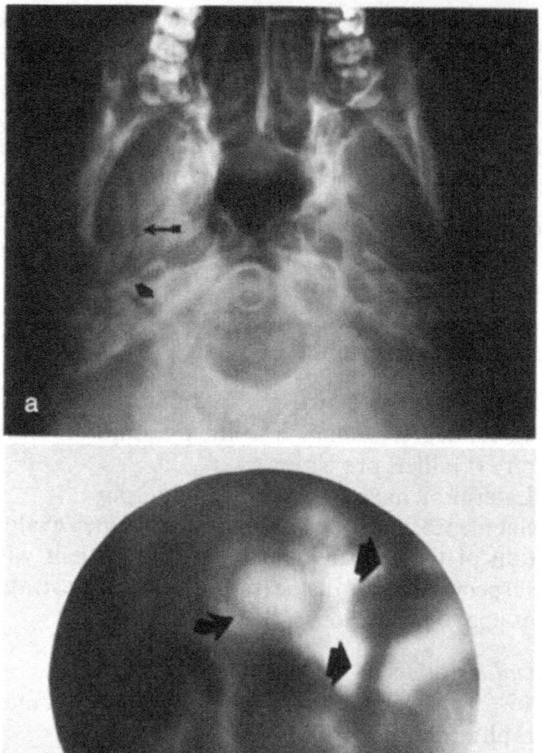

Fig. 5.21 a–c. Sixteen-year-old male brought to hospital after falling off motorcycle. He had a right facial nerve palsy, vertigo and complete neurosensory hearing loss. **a** Submentovertex plain film demonstrating a basilar skull fracture through the sphenosquamosal suture (*arrow*) extending transversely across the temporal bone (*arrow-head*). **b** Stenvers tomogram showing fracture across internal auditory canal (*arrowheads*); posterior semicircular canals (*arrow*). **c** Stenvers tomogram showing fracture through geniculate (*arrow*) and cochlea (*arrowhead*)

5.2.2 Conductive Hearing Loss

Conductive hearing loss can be a sequel of minor trauma to the ear without fracture. The etiology of the hearing loss can be secondary to a hematoma (Fig. 5.22) or edema in the middle ear to external auditory canal, rupture of the tympanic membrane or ossicular injury (ossicular dislocation or ossicular fracture). Wright [36] states that severe ossicular abnormalities can be seen in patients with minor head trauma and that there is no correlation between the severity of the injury and the degree of distur bance of the ossicular chain. In our series and Wright's [35] series, the most frequent dislocated ossicle is the incus (Figs. 5.23, 5.24, 5.25).

More severe trauma can cause temporal bone fractures which may result in permanent conductive hearing loss. Vignaud [32] states that any patient who has a conductive hearing loss for more than 21 days following temporal bone trauma requires complex motion tomography to evaluate the external and middle ears. Twenty-one days allows time for fluid or a hematoma to resolve. A hearing loss that remains longer is usually secondary to some anatomical derangement which complex motion tomography should define. The abnormality may be a fracture through the external auditory canal or an ossicular chain derangement. In addition, the tomography may reveal that the fracture extends to the dura mater through the mastoid or tegmen tympani (Fig. 5.17).

5.2.3 Facial Nerve Injury

The seventh cranial nerve enters the medial end of the internal auditory canal with the eighth cranial nerve. This petrous portion of the seventh cranial nerve is in the anterosuperior portion of the internal auditory canal. At the lateral end of the internal auditory canal, the seventh cranial nerve enters the bony facial nerve hiatus and extends slightly laterally and anteriorly to the geniculate ganglion where the greater and lesser superficial petrosal nerves arise. Then, the seventh nerve travels posteriorly, and slightly laterally, in its own canal (fallopian canal) along the medial wall of the tympanic cavity. After a course of approximately 6 mm this tympanic portion of the seventh cranial nerve makes an inferior turn of approximately 60° called the "genu" and becomes the mastoid portion of the nerve. The nerve now has an inferior course and its exit from the temporal bone is at the stylomastoid foramen. Trauma to the temporal bone can fracture any portion of the seventh cranial nerve canal. Involve-

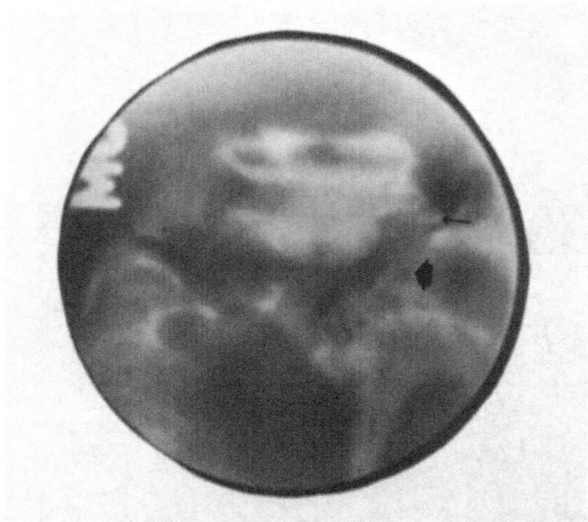

Fig. 5.22. Female patient presented with traumatic conductive hearing loss following blunt trauma directly to the left ear. Semiaxial tomogram at the level of the incus (*arrow*); soft tissue (*arrowhead*) density in the left middle ear representing a hematoma. The hearing returned to normal within 3 weeks

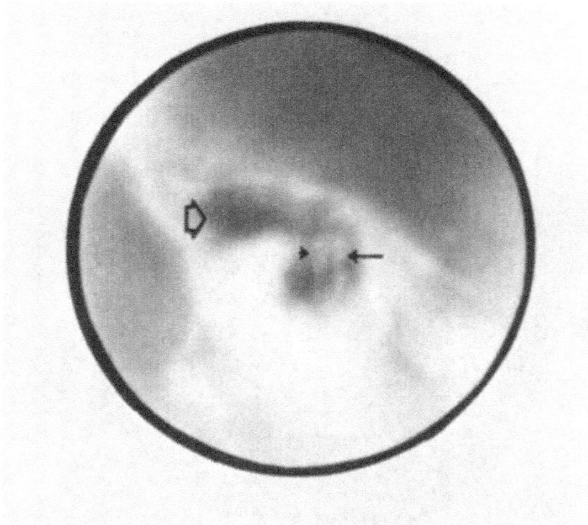

Fig. 5.23. Normal right inclined lateral tomogram demonstrating normal malleus (*long arrow*), incus (*small arrowhead*), mastoid antrum (*open arrowhead*)

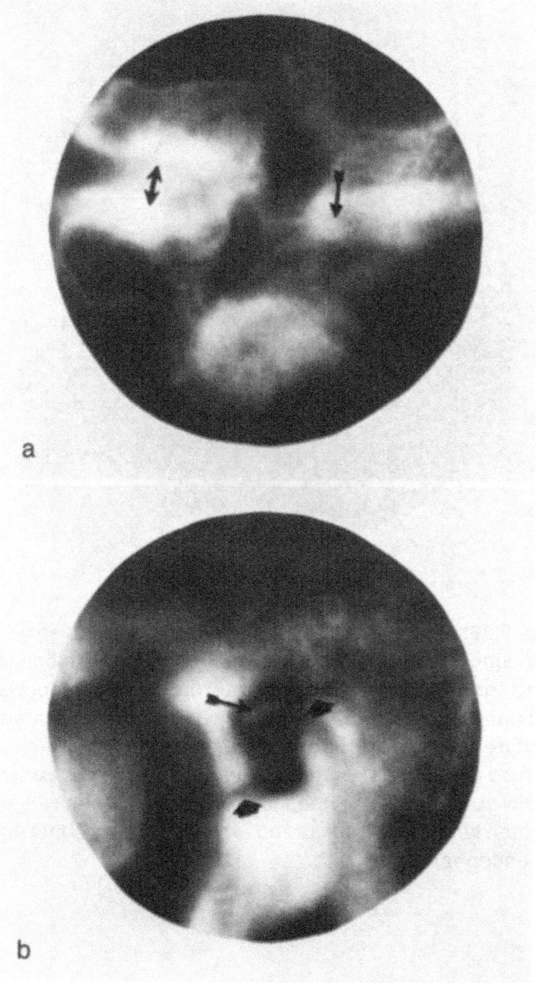

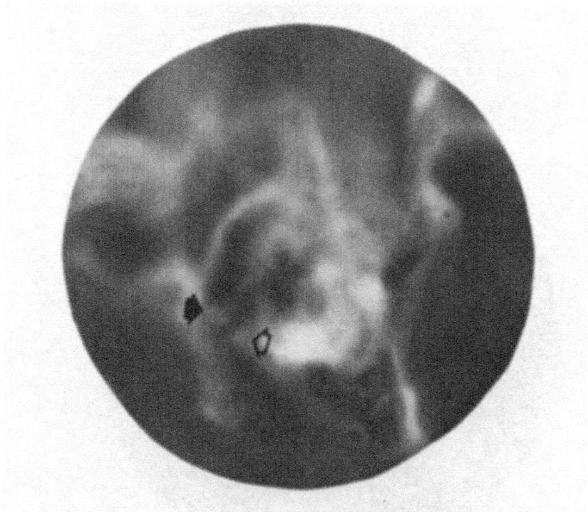

Fig. 5.25. Patient with a conductive hearing loss approximately 1 month following head trauma. Inclined lateral tomogram revealing an ossicular dislocation: malleus (*closed arrowhead*), dislocated incus (*open arrowhead*), with separation of the malleus and incus

◁ **Fig. 5.24 a, b.** Seventeen-year-old male who was struck on the head with a club during a fight. **a** Semiaxial tomogram through the middle ear: internal auditory canal (*small double-headed arrow*), bony density (*arrow*) superiorly and medially in the external auditory canal representing the dislocated incus. **b** Lateral tomogram through the external auditory canal showing fractures (*arrowheads*) and the incus (*arrow*) dislocated in the external auditory canal

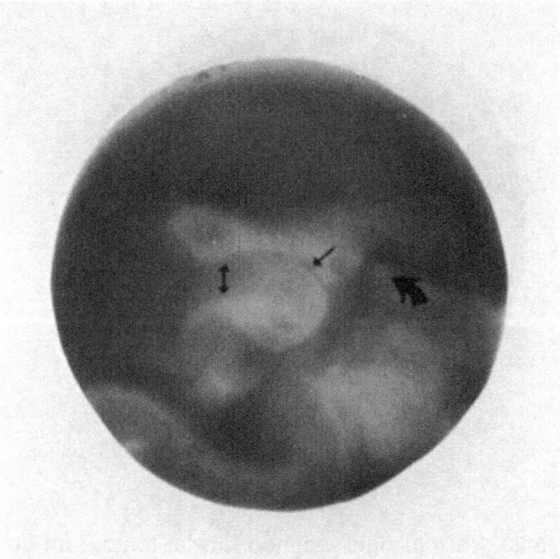

Fig. 5.26. Same patient as in Fig. 5.19. Facial nerve palsy secondary to a fracture extending through the facial nerve canal (*small arrow*) immediately proximal to the geniculate ganglion; internal auditory canal (*double-headed arrow*), malleus (*large arrow*)

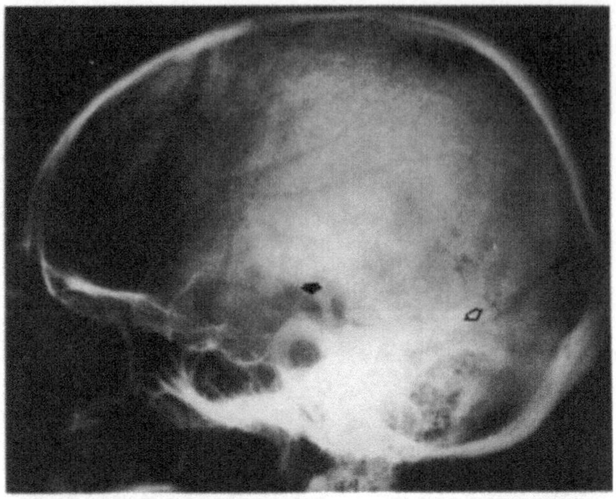

Fig. 5.28. Female patient entered the hospital immediately after head trauma. Lateral plain skull radiograph shows a fracture near the lambdoidal suture (*open arrowhead*) extending into the mastoid. Note pneumocephalus (*closed arrowhead*) with gas outlining gyri

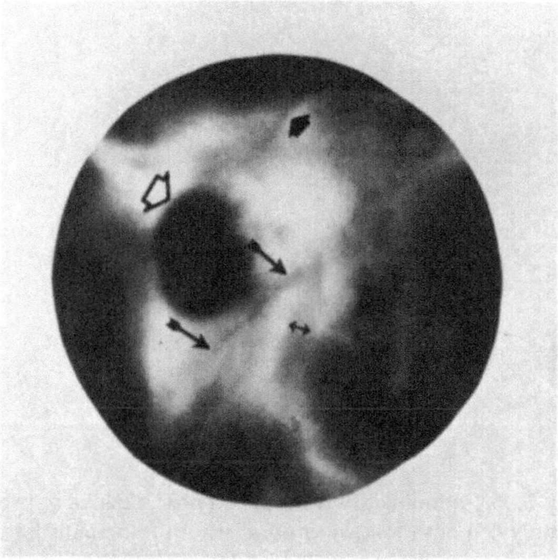

Fig. 5.27. Sixteen-year-old male patient entered hospital after blunt trauma to the head with an immediate facial nerve palsy. Lateral tomogram shows a longitudinal fracture (*arrows*) extending through the mastoid portion of the facial nerve canal (*double-headed arrow*). The fracture extends to the tegmen tympani (*closed arrowhead*); external auditory canal (*open arrowhead*)

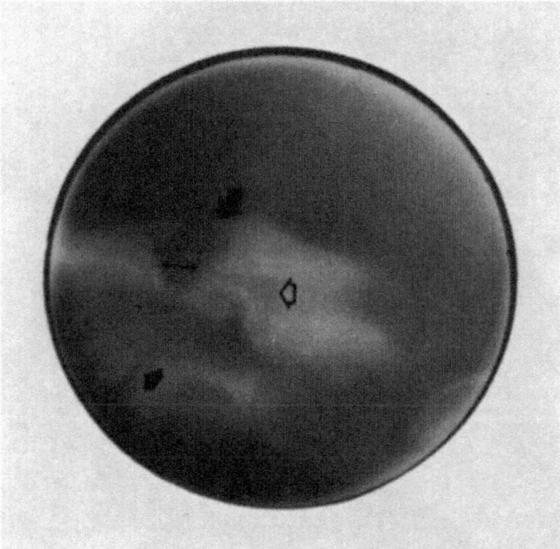

Fig. 5.29. A 55-year-old male with a long histiry of pulsating tinnitus and contuctive hearing loss following head trauma as a teenager. Anteroposterior tomogram through the vestibule (*open arrowhead*) demonstrates a fracture through the floor of the external auditory canal (*closed arrowhead*). A soft tissue density fills the epitympanic space (*double-head arrow*) with a defect in the tegmen tympani (*large curved arrow*). Surgery confirmed an encephalocele

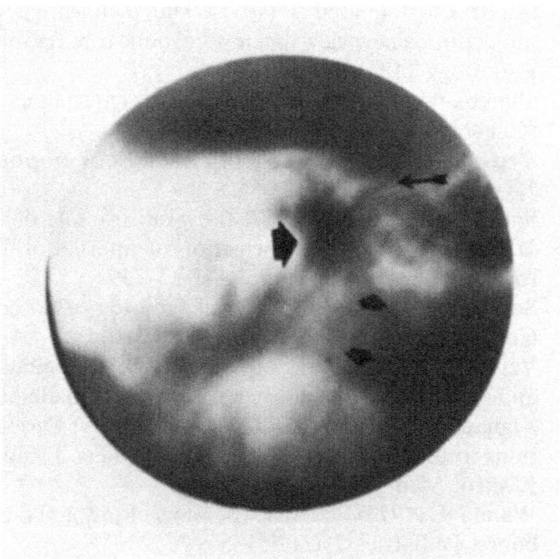

Fig. 5.30. Fifty-year-old female entered the hospital with recurrent episodes of meningitis extending over approximately 35 years and following head trauma. Semiaxial tomograms through the mastoid antrum (*large arrowhead*) reveals a fracture extending to the tegmen (*arrow*); external auditory canal (*small arrowheads*)

ment of the petrous portion of the seventh cranial nerve is usually by a transverse fracture (Figs. 5.18, 5.21, 5.26), whereas trauma to the tympanic or mastoid portions of the nerve is usually by a longitudinal fracture (Fig. 5.27).

The clinical evaluation of the patient can usually determine the exact segment of the facial nerve which is injured. Tests for lacrimation and taste are frequently necessary to find out the position of the facial nerve injury so that the appropriate tomographic evaluation can take place. In young children, these tests may be difficult to perform and may be unreliable.

5.2.4 Sequelae of Temporal Bone Trauma

Immediately after a temporal bone fracture there may be CSF otorrhea. The fracture leaves an open pathway from the meninges to the external auditory canal, acting as an avenue for infection with the potential for meningitis (Fig. 5.28).

Another potential sequel of temporal bone fracture is a traumatic meningocele or encephalocele (Fig. 5.29). The authors have examined two patients with traumatic encephaloceles in patients who have suffered temporal bone fractures as children. The encephalocele presents as a soft tissue mass in the mastoid, mastoid antrum or attic, with the tegmen tympani antra being absent. Presumably the mechanism for this process is similar to that of a leptomeningeal cyst. After the fracture through the tegmen and dura, continual CSF pulsations against the arachnoid herniate the arachnoid through the fracture. The fracture continually widens, giving the radiological impression that the tegmen is absent.

It has been reported by Potter that temporal bone fractures heal by fibrous union rather than bony union [23]. It is believed that this fibrous tissue is not as effective a barrier to infection as bone. Therefore, patients who have experienced temporal bone fractures are susceptible to meningitis during an ear infection. The susceptibility to meningitis remains increased throughout the life of the patient (Fig. 5.30).

References

1. Bloem JJAM, Von dam Meulen JL, Ramselaar JM (1975) Orbital roof fractures; Proc 2nd Int. Symp. on orbital disorders. Mod Probl Ophthalmol 14:510–512
2. Converse JM, Smith B, Wood-Smith D (1975) Deformities of the mid face resulting from malunited orbital and naso-orbital fractures. Clin Plast Surg 2(1):107–130
3. Cooper RL (1977) "Blow-in" fracture of the orbit with partial visual loss and choroidal folds. Med J Aust 1(4):100–101
4. Crumley RL, Leibsohn J, Krause CJ et al (1977) Fractures of the orbital floor. Laryngoscope 87(6):934–947
5. deLacey GJ, Wignall BK, Hussain S et al (1977) The radiology of nasal injuries: problems of interpretation and clinical relevance. Br J Radiol 50:412–414
6. Dodd GD, Jhig BS (1977) Traumatic lesions involving the nasal bones and nasal cavity in radiology of the nose, paranasal sinuses and nasopharynx. Williams & Wilkins, Baltimore, pp 33–42
7. Facer GW (1975) Management of nasal injury. Postgrad Med 57(6):123–126
8. Frey KW (1971) In: Jensen J, Rowsing H (eds) Fundamentals of ear tomography. Thomas, Springfield, Chap 13
9. Gerlock AJ, Sinn DP (1977) Anatomic, clinical, surgical and radiographic correlation of the zygomatic complex fracture. AJR 128:235
10. Goode RH, Spooner TR (1972) Management of nasal fractures in children. Clin Pediatr (Phila) 11:526–529
11. Gozum E (1976) Blow-out fractures of the orbit. Otolaryngol Clin North Am 9(2):477–487
12. Griffin JM, Hartley JH, Crow RW et al (1976) Diabetes insipidus caused by craniofacial trauma. J Trauma 16(12):979–984
13. Harwood-Nash DC (1972) Optic Gliomas and pediatric neuroradiology. Radiol Clin North Am 10(1):83–100

14. Jacobs GB, Rubin RC, Jotkowitz S et al (1977) Brain abscess associated with facial trauma. Int Surg 62(4):236–37
15. Keyes KS (1977) Dental aspects of maxillofacial injuries. Laryngoscope 87(6):954–956
16. Lloyd GAS (1975) Radiology of the orbit. Saunders, Philadelphia, pp 60–90, 180–188
17. McGrail JS (1976) Management of maxillary fractures. Otolaryngol Clin North Am 9(1):223–232
18. McLennan JE, Mickle JP, Treves S (1976) Radionuclide cisternographic evaluation and follow-up of posttraumatic subconjuntival CSF loculation. J Neurosurg 44:496–499
19. Moran WB (1977) Nasal trauma in children. Otolaryngol Clin North Am 10(1):95–101
20. Patten BM (1968) Human Embryology. McGraw-Hill, New York, pp 335–344
21. Pendergrass EP, Schaeffer JP, Hodes PJ, (1956) The head and neck in roentgen diagnosis. 2nd edn Thomas, Springfield
22. Potter GD (1973) The ear, the surgeon and the radiologist–Hickey Lecture AJR 118:501–510
23. Potter GD (1962) The lateral projection in tomography of the petrous pyramid. AJR 104:194–200
24. Prasad SS (1975) Blow-out fracture of the medial wall of the orbit. Proc 2nd Int. Symp. on orbital disorder. Mod Probl Ophthalmol 14:510–512
25. Rothman SG, Allen WE, Kier EL (1973) Stereo roentgenography in cranio-facial injuries. Radiol Clin North Am 11(3):683–696
26. Schatz CJ, Vignaud J (1976) The inclined lateral projection: a new view in temporal bone tomography. Radiology 118:355–361
27. Shambaugh GE (1967) Surgery of the ear. Saunders, Philadelphia, Chapter 1
28. Slepyan DH (1976) A case of orbital floor eruption. J Trauma 16(4):320–327
29. Smith B, Regan WF (1957) Blow out fracture of the orbit; mechanism and correction of internal orbital fracture. Am J Ophthalmol 44:733–739
30. Sutton D (1975) A textbook of radiology. 2nd edn. Churchill Livingstone, Edinburgh, p 1011
31. Valvassori GE, Buckingham RA (1975) Tomography and cross sections of the ear. Saunders, Philadelphia
32. Vignaud J, Sutton A, Donic J et al. (1969) Dislocations traumatiques de la chaine des osselets. J Radiol Electrol Med Nucl 50:803–806
33. Waite DE (1973) Pediatric fractures of jaw and facial bones. Pediatrics 51(3):551–559
34. Waring GO, Flanagan JC (1975) Pneumocephalus, a sign of intracranial involvement in orbital fracture. Arch Ophthalmol 93:847–850
35. Wright WJ, Taylor C, Bizal J (1969) Tomography and the vulnerable incus. Ann Otol Rhinol Laryngol 78:263–276
36. Wright WJ (1974) Trauma of the ear. Radiol Clin North Am 12:527–532
37. Yarington CT (1977) Maxillofacial trauma in children. Otolarngol Clin North Am 10(1):25–32

6 Nuclear Medicine and Ultrasound in Pediatric Trauma

Gary F. Gates

The role of trauma as leading cause of death and disability in children is universally appreciated. Similarly, the contribution of diagnostic radiology to the management of an injured child is well understood. In recent years, nuclear medicine and diagnostic ultrasound have begun to have an impact on the assessment of the traumatized patient. These newer diagnostic techniques are not merely duplications of radiographic examinations: nuclear medicine studies allow for unique assessment of organ function while ultrasonography can determine the internal morphology of a soft tissue organ or mass. The radiation exposure to the patient is low as in nuclear medicine, or nonexistent as with ultrasonography. Furthermore, these examinations can be performed rapidly and require little, if any, patient cooperation, and these are features of importance when dealing with traumatized children.

The purpose of this chapter will be to show the clinical utility of these virtually (if not literally) noninvasive diagnostic tests. Webster's dictionary [57] defines *trauma* as "an injury (as a wound) to living tissue caused by an extrinsic agent," which is then illustrated by the example "surgical trauma"! Thus, some of the undesirable consequences of surgery as well as radiation therapy will be discussed in addition to the usual examples of trauma (e. g., automobile accidents). This is not intended as a criticism of these therapeutic modalities, but rather to serve as an illustration of the usefulness of nuclear medicine and ultrasonography in the patient who has been traumatized, regardless of etiology.

6.1 Brain

Radionuclide scintigraphy of the brain is an effective means of assessing a child who has sustained a head injury. We use ^{99m}Tc-DTPA (diethylenetriaminepentaacetic acid) for cerebral scintigraphy since, unlike ionic pertechnetate, perchlorate need not be administered to block the choroid plexus; furthermore, adequate static delayed images can be obtained in 30–60 min. Dynamic scintigraphy (i. e., scintiangiography) is an important portion of the examination and follows the course of the intravenously administered tracer as it is mixed with the blood perfusing the brain. This important procedure does not increase the radiation exposure to the patient, yet extracts additional valuable information from the already injected radionuclide.

Radionuclide scintigraphy has been used successfully to detect subdural hematomas. This potentially life-threatening lesion is believed to result from tears in the cortical veins as they pass through the subdural space; the subsequent bleeding spreads over the cerebral convexities and eventually forms a solidified clot. The hematoma becomes encapsulated by a pseudomembrane which organizes over its surface and contains many immature capillaries. The encapsulated clot eventually liquifies and may be gradually absorbed. On occasion, the liquified contents may expand in size due to, either singly or in combination, osmosis across a semipermeable membrane, continued exudation from newly formed capillaries, or persistent leakage of blood [14].

Subdural hematomas are usually seen on anterior and posterior static scintigrams as an increase in width of the peripheral crescent of tracer activity which is less well identified on lateral projections. However, this crescent pattern is not pathognomonic of subdural hematomas as it has been seen in a variety of conditions including: scalp or skull lesions (e. g., scalp vein infusion sites, cephalohematomas, subdural taps through a fontanel, scalp contusion, skull fractures, craniotomy sites, and inflammatory conditions); epidural collections; subdural effusions due to infections or hygromas; pachymeningitis; cerebral contusion or infarction; and peripheral metastases [7, 12, 28]. The major diagnostic problem in the case of an injured patient, however, is the differentiation of a possible subdural hematoma from scalp, skull, or brain trauma.

On occasion, a subdural hematoma may also be seen as a circumferential rim of increased radionuclide uptake around a central region devoid of tracer (i. e., "doughtnut" or "rim" sign). This is due to a medial rim of increased activity which is attributed to altered and displaced vascular structures as well as tracer accumulation within the inner membranes [14]. This bizarre scintigraphic appearance may be seen on lateral as well as anterior and posterior views and should not be mistaken for scalp or skull lesions (although it may also be associated with epidural hematomas or subdural empyema).

While the scintigraphic features of subdural hematomas may also be seen in other conditions, the radionuclide study is still useful as a screening test due to its high sensitivity. Cowen et al. [13] reviewed the literature up to 1968 and reported an overall 81% detection rate for subdural hematomas; since then, this detection rate has been revised upward to 90% [14]. A variety of factors are important in determining this accuracy, however:

1) Delayed scans have an improved accuracy compared with studies obtained immediately following radionuclide injection.
2) Although there appears to be a correlation between the size of a subdural hematoma and the width of the crescent on a brain scan [22], size alone does not appear to be the determining factor in development of an abnormal scan [14].
3) Acute subdural hematomas are not detected as readily as chronic ones.
4) Subdural hematomas present for at least 10 days were detected with an accuracy of 86% in Cowan's series [14]; contrariwise, only 50% of lesions less than 10 days in duration were detected.
5) In the presence of a subdural hematoma, cerebral scintiangiography may show an inward displacement of peripheral activity throughout the dynamic study. However, a subdural process cannot be excluded solely on the basis of normal scintiangiography; lesions producing less than 2 cm inward displacement of cerebral vessels on contrast angiography were associated with normal dynamic studies in Cowan's series [14]. Overall Cowan had only a 47% accuracy in detecting subdural hematomas on dynamic scintigraphy although others have reported an accuracy approaching 100% [30].
6) The presence of a thick membrane encapsulating the hematoma usually correlates with an abnormal scan. However, abnormal scans can occur in the absence of a membrane, and patients with well developed membranes may have normal scans [22]. Tracer activity has been localized in the subdural membrane as well as in the hematoma fluid; furthermore, radionuclide has been detected in the subdural fluid of patients in whom a membrane was lacking [3].
7) Subtemporal, interhemispheric, or posterior fossa subdural hematomas may be difficult to detect and do not show the typical crescent of activity.
8) Recognition of bilateral subdurals is more difficult than detecting a unilateral process since the two sides may appear similar (albeit thickened). Dynamic scintigraphy may be quite helpful in this circumstance.

Detection of subdural hematomas in children has been less successful than in adults. The membrane of the subdural hematoma, which is probably at least in part responsible for abnormal tracer accumulation, is poorly developed in children [45]. Subdural collections are frequently bilateral in the pediatric patient [45, 59] and located somewhat higher over the cerebral convexities [59]. Conway and Vollert [11] reported a 72% incidence of bilateral subdural hematomas in children compared with 16% in adults. Although one side may be more severe than the opposite, the bilaterality makes the diagnosis more difficult and probably accounts for the overall 60% accuracy of subdural hematoma detection in children [11] compared with the 80%–90% accuracy reported in adults.

The child in Fig. 6.1 had the typical scintigraphic features of a subdural hematoma: a prominent peripheral crescent of radionuclide uptake on anterior and posterior views with virtually normal lateral

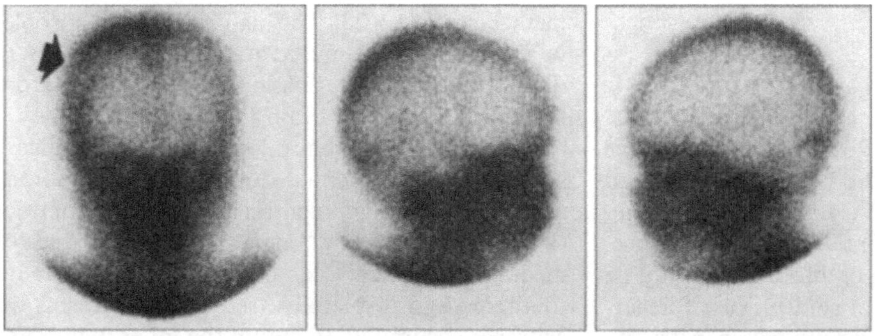

Fig. 6.1. A 16-month-old girl with a right subdural hematoma following head trauma. *Arrow*, peripheral crescent of ^{99m}Tc-DTPA activity on anterior view. Right lateral view has slightly increased uptake compared with the left side

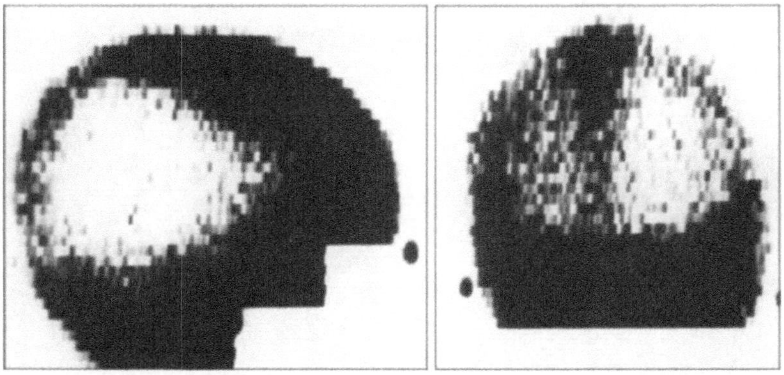

Fig. 6.2. Infiltration of a scalp vein infusion site resulted in peripheral tracer uptake in this 6-mounth-old girl undergoing brain scanning. Scalp trauma may result in a radionuclide scan having features similar to a subdural hematoma

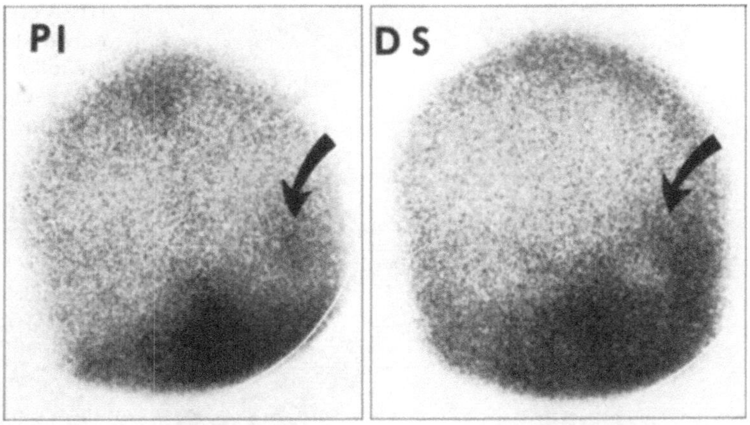

Fig. 6.3. Supraorbital skull fracture identified on ^{99m}Tc-DTPA brain scintigraphy in this 15-year-old girl. The abnormal region (*arrows*) accumulated radionuclide both on immediate postinjection (*PI*) and delayed static (*DS*) views, presumably due to hyperemia

views. Severe scalp trauma or infiltrated scalp vein infusion sites may also result in an abnormal brain scan (Fig. 6.2). Skull trauma such as the left supraorbital ridge fracture shown in Fig. 6.3 or the craniotomy site in Fig. 6.4, may also result in an abnormal brain scintigram. As opposed to subdural hematomas, however, patients with scalp or skull trauma will usually show decreasing tracer accumulation on delayed scintigrams instead of a progressive increase. Much of not all abnormal tracer uptake in sites of skull or soft tissue trauma is probably due to the associated hyperemia around the lesion. This hyperemic effect is illustrated in Fig. 6.5 where a brain scintigram shows orbital uptake due to a recent enucleation for a retinoblastoma; bone scintigraphy on the following day showed normal uniform osteoblastic activity in both orbits.

Patients with acute epidural hematomas are infrequently studied by radionuclide techniques since CT is usually the primary investigative technique. These hematomas usually result from a laceration of a meningeal artery although a venous origin of bleeding may occur. Brain scanning often shows features similar to those associated with subdural hematomas: displacement of vessels away from the inner table of the skull on dynamic scintigraphy, static views revealing the crescent pattern of radionuclide uptake [47, 58]. Lin [39] and Buozas et al. [9] have reported a separation of the superior sagittal sinus from the skull during dynamic scintigraphy in patients with epidural hematomas. Lin [39] draws attention to an interesting characteristic of these vertex hematomas: a primary venous origin of the hemorrhage.

Cerebral contusions as well as cerebral hematomas can result in an abnormal brain scan (Fig. 6.6). Both conditions often produce a region of well circumscribed radionuclide uptake in the brain sub-

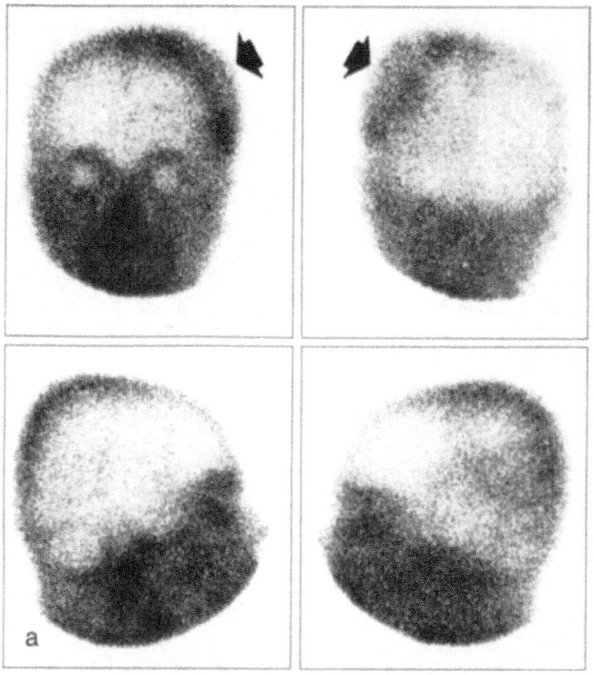

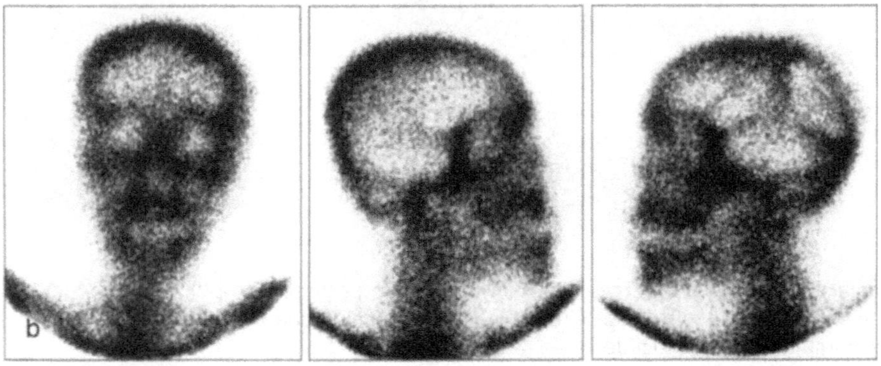

◁

Fig. 6.4 a, b. A 13-year-old boy with a glioblastoma had craniotomy for removal of tumor. Seven days later, ^{99m}Tc-DTPA brain scintigraphy was performed (**a**) and showed calvarial uptake of radiotracer (*arrows*). Bone scan on the following day (**b**) using ^{99m}Tc-pyrophosphate showed the reactive changes of osteoblastic hyperactivity around the bone flap site, especially on the left lateral view

stance although multiple regions may occur in some patients. Delayed scanning improves the accuracy in identifying both contusions and hematomas; the overall accuracy for detecting cerebral hematomas is around 75% while that for cerebral contusions may be somewhat higher [14].

From the time of trauma until the appearance of a positive scan there is a delay of probably 1–2 weeks for cerebral hematomas. Sugitani et al. [52] studied the time sequence of tracer appearance in experimentally produced cerebral hematomas in rats; radionuclide uptake was greatest during the 1st to 2nd weeks, a time period during which newly forming capillaries appeared. Brain scans which are abnormal due to cerebral contusion usually return rapidly to normal, especially when 6 to 10 weeks have passed [25].

The differentiation of an intracerebral hematoma from a subdural hematoma may be difficult, especially if the intracerebral hematoma is either close to the brain surface or in the temporal lobe; not uncommonly the two conditions may coexist. If an abnormal region of radionuclide uptake occurs in the hemisphere opposite from the side of trauma, one must suspect the presence of a contrecoup contusion. Brain scanning alone may not separate cerebral contusions from intracerebral hematomas, but in either circumstance an abnormal study is of great value and often leads to further studies.

Direct injury to the carotid arteries may be assessed by dynamic scintigraphy (Fig. 6.7). Penetrations of the neck or transoral trauma may produce such injuries. Usually, contrast angiography is indicated at the time of acute injury while radionuclide studies are reserved for follow-up assessment.

Cerebrospinal fluid (CSF) rhinorrhea is a complication in 30% of basal skull fractures [38] as well as in

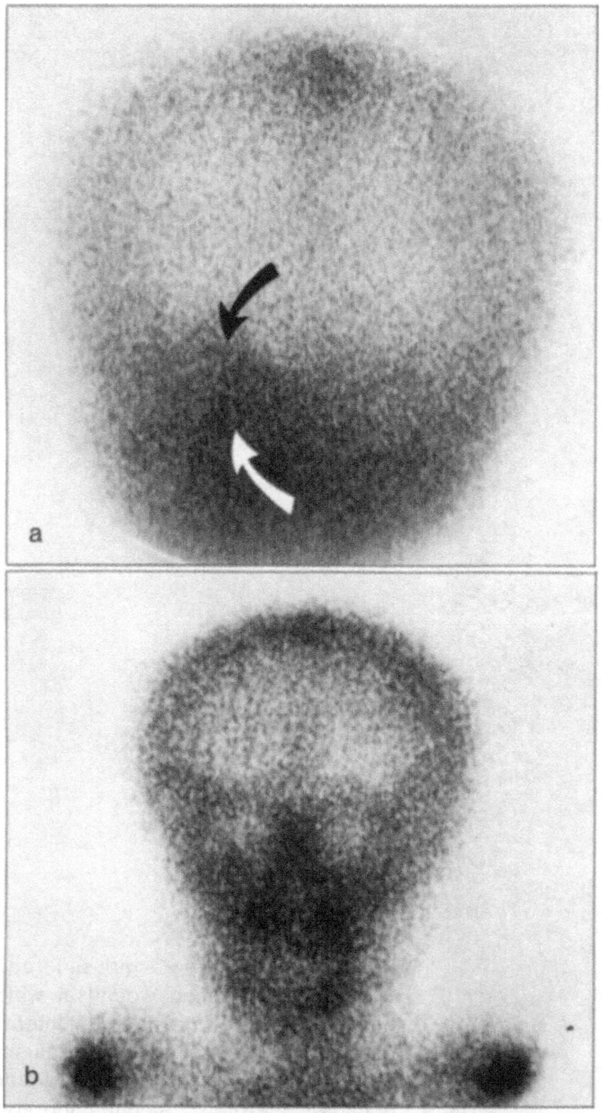

Fig. 6.5 a, b. A 3-year-old boy a right retinoblastoma had an orbital enucleation. **a** ^{99m}Tc-DTPA brain scintigram 4 days later showed orbital hyperemia (*arrows*); **b** ^{99m}Tc-pyrophosphate bone scan on following day showed little if any bony orbital changes

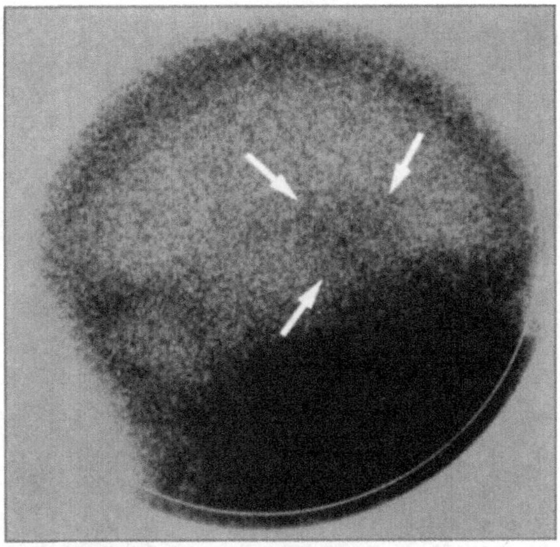

Fig. 6.6. An 8-year-old boy with a cerebral contusion had a focal region of ^{99m}Tc-DTPA uptake shown on a right lateral view (*arrows*)

circumstances when fractures pass through the frontal or ethmoid sinuses. CSF otorrhea may similarly occur following petrous bone fractures in patients with ruptured tympanic membranes. The CSF leakage through the torn meninges usually manifests as a bloody discharge within 48 h following cranial trauma. The leakage ceases spontaneously within a week in 90% of cases, but may be complicated by pyogenic meningitis in up to 25% of patients who are not placed on prophylactic antibiotics [41]. Associated clinical and/or radiological features may include: anosmia, periorbital edema, neurological defects, intracranial air, and air-fluid levels within a sinus.

The site of apparent CSF leakage on physical examination may not accurately indicate the precise location of a fistula. Likewise, skull radiography may not always uncover a bony defect, especially in instances of small, linear, nondisplaced fractures. The role of nuclear medicine in such circumstances is twofold: *detection* and *localization* of the CSF fistula. ^{111}In-DTPA or ^{131}I human serum albumin are the radiopharmaceuticals most commonly used for radionuclide cisternography. Following intrathecal injection of the radionuclide, imaging is started within 1–2 h and continued thereafter as needed. The patient's head is placed in a position that augments the leakage. Anterior and lateral scintigrams are usually obtained. Pledgets may also be placed in the nose near the cribriform plate, the middle turbinate, and at the eustachian tube orifice in order to help further localize the route of CSF leakage. Nearly all CSF leaks can be diagnosed by the combination of these two radionuclide techniques.

Under favorable conditions the fistula may be visualized as a linear stripe of radioactivity extending outward from the CSF space. The study should be continued for 24 h since many fistulas may not be seen on early scans. Magmaes and Solheim [42] advocate controlled "over pressure" cisternography to detect leaks which occur only intermittently: this technique is performed by infusing "artificial" CSF at a rate of up to 5 ml/min. However, demonstration of a fistula is not the sole requirement for localiza-

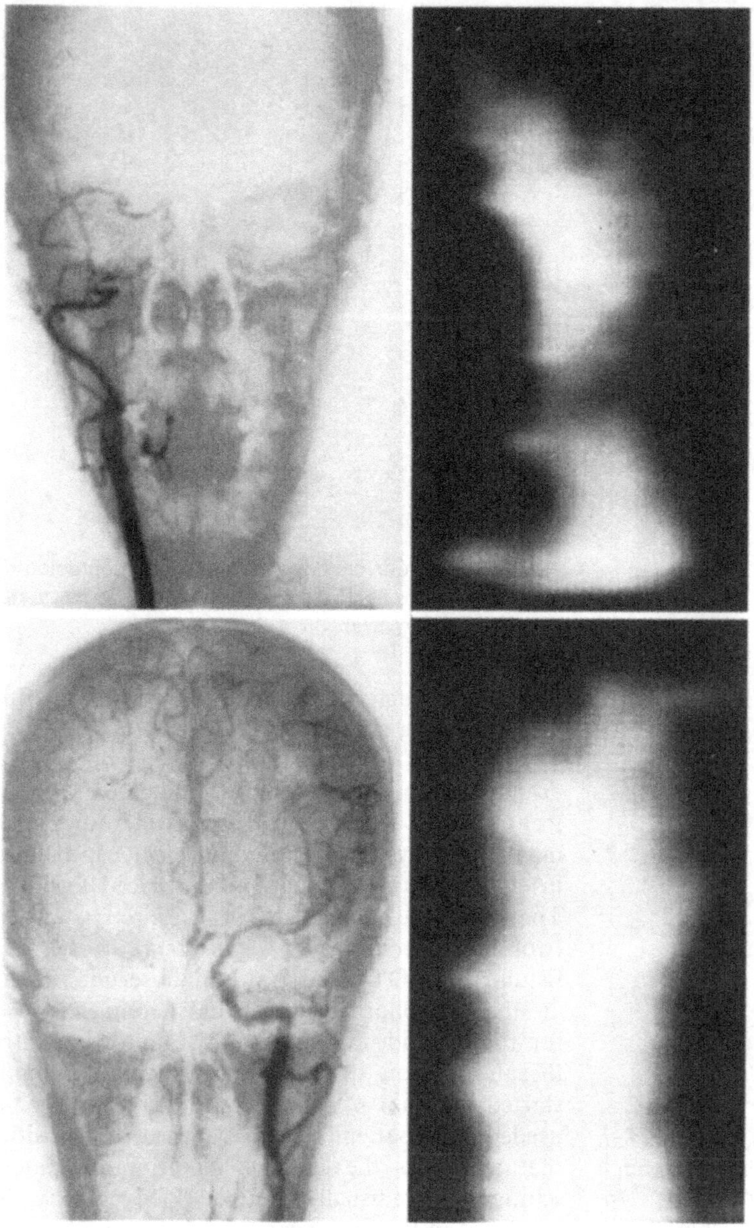

◁
Fig. 6.7. An 8-year-old girl suffered a transoral penetrating wound at which time a stick penetrated the right internal carotid artery resulting in its occlusion (angiograms). Eight months later radionuclide carotid scintiangiography showed a marked narrowing in the caliber of the right carotid (*above:* scintigram) whereas the left was normal (*below:* scintigram)

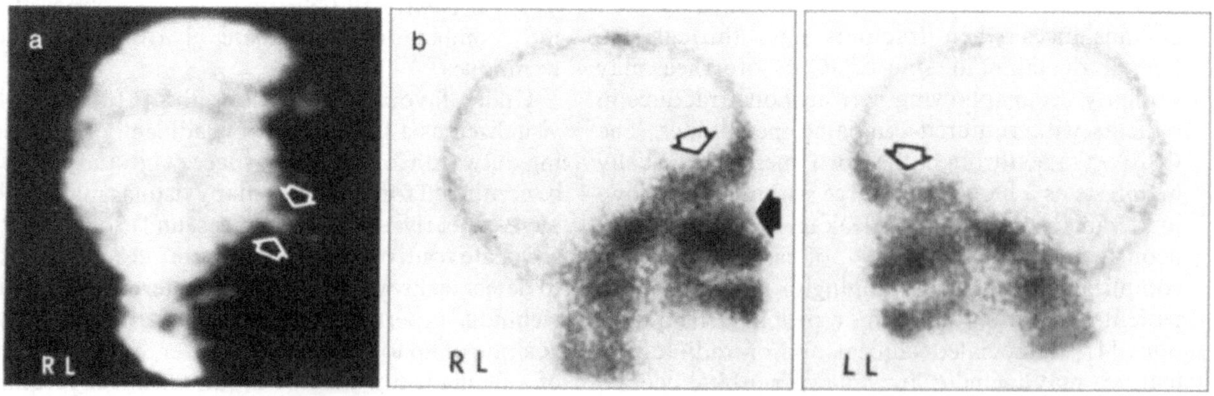

tion of a site of leakage; prominent basal cisternal pouches or sphenoidal collections may pinpoint the site without actually showing the fistulous tract [41] (Fig. 6.8). Documentation of nasal pledget activity or visualization of pharyngeal, middle ear, or nasal activity by radionuclide cisternography may be the only means of localizing CSF leaks in some patients and always provides valuable information for either further radiographic investigations or neurosurgical repairs.

6.2 Lungs

Chest injuries may damage either the rib cage (see later section on "Bone") or the soft tissue organs contained within. Cardiac contusions can be detected by myocardial scintigraphy using ^{99m}Tc-pyrophosphate [55] while changes in global cardiac function may be assessed by nuclear angiocardiography. Although pericardial effusions of greater than 200 ml are detected by blood pool scanning, echocardiography is currently preferred since it is more sensitive in detecting small effusions.The perfusion lung scan, performed with either ^{99m}Tc macroaggregated albumin (MAA) or similarly labeled albumin microspheres (MSP), is the easiest and probably most consistantly reliable radionuclide technique of assessing the lungs following chest trauma. Often, the results of ventilation scintigraphy using either radioactive gases (e. g., ^{133}Xe or ^{81m}Kr) or radioactive aerosols (e. g., ^{99m}Tc-sulfur colloidal aerosol) are also of major importance in evaluating the injured patient.

Pulmonary contusion may follow blunt thoracic trauma. Radiographic abnormalities may develop within 6 h of injury, start to improve by 1–2 days, and be totally resolved by 7–10 days. Clinical symptoms include hemoptysis, fever, and dyspnea. Lung scanning with either MAA or MSP may reveal a perfusion defect even though a radiographically detectable infiltrate may be lacking. These are often peripheral, pleural based defects and must be distinguished from pulmonary thromboemboli which usually present later in the posttraumatic course [44]. Pulmonary embolization, of course, may occur after trauma or surgery to the extremities or following prolonged leg immobilization in a cast, as is shown in Fig. 6.9. In addition, we have had pulmonary embolization occur secondary to the placement of central venous (i. e., umbilical venous) catheters in neonates.

Pulmonary fat embolism may also occur 1–4 days following lower extremity fractures. Clinical symptoms include hypoxemia, urine fat droplets, tachypnea, tachycardia, fever, and petechiae. Lung scan-

Fig. 6.8 a, b. CSF rhinorrhea in an 8-year-old boy persisted for 30 days following his falling from a tree. **a** Radionuclide cysternography with ^{131}I-human serum albumin showed an outward extention of tracer from the base of the skull on the right lateral view (*arrows*). Nasal pledgets revealed 14 times as much radiotracer in the right nostril as in the left. **b** Bone scintigraphy revealed increased tracer uptake in the floor of anterior fossa on the right compared with the left (*open arrows*). Some increased right ethmoid uptake was also seen (*solid arrow*). A right-sided cribifrom plate fracture was detected at surgery

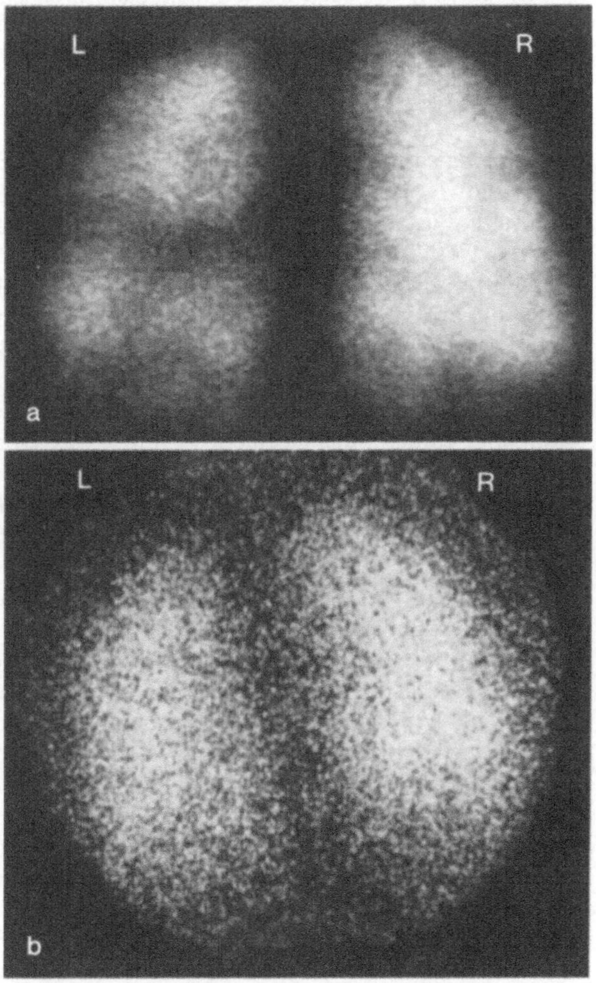

Fig. 6.9 a, b. A 9-year-old boy had onset of chest pain and dyspnea after leg had been in cast for several weeks following orthopedic surgery. **a** Perfusion scintigram with ^{99m}Tc microspheres (posterior view) showed multiple, bilateral defects. **b** ^{133}Xe ventilation study (posterior view) was normal. These features are due to multiple pulmonary emboli

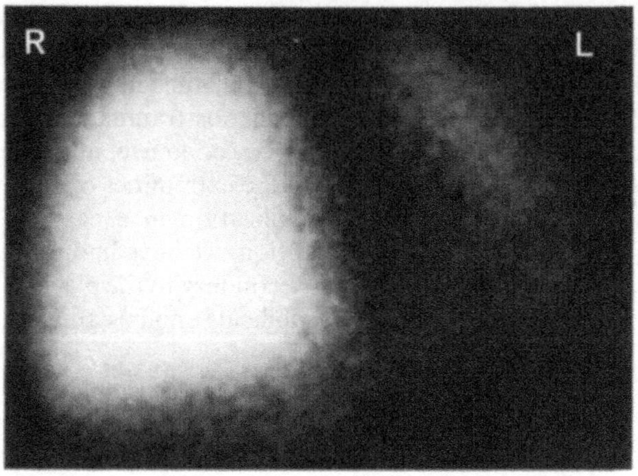

Fig. 6.10. An 8-month-old girl aspirated a piece of carrot which partially occluded the left main stem bronchus, producing an abnormal perfusion lung scan (anterior view). (Courtesy by Gates, G.: Radionuclide Scanning in Cyanotic Heart Disease. Springfield: Thomas 1974)

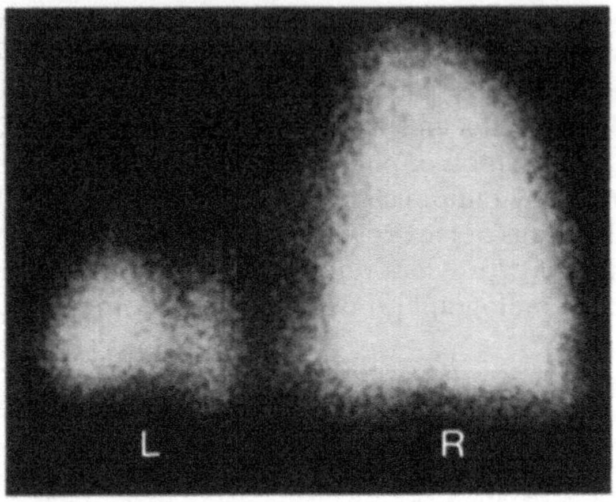

Fig. 6.11. A 12-year-old boy with Wilms' tumor metastatic to the left lung had megavoltage radiation therapy directed to the area. A perfusion lung scan afterward showed a large defect in the treated region (posterior view)

ning reveals multiple small perfusion defects which clear slowly (up to a month) [44]. The perfusion scintigraphic appearance of "shock lung" may be similar to that of fat embolism.

The presence of pleural fluid may considerably alter the appearance of a perfusion lung scan. The posterior view of a supine patient may show markedly reduced tracer content in the lung on the affected side due to: interposition of fluid between lung and camera, displacement of lung away from the detector, or actually reduced pulmonary perfusion. An anterior scan will allow for a more meaningful evaluation of relative pulmonary perfusion.

Aspirated foreign bodies result in marked perfusion abnormalities (Fig. 6.10). Regional alveolar hypoxia following endobronchial occlusion results in decreased arterial perfusion to the affected lung area. This hypoventilation produces active pulmonary arterial constriction with elevation of pulmonary artery pressure in the hypoxic lung [2]. Perfusion scintigraphy reveals a considerable maldistribution of pulmonary arterial perfusion secondary to the redistribution of flow away from hypoxic lung segments [20]. The main value of lung scanning is in circumstances where the presence of an endobronchial foreign body may be suspected on clinical grounds but not confirmed by an abnormal chest radiogram. The identification of a perfusion defect (or ventilation defect if ventilatory scanning is performed) will direct the bronchoscopist to the affected lung region. However, pulmonary scintigraphy (perfusion or ventilation) may also be abnormal following aspiration of blood or secretions by severely injured patients. Perfusion scintigraphy may also be utilized after bronchoscopy; if a scan is normal 1–3 days following bronchoscopy, retention of aspirated material large enough to block a lobar or segmental bronchus partially is highly unlikely [33]. However, residual perfusion defects – some of which involved an entire lung – have been present from 4–19 days following presumed removal of the aspirated material [33].

Radiation therapy to the lung, chest wall, or nodal regions may also result in pulmonary injury. Perfusion scintigraphy often reveals a sharply demarcated, nonsegmental region of decreased perfusion corresponding to the patient's radiation portals [26] (Fig. 6.11). The scintigraphic study is much more sensitive in demonstrating radiation damage to the lung than conventional chest radiography [44].

Mechanical impingements upon major bronchi following vertebral spine surgery can be well shown by ventilation scintigraphy, as shown in Fig. 6.12. This young girl with scoliosis (who previously had an esophageal ring) underwent surgery for placement of a Harrington rod which resulted in a drastic change in the contour of her chest and in a reduction in its anterior-posterior dimensions. Scintigraphy with both ^{133}Xe and radioaerosols revealed ventilation abnormalities due to mechanical impingement of the airways which occurred secondary to the narrowing of her already thin chest.

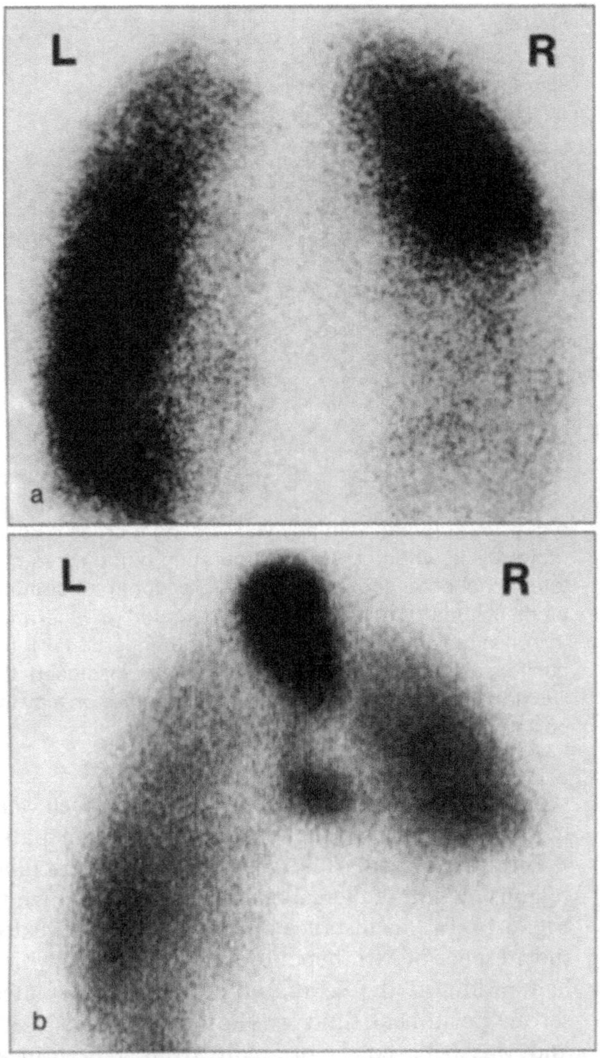

Fig. 6.12 a, b. A 15-year-old girl with scoliosis had a Harrington rod so placed that her chest diameter was narrowed, resulting in impingement upon the airways to the right lower lobe (RLL). **a** ^{99m}Tc-macroaggregated albumin scintigram (posterior) showed poor RLL perfusion. **b** Radioaerosol scintigraphy (^{99m}Tc-sulfur colloid aerosol) demonstrated poor ventilation to the RLL (posterior)

6.3 Abdomen

The liver, spleen, and pancreas are particularly susceptible to either blunt or penetrating upper abdominal trauma. Scintigraphy of the liver and spleen (using radiolabeled colloids) and pancreatic ultrasonography are particularly effective in evaluating these respective organs. Both require little patient cooperation and in some circumstances obviate the need for angiography.

6.3.1 Liver

The liver is the organ most commonly injured following a penetrating abdominal wound [10, 29] but in blunt abdominal trauma it is injured only about half as frequently as the spleen [29, 40]. The high incidence of hepatic injury is a result of its size, relative fixation, and poor eleasticity and compressibility [23, 34]. About 30% of all deaths following closed abdominal trauma are due to liver damage [17, 35, 46, 56].

Hepatic scintigraphy depends upon the phagocytosis of an intravenously administered radiocolloid (usually ^{99m}Tc-sulfur colloid) by the liver's functioning reticuloendothelial cells. These cellular components may be damaged following liver trauma and thereafter be unable to accumulate selectively the administered tracer. Consequently, one or more focal defects, corresponding to areas of hepatic injury, will appear on the scan. In themselves these defects are indistinguishable from other liver abnormalities, including neoplasms. However, the clinical setting usually clarifies the situation: in doubtful cases, hepatic ultrasonography may be useful in distinguishing hematomas (i. e., sonolucent defects) from neoplasms (i. e., solid echogenic defects). Hepatic displacement (by an adjacent hematoma) can be another sign of intra-abdominal injury.

Gilday and Alderson [23] reviewed 162 patients with closed abdominal trauma who had liver scans. No false negative studies were reported; there was a 7% false positive rate. These results are nearly ideal for a screening test: a negative study is truely negative while a positive study has a 93% chance of indicating an abnormality. Besides determining the presence of an hepatic injury, liver scanning is very useful in localizing the abnormality and determining its extent, especially in the right lobe, which is the most common site of liver injury following blunt abdominal trauma. Serial follow-up scans are a convenient, easy and accurate means of assessing the healing process following trauma.

A variety of scintigraphic images may result following hepatic trauma. Figures 6.13 and 6.14 show differing hepatic defects following blunt abdominal trauma. Such defects may result from either a liver contusion or a frank hematoma. On occasion the liver may actually "fracture" along the line of the falciform ligament (from which it is suspended beneath the anterior abdominal wall); this injury produces a vertical transhepatic band of decreased activity extending through the region of the porta hepatics. The child in Fig. 6.15 sustained such a liver fracture; a surgical exploration revealed a fracture

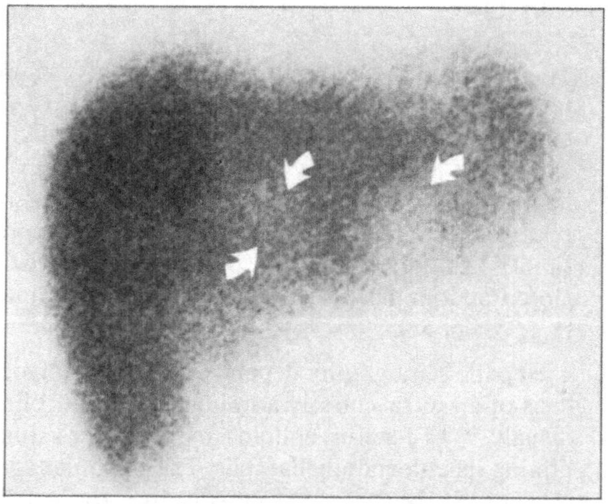

Fig. 6.13. Following an auto accident, a 5-year-old boy had a fractured femur and upper abdominal trauma. Anterior hepatic scintigram revealed multiple, mottled defects (*arrows*) corresponding to regions of liver contusion

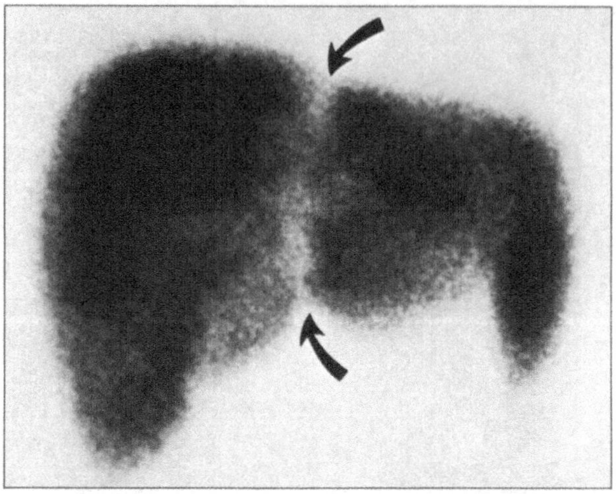

Fig. 6.15. A 15-year-old boy was driving a cross-country motor cycle when he struck supporting guide wires of a telephone pole and suffered severe upper abdominal blunt trauma. An hepatic scan revealed a laceration (*arrows*) through the liver near the insertion of the falciform ligament. Subsequent surgery disclosed the two hepatic components were joined together only by the portal vessels only

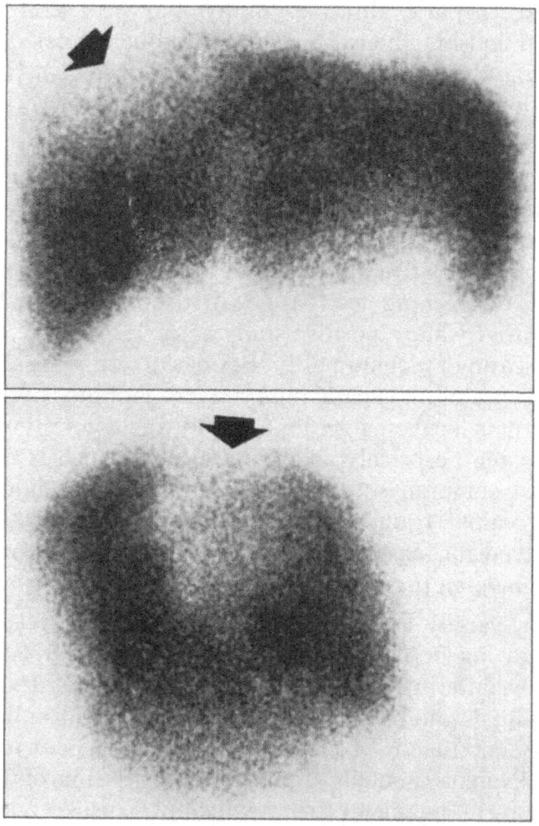

Fig. 6.14. A 6-year-old boy was struck by a car and suffered a severe hepatic injury. The anterior (*above*) and right lateral (*below*) liver scintigraphic views revealed a large right lobe defect (*arrows*) which extended deeply into the parenchyma

separating the liver into two components which were held together only by the vessels in the porta hepatis.

Intra-abdominal fluid may loculate in peculiar regions including the gallbladder fossa, as shown in Fig. 6.16. In this instance ultrasonography revealed the presence of extrahepatic, extrabiliary fluid which had produced the scintigraphic defect. Loculated serous peritoneal fluid was discovered at surgery and was believed to originate from a peritoneal reaction following traumatic rupture of the small bowel.

Combined liver-lung scanning is quite useful in evaluating a child for the possibility of a subdiaphragmatic abscess. Such infections may occur after penetrating abdominal wounds or following surgery for any cause. The dome of the right lobe of the liver and base of the right lung are normally in close approximation. A right subdiaphragmatic abscess results in a separation between these two contiguous organs (Fig. 6.17). However, right pleural fluid will cause a similar defect and, thus, a chest radiogram should be inspected prior to performing this test. Usually, a right subdiaphragmatic abscess will produce some identifiable abnormality on the liver scan while a right pleural fluid collection will not; nevertheless, a recent chest radiogram is invaluable in these circumstances.

Radiation therapy will also produce a liver scan defect, the sharp borders of which conform to the treatment portals (Fig. 6.18). This effect is seen

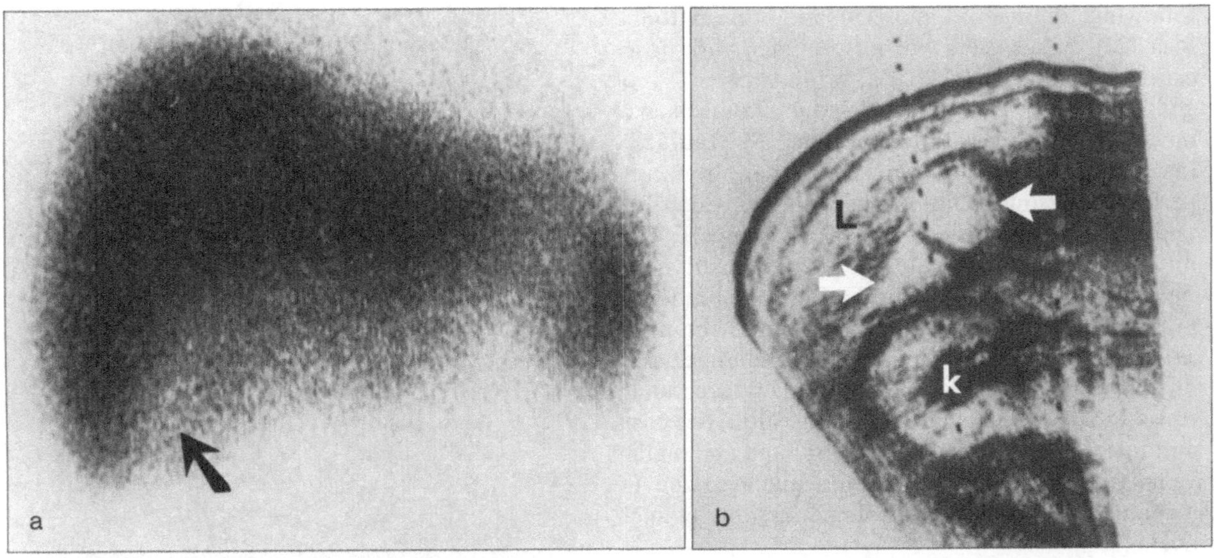

Fig. 6.16 a, b. Following blunt abdominal trauma, a 7-year-old girl had a liver scintigram (**a**) which revealed a somewhat prominent gallbladder fossa (*arrow*). A supine, transverse ultrasonic section (**b**) revealed a fluid collection (*lower, left arrow*) just lateral and below the gallbladder (*upper, right arrow*). The liver (*L*) and kidney (*k*) were normal. Serous fluid was discovered at surgery and presumed to originate from reaction following traumatic rupture of the small bowel

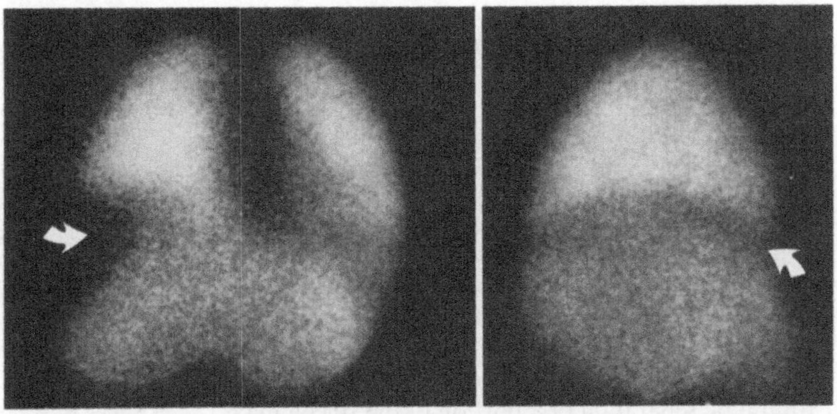

△
Fig. 6.17. A 6-year-old boy had a subdiaphragmatic abscess following a ruptured appendix. Combined liver-lung scintigraphy revealed an abnormal separation between the dome of the right hepatic lobe and the base of the right lung (*arrows*; anterior and right lateral views shown). This separation corresponded to the location of the abscess

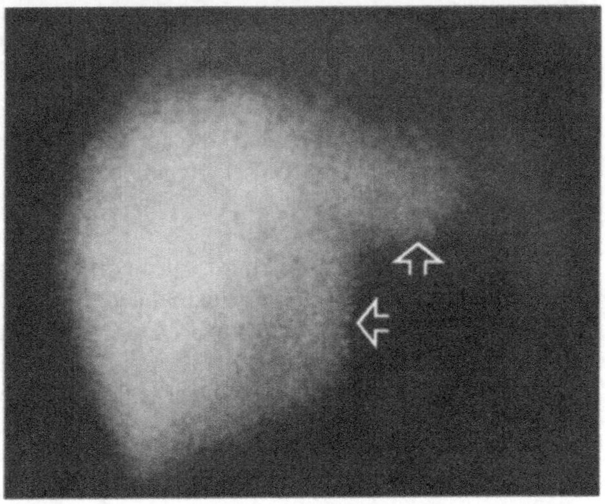

▷
Fig. 6.18. A 12-year-old boy had a left Wilms' tumor removed at surgery and megavoltage radiation directed to the previous tumor site. This radiation resulted in a "squared-off" defect in the left lobe, the boundaries of which exactly corresponded to the treatment portals (*arrows*)

following administration of 3500 rad or more to the liver [23]. Adult livers will recover even with doses exceeding 5500 rad [31, 36] while only 18% of children with such radiation-induced defects will have normal scans within 6 months [53]. Radiocolloid scans show a larger defect than do scans performed using radiopharmaceuticals which are taken up by hepatocytes (i.e., Rose Bengal). This differential uptake indicates the greater sensitivity of reticuloendothelial cells to radiation compared with polygonal cells [23]. Both polygonal and the more extensive reticuloendothelial cellular changes seen on appropriate liver scans are presumably secondary to veno-occlusive changes and congestion. Sclerosis and internal proliferation in central and sublobular veins with secondary congestion and hepatocytic atrophy are all seen on histologic sections of such livers [37].

Radionuclide hepatic scintigrams are also useful for assessing regrowth of liver following partial hepatectomy. Penetrating hepatic wounds such as are caused by bullets, knives, or needle biopsies may also produce focal defects on liver scans.

6.3.2 Spleen

The spleen is also visualized along with the liver following administration of ^{99m}Tc-sulfur colloid. The reticuloendothelial component of the spleen normally accumulates up to 10% of an administered dose of sulfur colloid (85% goes to the liver, 5% to bone marrow) which accounts for its visualization during "liver" scanning. Significant splenic trauma usually appears on a scan as either a complete disruption of the organ's integrity or a "wedge-shaped" defect within its substance. A complete traumatic separation of a portion of the spleen may occur, resulting in two functioning components separated by a variable distance. Splenic contusion or subcapsular hematomas may have a variable appearance by comparison with the lacerated spleen. Gilday and Alderson [23] reviewed the accuracy of scanning in detecting splenic trauma in 136 patients. Of the studies, 1.5% were falsely negative compared with a false positive rate of 7.5%. Some of the false positive studies could have been errors in interpretation due to rib impressions on the spleen or incorrect assessment of the sometimes normal separation of the spleen and left lobe of the liver. These misinterpretations can be minimized by obtaining multiple views; these include anterior, posterior, left anterior oblique, and left lateral.

For several years there has been a growing realization that splenectomy in children, for whatever reason, may be followed by fulminating sepsis and death. Such a catastrophe is probably the result of an adversely affected immune response following surgery [21]. This has prompted many clinicians not to operate on patients with splenic traum or, when operation is unavoidable, to do only a partial

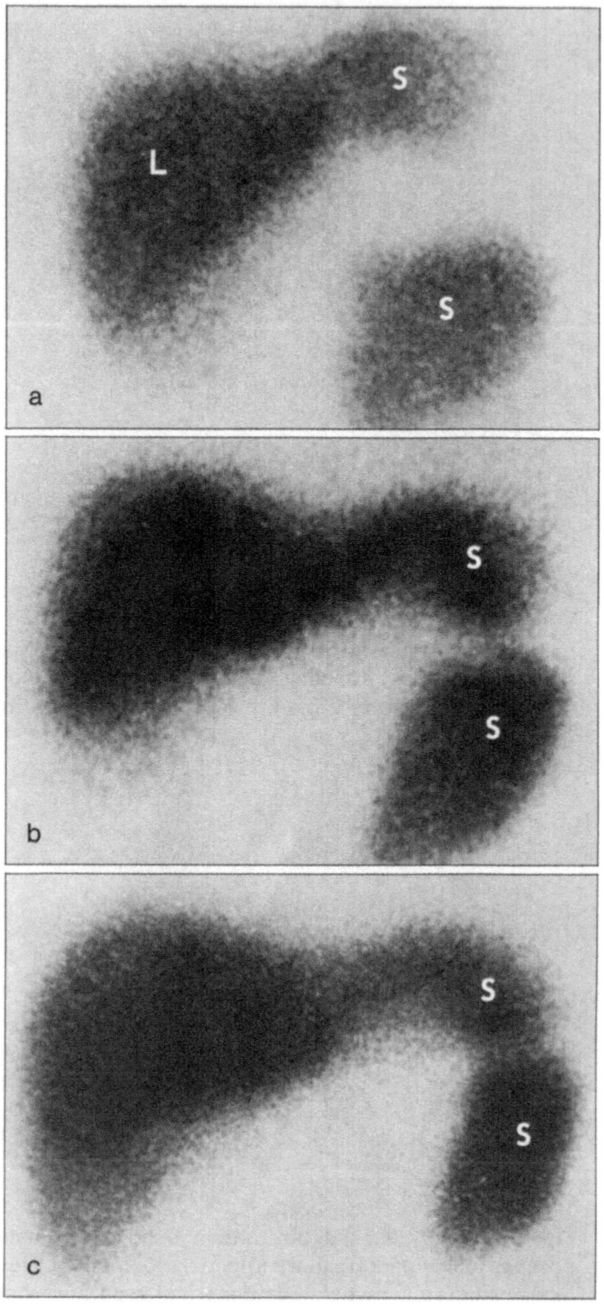

Fig. 6.19 a–c. An 8-year-old boy with fractured spleen had (**a**) radiocolloid scintigraphy showing the parenchymal disruption (*L*, liver; *S*, spleen). This and subsequent views are left anterior oblique projections. Repeat studies 1 (**b**) and 3 (**c**) month later showed a gradual healing of the defect. Surgery was not performed

splenectomy. Consequently splenic scanning has assumed a new role: besides detecting a laceration, serial scans are now advocated for determining the rate of splenic healing [18, 21] (Fig. 6.19). Fisher et al. [18] have shown that scintigraphic defects can persist for long periods of time in asymptomatic patients although the defects are usually smaller than the original disruption. However, a defect of increasing size must be viewed with suspicion as representing either a pseudocyst or recurrent bleeding within a hematoma.

6.3.3 Pancreas

Blunt abdominal trauma may injure the pancreas which is easy to understand considering the position of this soft tissue organ draped across the vertebral spine. It is not practicable to perform ^{75}Se-selenomethionine pancreatic scans on an emergency basis. However, ultrasonography is a rapid and feasible means of directly assessing pancreatic size and structure.

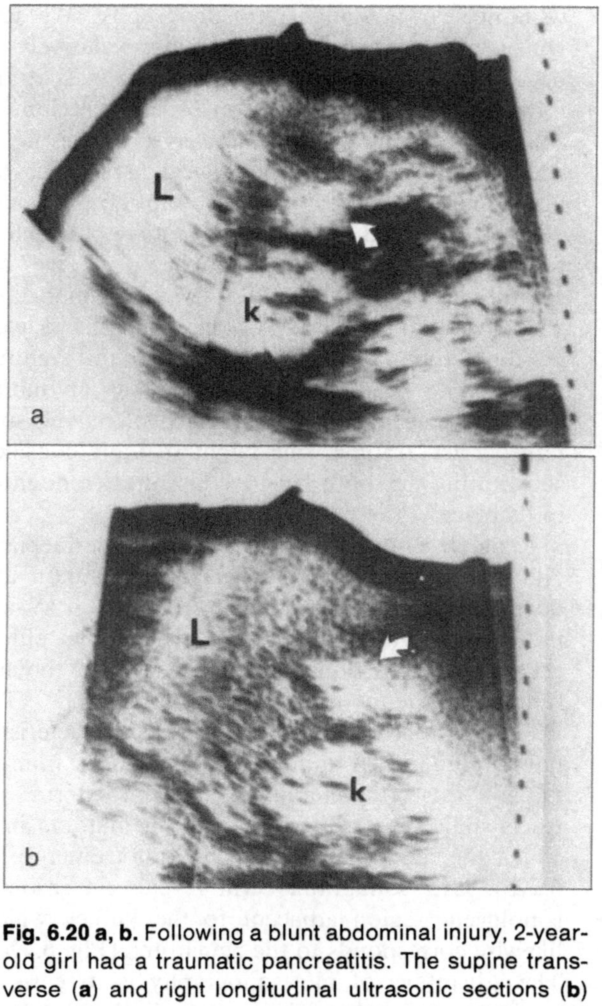

Fig. 6.20 a, b. Following a blunt abdominal injury, 2-year-old girl had a traumatic pancreatitis. The supine transverse (**a**) and right longitudinal ultrasonic sections (**b**) showed an enlarged pancreas with reduced, but still remaining, internal echoes (*arrows*). Liver (*L*) and kidney (*K*) were normal

The head of the pancreas is anterior to the inferior vena cava while its body and tail cross the midline to be positioned anterior to the aorta. The extrahepatic portion of the portal vein is superior to the pancreatic head while the splenic vein is behind the neck and body. The superior mesenteric artery and vein are anterior to the pancreas. Frequently the liver is the only structure interposed between the abdominal wall and the pancreas.

Acute pancreatitis (whatever the cause) is ultrasonically identified by a swelling of the organ associated with diminished internal echoes (Fig. 6.20). Serial examinations are quite useful in following the course of pancreatitis since a return of a normal echo pattern and a more distinct organ outline are characteristic of a resolving acute inflammatory process. Chronic, inactive pancreatitis, however, may be ultrasonically indistinguishable from a normal pancreas.

Pseudocyst formation is a recognized complication of pancreatitis. Ultrasonography is the imaging test of choice for identifying such a process and following its course (Fig. 6.21). These cysts may vary in size from tiny to huge; they appear as sonolucent, transonic midepigastric masses.

6.4 Renal

Renal injuries frequently occur after thoracoabdominal trauma although such abnormalities are less prevalent than splenic or liver damage. A significant number of patients with renal trauma have simultaneously sustained a splenic injury; the association of renal with hepatic lacerations is less common [6]. A variety of methods are available for studying children suspected of having sustained renal trauma [6, 48]. Ultrasonography is probably the easiest and quickest imaging test available and is useful in detecting hematomas, urinomas, and so on. However, echography cannot assess renal function. It is in this latter area that nuclear medicine makes its greatest contribution – assessment of function.

A variety of radiopharmaceuticals are available for scintigraphic imaging of the kidneys. They can be grouped into two categories: (1) ^{131}I-orthoiodohippurate, and (2) ^{99m}Tc-labeled agents such as DTPA. ^{131}I-orthoiodohippurate is generally considered the most sensitive radionuclide test available for assessing renal tubular function. Computer

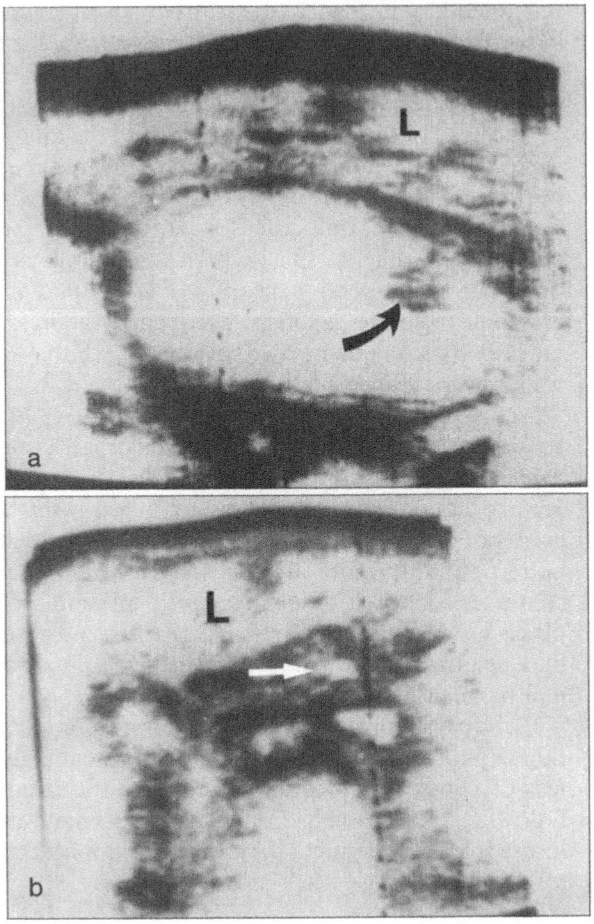

Fig. 6.21 a, b. A 15-year-old boy was involved in motorcycle accident at which time one handlebar was forcefully driven into his upper, mid abdomen. He had a pancreatic contusion with traumatic pancreatitis which developed into a large pseudocyst (**a**, supine transverse section). A Penrose drain was placed (*arrow* in **a** points to drain) but the cyst was slow to decompress. Eventually, cyst contents drained and a repeat scan (**b**, same orientation) showed only a 1 × 2 cm cyst remaining (*arrow*) compared with the original 6 × 11 cm. Transition between an edematous, enlarged pancreas and early pseudocyst formation may be difficult to detect without serial studies

analysis of the renal tubular clearance of hippurate can result in an accurate estimation of effective renal plasma flow [49]. Such quantitative information is vital when evaluating serial studies that are being performed to determine return of function. Sequential renal images can also be obtained at the same time when using hippurate. ^{99m}Tc-DTPA is used to perform renal scintiangiography and static imaging; computer analysis of its clearance allows for an estimation of the glomerular filtration rate [5]. The images resulting from use of DTPA are generally superior to those obtained by using hippurate. However, the determination of glomerular filtration rate is more difficult than estimation of effective renal plasma flow since multiple blood samples are required, which is not the case with the hippurate study.

As each institution must come to grips with the variety of imaging techniques available and ultimately make a choice based on efficiency in handling traumatized patients, the following procedural sequence has evolved at Childrens Hospital of Los Angeles. ^{131}I-orthoiodohippurate renography is performed as the initial examination; this produces serial 4-min renal scintiphotos plus an estimation of effective renal plasma flow for each kidney. If the 24-min study is normal, no further examination is recommended. If a hippurate test is abnormal, two additional studies may be performed: ultrasonography and/or ^{99m}Tc-DTPA scintigraphy. Ultrasonography is an ideal complementary test to perform with nuclear imaging: ultrasonography is a test which yields information pertaining exclusively to organ morphology, while nuclear medicine tests are focused on organ function. Consequently, regions of abnormality on hippurate scans can be easily evaluated for accompanying morphological disturbances by ultrasonography. ^{99m}Tc-DTPA scintigraphy may also be performed, the major advantage of which is the ability to do scintiangiography. This gives an overall idea of renal blood flow which is important when evaluating an injured kidney that has little or no renal tubular function. Although intravenous urography is commonly performed as an initial screening test in patients suspected of having sustained renal trauma, one might strongly consider substituting the more sensitive hippurate renogram in its place.

Renal laceration with a secondary perinephric and retroperitoneal hematoma is a common abnormality following renal trauma. ^{131}I-orthoiodohippurate renography will show either generalized or regionally diminished renal tubular function in the involved kidney (Fig. 6.22a). ^{99m}Tc-DTPA scintigraphy often reveals a characteristic halo of diminished radioactivity around the injured kidney; this circumferentially diminished ring of tracer activity corresponds to the hematoma into which the radiopharmaceutical cannot enter (Fig. 6.22b). Ultrasonography will reveal a transonic, sonolucent region adjacent to the kidney which likewise corresponds to the hematoma (Fig. 6.22c). The advantage of ultrasonography is its ease of performance, lack of ionizing radiation, and its ability to determine accurately the dimensions of a lesion; all three are especially important in injured

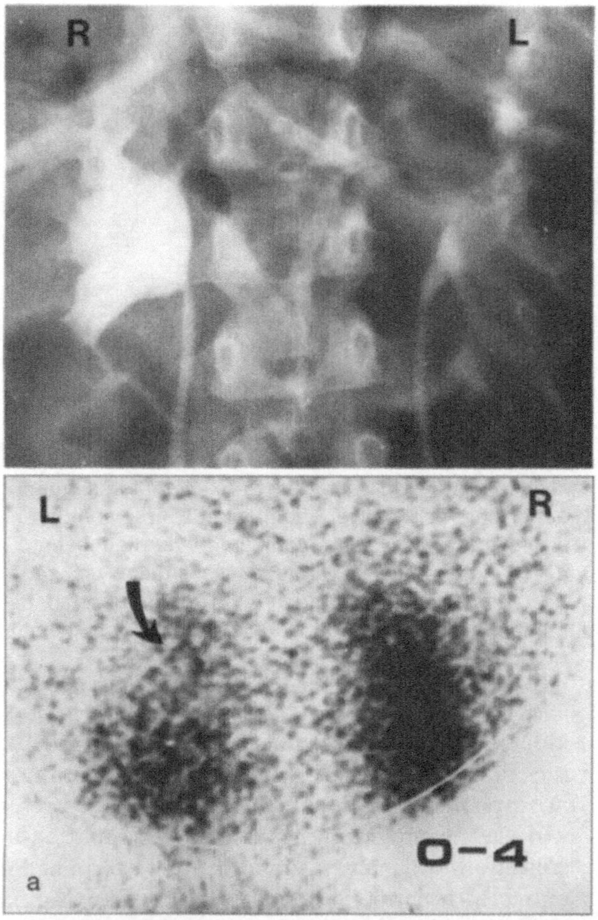

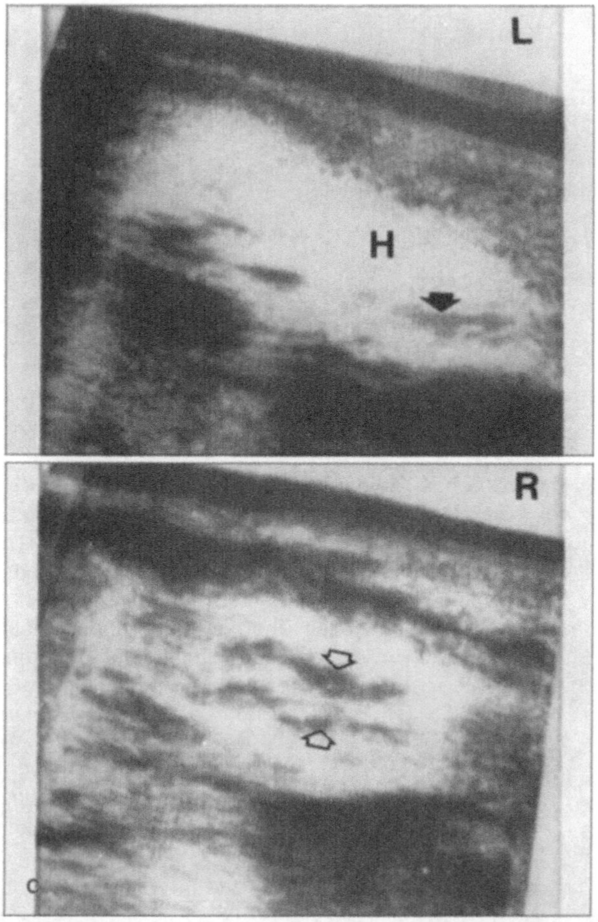

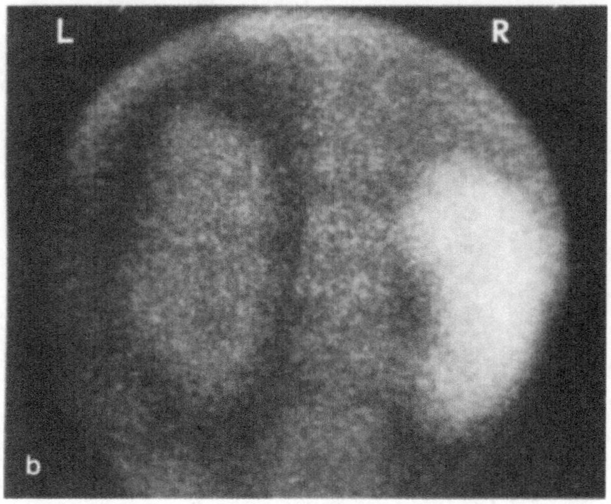

Fig. 6.22 a–c. A $2^1/_2$-year-old girl was hit by a car. An intravenous pyelogram showed reduced renal function on the left while an ^{131}I-orthoiodohippurate renogram (posterior view) (**a**) revealed the left upper pole (*arrow*) to have less function than the lower pole; the right kidney functioned normally. Numbers on renogram indicate time in minutes following tracer injection during which time the scintiphoto was exposed. A perirenal hematoma or abscess (**b**, different patient) will show a tracer-free "halo" around the poorly functioning kidney (^{99m}Tc-DTPA). Ultrasonography (**c**, same patient as in **a**; prone longitudinal sections of left and right kidneys) showed an echo-free area posterior to the left kidney which was due to a hematoma (*H*) which displaced the central, linear pelvic echoes anteriorly (*clossed arrow*). The right kidney was normal; the slight separation of the central echoes (*open arrows*) was due to a mild ureteropelvic junction obstruction

children which often accounts for its use as a follow-up procedure.

Renal contusion without hematoma formation is shown in Fig. 6.23. This child's intravenous urogram showed a region of diminished function which was well identified on the hippurate renogram. At that point a hematoma was considered. Ultrasonography was normal, however; this finding eliminated a hematoma from practical consideration and lead the diagnosis toward a contusion.

Renal surgery may also be associated with unforeseen complications. The child shown in Fig. 6.24 had a renal transplantation and soon thereafter had an episode of fever, chills, and tenderness near the

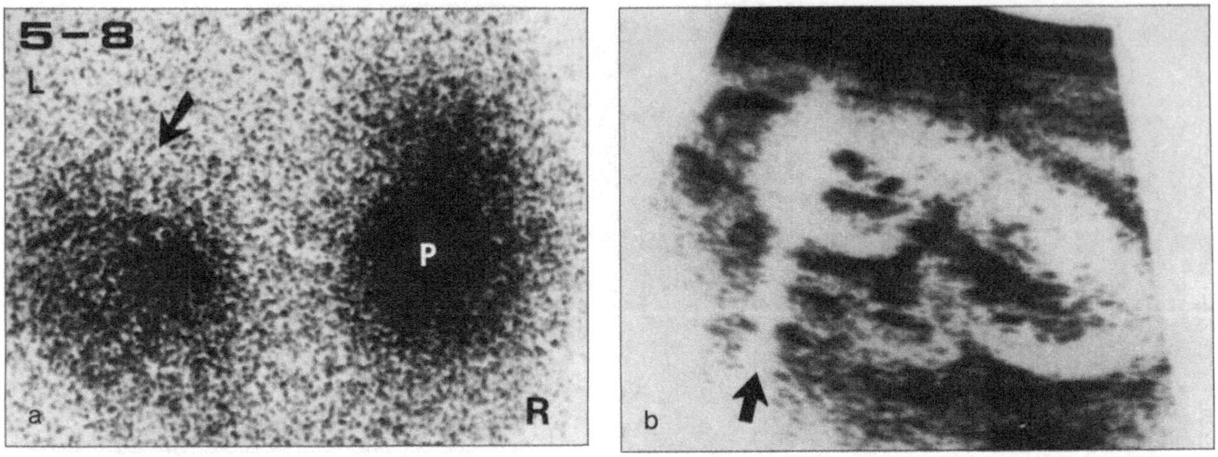

Fig. 6.23 a, b. A 15-year-old girl fell out of a tree fracturing her spleen and injuring her left kidney. A hippurate renogram (**a**) showed poor function of left upper pole. The effective renal plasma flow was estimated (by method of Schlegel and Hamway [49]) to be 373 ml/min on the right and 193 ml/min on the left. There was prominence of the right renal pelvis (*P*). **b** Prone longitudinal ultrasonic sections failed to reveal a frank hematoma although upper pole echoes were somewhat sparse compared to the lower pole. A renal contusion was diagnosed. The *arrow* in **b** points to an acoustic shadow caused by overlying rib and should not be misinterpreted as a hematoma when the sonolucent stripe crosses the superior pole

kidney. Two major circumstances were considered: rejection versus abscess formation. Hippurate renography showed adequate function to be present while ultrasonography revealed a perinephric fluid collection which was subsequently determined to represent a perinephric abscess. Not all extrarenal fluid collections in transplanted patients need represent abscesses, however. Hematomas, urinomas, or lymphoceles (the latter shown in Fig. 6.25) may also be detected by ultrasonography as transonic, sonolucent fluid masses.

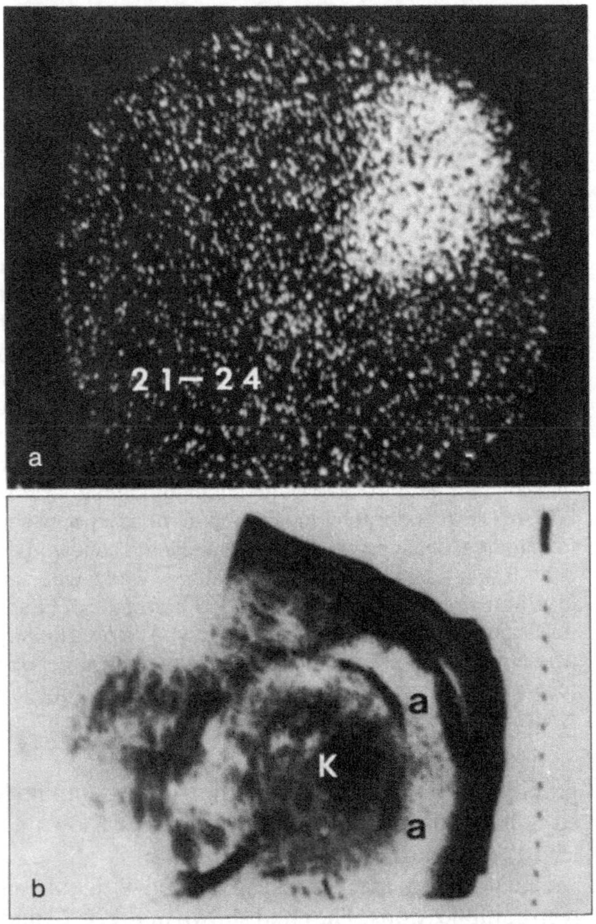

◁

Fig. 6.24 a, b. A 4-year-old boy with a renal transplant had a painful kidney region 2 weeks after surgery. A hippurate renogram (**a**) showed an adequate effective renal plasma flow (72 ml/min) which had steadily improved since surgery (normal value for both kidneys in person of this size is 237 ml/min). Supine transverse ultrasonography (**b**) revealed a perinephric fluid collection around the kidney (*K*) which corresponded to an abscess (*a*). 300 ml pus was subsequently drained at surgery

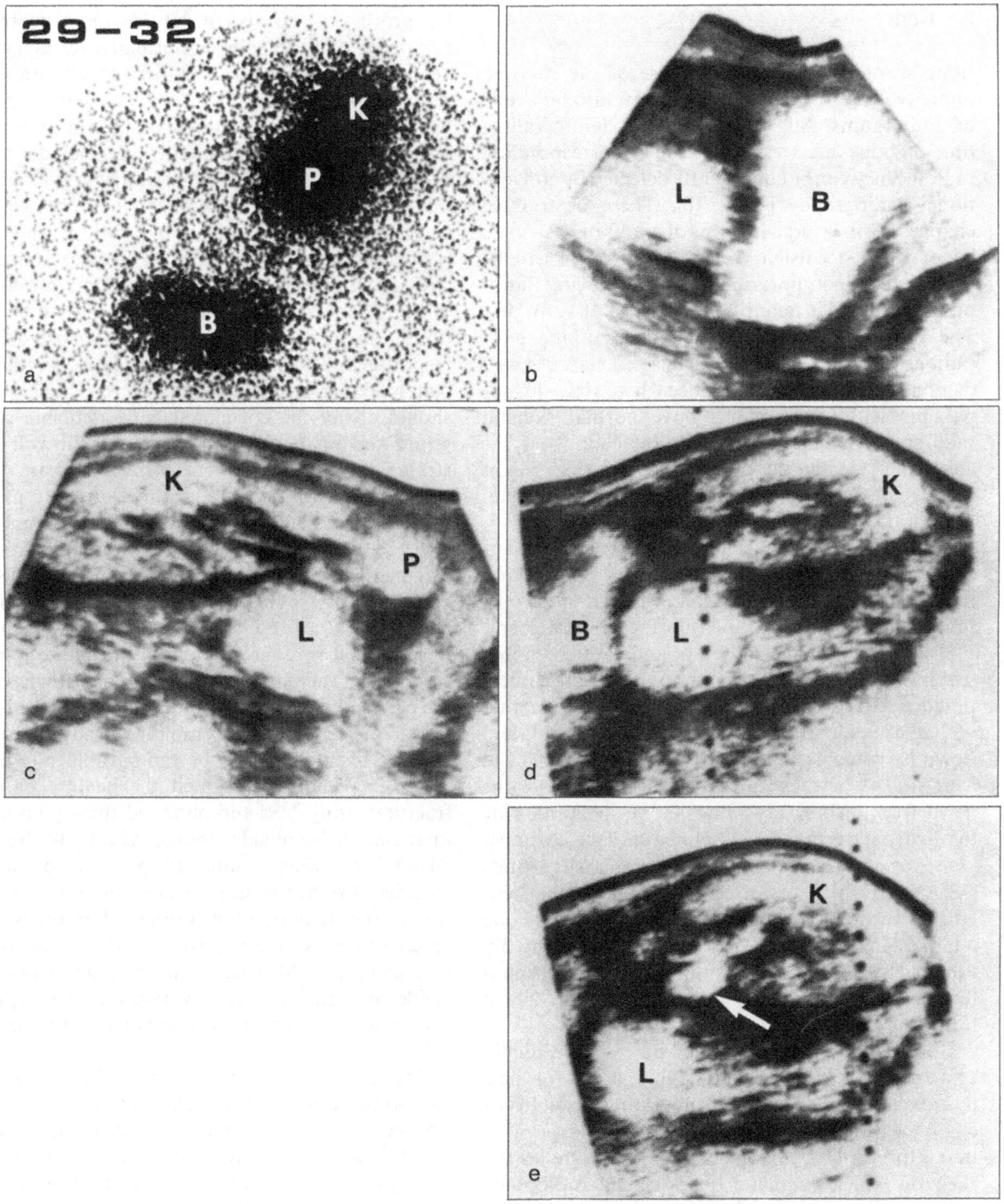

Fig. 6.25 a–e. A 19-year-old male with a renal transplant had a hippurate renogram (**a**) during which an effective renal plasma flow of 203 ml/min was computed (normal for a person of this body size having both kidneys is 565 ml/min). The renal pelvis (*P*) was prominent and the drainage from the kidney (*K*) to bladder (*B*) was slow. Ultrasonography revealed a fluid-filled cyst interposed between kidney and bladder. The cyst was a lymphocele, often formed by weeping lymphatics from the donor kidney or recipient site. **b, c** Supine, longitudinal sections obtained medially and laterally, respectively; **d, e** supine transverse sections obtained cranially and caudally, respectively. The kidney (*K*), bladder (*B*), and lymphocele (*L*) were well seen. The renal pelvis (*P, arrow*) was dilated, which correlated with the renogram

6.5 Bone

Bone scanning developed because of the need to improve upon the sensitivity of conventional skeletal radiograms. Approximately 50% demineralization of bone must occur before a corresponding radiolucency can be consistently detected by conventional radiography [4, 8, 16]. These destructive changes are measured in terms of grams of destroyed bone, yet a coexistent reparative process can be identified by incorporation of a bone-seeking radiopharmaceutical in quantities as small as 10^{-13} g [19]. The increased sensitivity of bone scanning over radiography in detecting skeletal metastases is well demonstrated in clinical practice where 10%–40% of patients with such lesions have normal skeletal radiograms at the time a radionuclide study is abnormal [15]. On the other hand, less than 5% of bone scans are normal at a time when skeletal radiograms reveal localized abnormalities.

Several radiopharmaceuticals have been advocated in the past as clinically suitable bone-seeking radiopharmaceuticals including: calcium 47, strontium 85, strontium 87m, and fluorine 18. At present, ^{99m}Tc-phosphate labeled compounds are the bone-seeking agents most commonly used in clinical practice. All of these radiopharmaceuticals interact with hydroxyapatite $[Ca_{10}(PO_4)_6(OH_2]$ crystals laid down by osteoblasts in newly forming bone. ^{47}Ca, ^{85}Sr, and ^{87m}Sr substitute for stable calcium in the newly forming bone crystal while ^{18}F substitutes for the hydroxyl group. The technetium-labeled phosphates appear to act through the phosphorus groups [32]. Nearly 50% of an administered technetium-labeled phosphate complex is deposited within bone 3 h after injection while much of the rest is rapidly excreted by the kidneys. Scanning with the phosphate compounds is usually performed within 2–4 h following their administration.

Bone is not a static organ but is continually undergoing remolding and laying down of new hydroxyapatite crystals. Proliferating osteoblasts cause the hydroxyapatite crystals to be incorporated into a preformed osteoid matrix. Since the entire skeleton will accumulate bone-seeking radiopharmaceuticals to various degrees, a subsequent scan will reflect regional versus generalized osteoblastic activity. Bone vascularity is also a governing factor in determining radionuclide uptake. Regions with poor blood flow have less uptake than would be expected despite the presence of a lesion that would otherwise result in increased accumulation [50].

Destructive bone lesions (e. g., fractures, infections, or tumors) often appear osteolytic on radiograms but in the vast majority of cases an osteoblastic process is coexistent. It is· this osteoblastic response, and not the abnormality itself, which accounts for the localized tracer accumulation. On rare occasions bone may be affected by a purely destructive process which elicits little if any osteoblastic response. Such conditions include a few neoplasms (e. g., breast, lung, and thyroid carcinoma; reticulum cell sarcomas; neuroblastomas), osteomyelitis (less than 24 h in duration), and acute bone infarctions (e. g., sickle cell disease). It must be stressed, however, that the overwhelming numbers of bony abnormalities (including the listed "exceptions" on many occasions) evoke an osteoblastic response and subsequently actively accumulate a bone-seeking agent. Furthermore, bone scans should always be correlated with available radiograms and a patient's clinical history; this will often straighten out an otherwise perplexing scan.

Patients with known fractures are not usually studied by skeletal scintigraphy unless a complication occurs such as nonosseous union of the fracture fragments, delayed union, avascular necrosis, or osteomyelitis. Cellular repair at a fracture site starts within 24–48 h following injury [43, 54]. At first, a fibrocallus forms across the fracture site to join the fragments. Thereafter, cartilage is laid down within the callus and eventually undergoes transformation into bone. Following remolding and repair the fracture eventually may be radiographically undetectable. Wendeberg studied the healing of tibial fractures using ^{85}Sr and observed three phases: (1) increased radionuclide uptake within the fracture 24–48 h following trauma; (2) peak activity at 6–8 months; (3) accentuated tracer uptake within a fracture could persist for as long as 9 years. Nonosseous union is characterized by decreased radionuclide uptake [51] whereas delayed union [43] or a viable bone graft [1, 51] may have increased uptake. Avascular necrosis has decreased tracer localization [43].

The child in Fig. 6.26 had multiple fractures following an automobile accident. The bone scan was performed to detect any additional fractures which might not have been detected by skeletal radiography. The multiple sites of increased tracer uptake shown in the illustration corresponded to the fractures. A similar pattern of tracer uptake was seen in the child shown in Fig. 6.27. However, this patient was referred from the emergency room for bone scanning because of a tender right leg; the clinical diagnosis was "possible osteomyelitis." The scan revealed multiple, extensive regions of abnormal tracer uptake in many long bones and one rib. This pattern is compatible with chronic child abuse. Following this scan, the entire clinical situation was

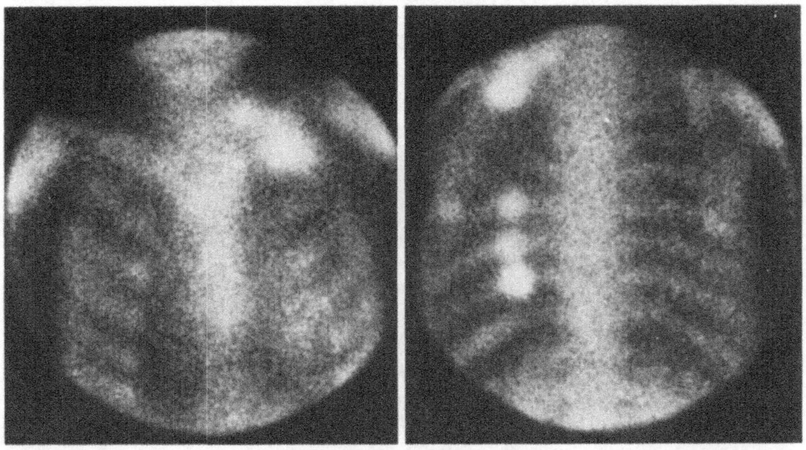

Fig. 6.26. Multiple sites of osteoblastic hyperactivity seen in the ribs and left clavicle of this 8-year-old girl who had many fractures following an automobile accident. Anterior (*left*) and posterior (*right*) ^{99m}Tc-pyrophosphate scintigrams are shown

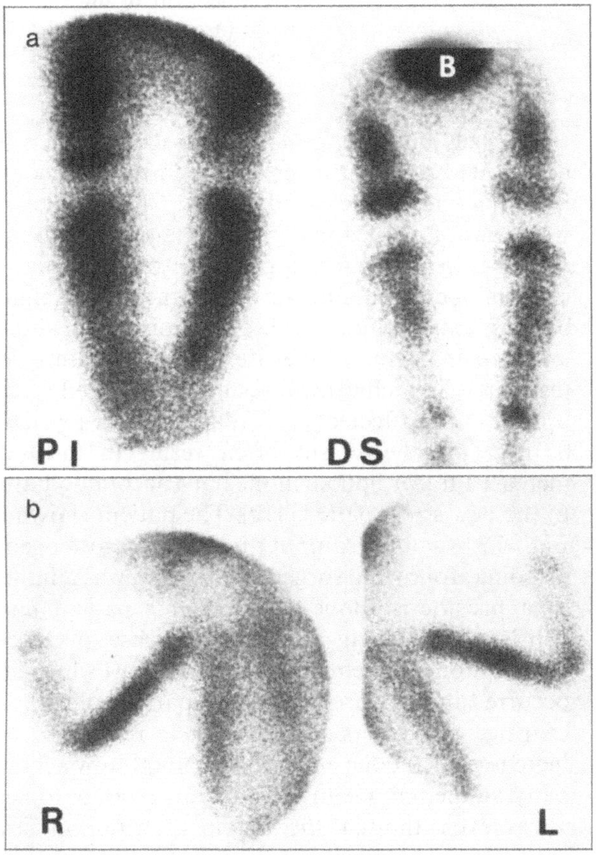

Fig. 6.27 a, b. A 6-month-old girl was referred from the emergency room for a bone scan. Clinical diagnosis was "possible osteomyelitis" of right leg. **a** An immediate postinjection (*PI*) scintigram showed diffuse hyperemia in many regions of both lower extremities which persisted as areas of osteoblastic hyperactivity on the delayed static (*DS*) scintigram. **b** Views of both arms revealed similar features. These changes were ultimately attributed to chronic child abuse

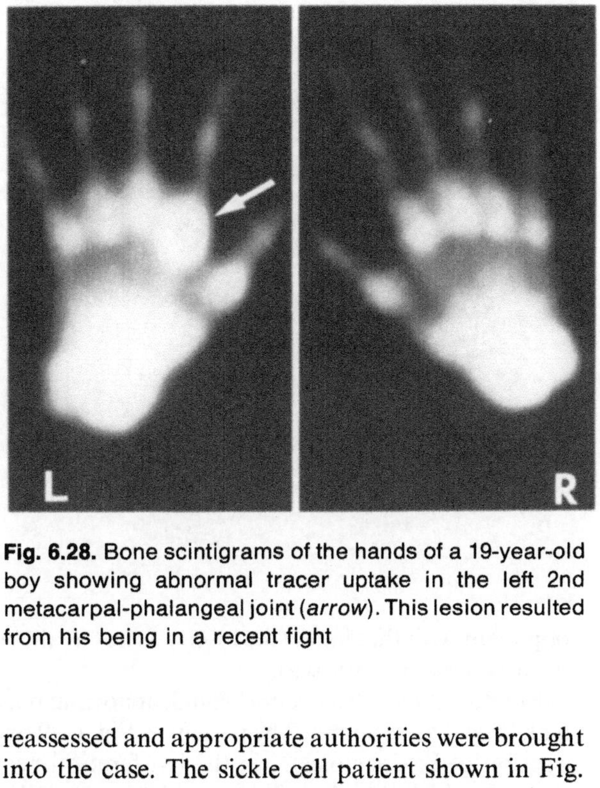

Fig. 6.28. Bone scintigrams of the hands of a 19-year-old boy showing abnormal tracer uptake in the left 2nd metacarpal-phalangeal joint (*arrow*). This lesion resulted from his being in a recent fight

reassessed and appropriate authorities were brought into the case. The sickle cell patient shown in Fig. 6.28 complained of a painful left hand and a bone scan was ordered to assess the possibility of osteomyelitis (which will result in increased tracer uptake) versus bone infarction (which initially may be associated with decreased tracer uptake). The scintigrams showed abnormal radionuclide uptake in the region of the second, left metacarpal-phalangeal joint. The area was tender to palpation and slightly deformed; discreet questioning brought out the previously unknown fact that the patient had just recently been involved in a fight and had struck an

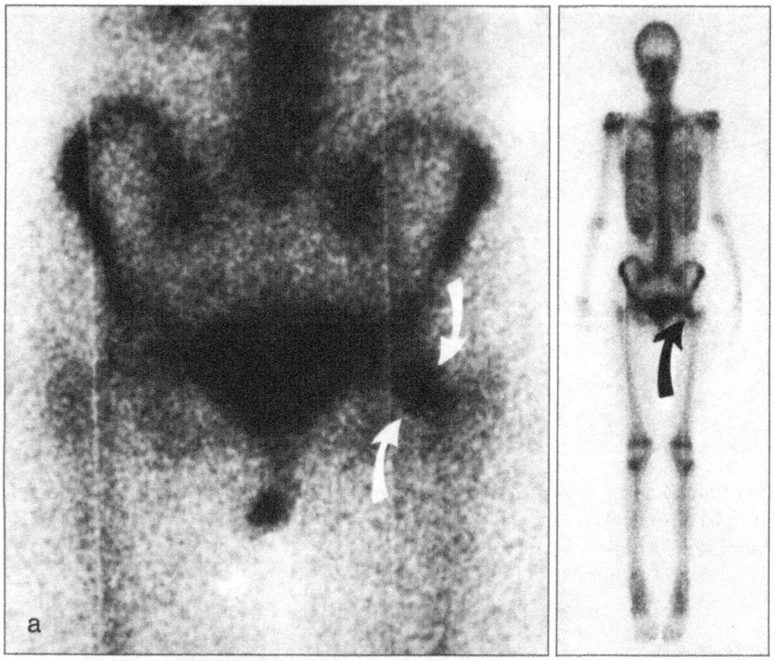

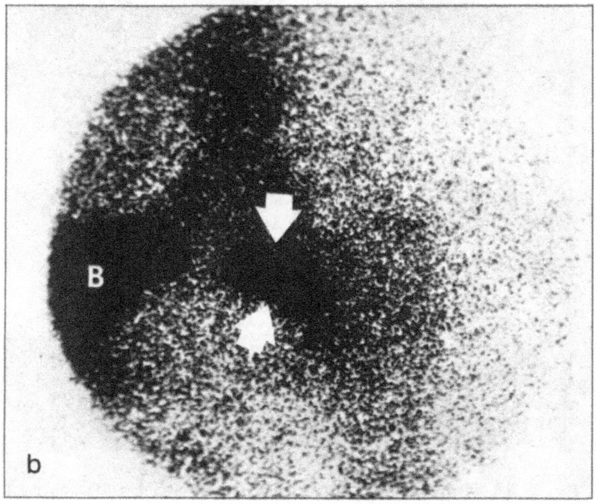

Fig. 6.29 a, b. A 17-year-old girl had a pathologic fracture through a region of histiocytosis X in left femoral neck shown by bone scintigraphy (**a,** total-body view as well as localized pelvic scintiphoto; *arrows point to fracture*). **b** A pinhole collimator view of the hip gave better define in of the femoral neck fracture (*arrows* indicate fracture; *B*, bladder)

opponent with that hand (the loser was not available for a complementary scan).

Fractures may also occur through abnormal bone with little if any trauma. The patient in Fig. 6.29 had a lesion of histiocytosis X in the left femoral neck through which a pathologic fracture occurred. The total-body scan showed the left femoral neck to be the only diseased area (Fig. 6.29a) while a pinhole collimator view of the region gave better anatomic detail (Fig. 6.29b). The girl in Fig. 6.30 had hyperparathyroidism secondary to chronic renal failure. She had several pathologic fractures including one thought to be a "brown tumor" in the left proximal tibia and another through an osteoporotic right ischium. There was no major traumatic event preceding these fractures in either of these cases.

Changes in stress patterns are accompanied by accelerated bone turnover which, in turn, is identified on a scan by increased uptake. Chronic pain or weakness of one leg may result in disproportionate weight-bearing by the opposite extremity; this results in increased uptake along the new weight-bearing axis including sacroiliac joint, hip, ilium, and proximal femur. Likewise, disuse of a painful leg (especially in a child) will result in decreased tracer uptake in the affected side. Adaptation to a weight-bearing prosthesis will often result in diffusely increased tracer uptake in the bone accommodating to the new stress pattern [19]. The patient shown in Fig. 6.31 had an amputation for an osteogenic sarcoma; following surgery, the stump was adapted to a prosthesis. Bone scans of this patient have consistently shown a diffuse increase in tracer uptake along the remaining femoral shaft which has occurred in response to the new pattern of weigthbearing. This uptake is most likely related to the increased metabolic activity and blood flow accompanying the remodeling of bone in response to new stress even though the stump's overall mineral content may be much less than that of the opposite, normal bone. Chronic low grade, repetitive trauma (as in games and athletics) may also produce unusual stress patterns resulting in fractures. The boy in Fig. 6.32 was a healthy athlete who had a "stress fracture" of the tibia. He was a cross-country runner and had not sustained any particular injury.

Bone surgery evokes a reparative osteoblastic response which may be indistinguishable from a

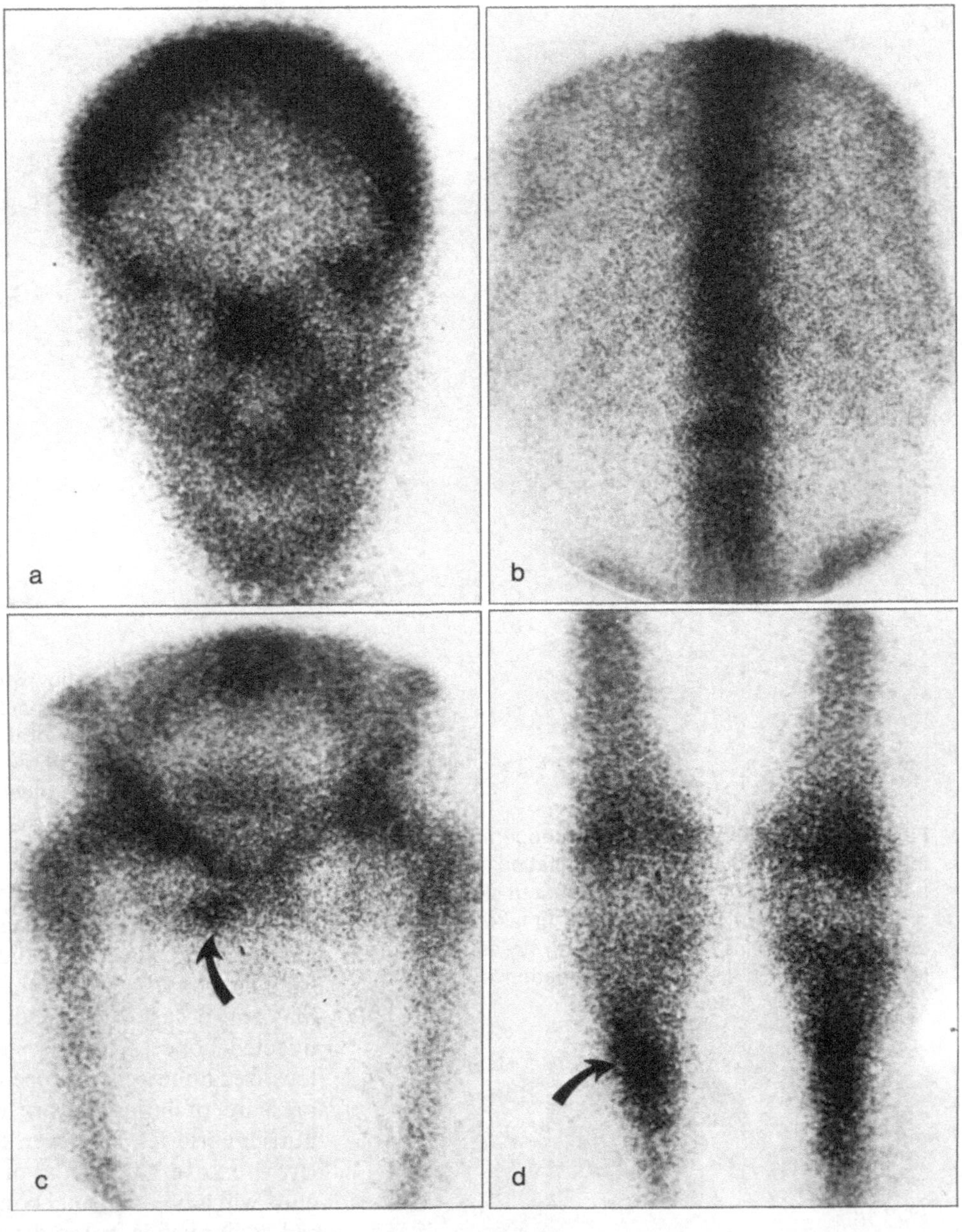

Fig. 6.30 a–d. A 19-year-old girl with chronic renal failure and secondary hyperparathyroidism had bone scintigraphy showing many typical features and complications of that condition. **a** shows typical accentuated calvarial uptake of ^{99m}Tc-pyrophosphate; **b** is a lumbar spine scintiphoto revealing lack of normal renal uptake of radionuclide. **c** An anterior pelvic view shows abnormal uptake in the right ischium (*arrow*) due to fracture through the generally diseased bone. **d** Anterior scintigrams of the knees shows abnormal regions of uptake, especially in the proximal right tibia (*arrow* points to a fracture site extending through a brown tumor) as well as a similar site on the left (pathologic fracture but lacking a localized brown tumor)

pathologic process (Fig. 6.33). Removal of large segments of bone will leave a gap in the normal osseous continuum on immediate postoperative studies (Fig. 6.34). Rib retraction following thoracotomy and surgical scars themselves not uncommonly account for unusual patterns of tracer uptake.

Osteomyelitis may be identified on bone scans as a region of increased tracer uptake even when skeletal radiograms are normal. Localized hyperemia will be identified if a scintigram of the abnormal area is obtained immediately following tracer administration (during which time a "blood pool" effect is dominant). However, such hyperemia may also

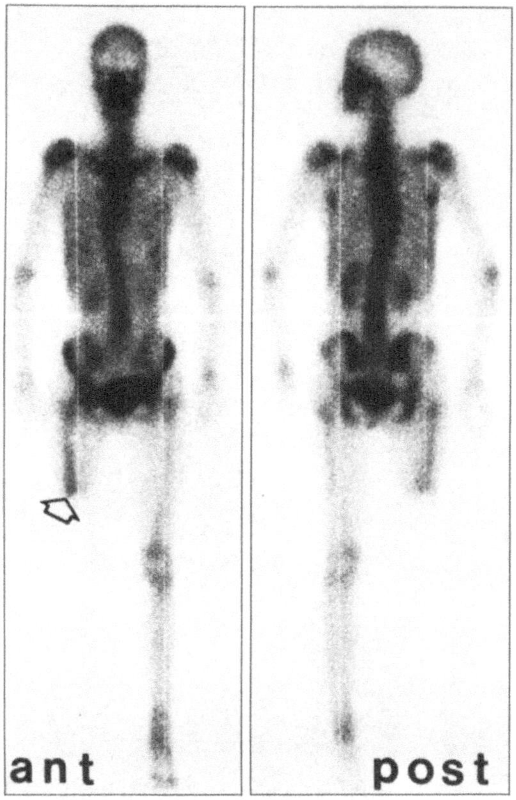

Fig. 6.31. A 17-year-old girl with a osteogenic sarcoma of the right distal femur had an amputation, a prosthesis being fitted to the stump. Many repeated skeletal scintigrams have shown increased tracer uptake in the stump due to patterns of new weight-bearing stress. There is no tumor recurrence. Notice also the patient's scoliosis

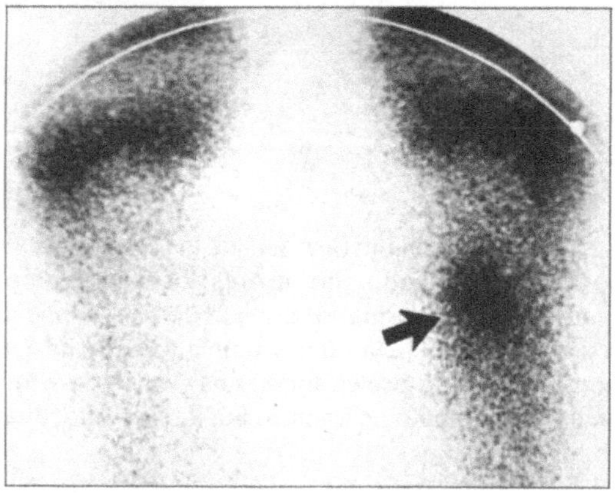

Fig. 6.32. A healthy 16-year-old boy, a cross-country runner, sustained a stress fracture of the proximal tibia (*arrow*). There was no particular trauma preceding the fracture

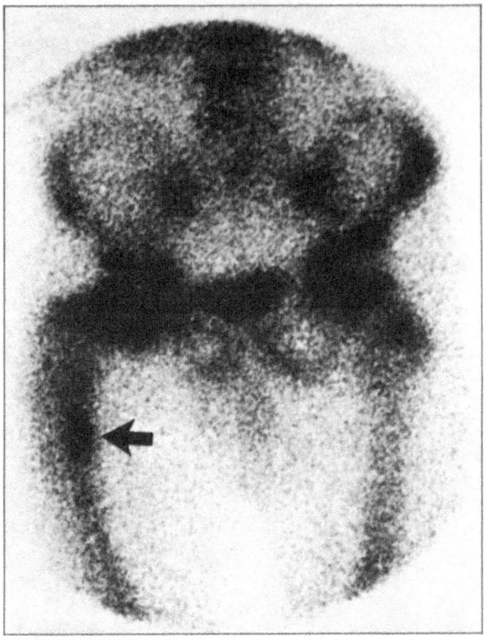

Fig. 6.33. A 6-year-old boy with Hodgkin's disease had orthopedic surgery for right-sided Legg-Perthes disease. Postoperative bone scintigram showed regional osteoblastic activity in the proximal right femoral shaft corresponding to a side of operative intervention, a finding not to be confused with neoplasm

occur with Ewing's sarcoma and osteogenic sarcoma [42], as well as fractures. Although bone scans may be abnormal in osteomyelitis as early as 24 h following onset of symptoms, scans obtained sooner may, on occasion, show diminished uptake in the infected bone [27]. This situation is attributed to localized bone ischemia occurring secondarily to the pressure of inflammatory debris compressing the nutrient arteries. However, the overwhelming majority (i. e., over 90%–95%) of patients with osteomyelitis will have abnormal bone scans showing increased radionuclide in the diseased region.

Osteomyelitis may follow various forms of trauma, ranging from the heel of a foot being caught in a bicycle chain sprocket (Fig. 6.35) to the results of a parent's enthusiastic piercing of a skin pustule with an unsterile needle (Fig. 6.36). An inflammatory process peculiar to tropical and subtropical zones (as Southern California and Florida) is shown in Fig. 6.37. This child had a puncture wound of the knee caused by running into the tip of a palm thorn. The sharp tip was embedded and broken off in the femur. Several months later the patient complained of a sore knee, and a bone scan showed increased tracer uptake in the joint. A palm-thorn granuloma in the femur was discovered at surgery and was the cause of the chronic arthritis. Palm-thorn granulomas

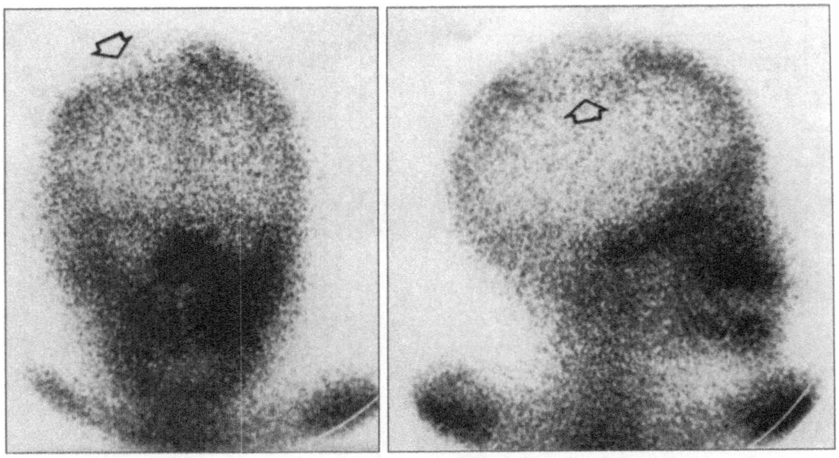

Fig. 6.34. A 10-year-old boy with Ewing's tumor metastatic to the skull had the tumor removed at surgery, with radiation therapy to the area afterwards. A postoperative scan showed a well circumscribed margin of diminished activity corresponding to the operative and radiation site (*arrows*)

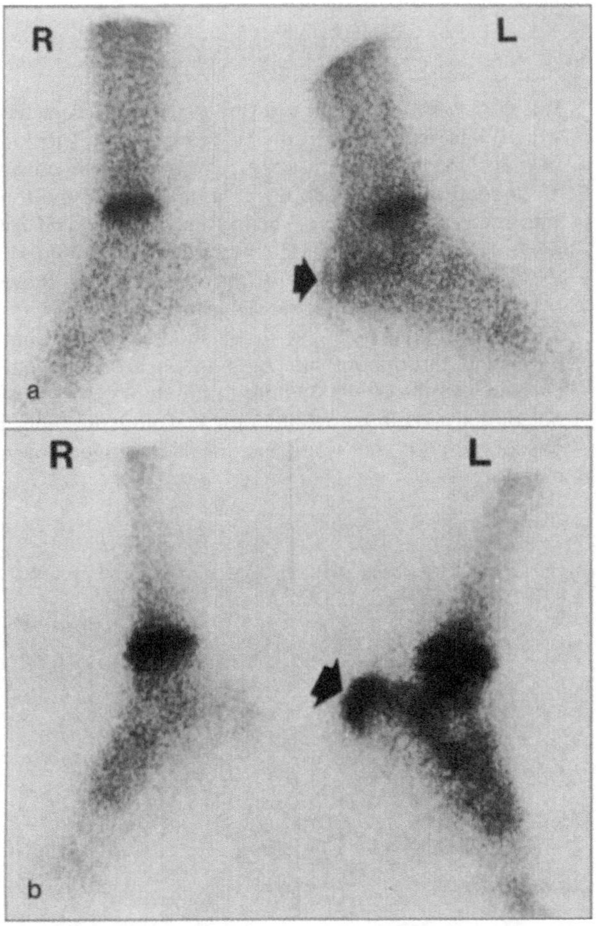

Fig. 6.35 a, b. A 7-year-old girl caught her heel in a bicycle chain sprocket and sustained a considerable soft tissue injury which became infected and ultimately extended to the calcaneus (which was not fractured). An immediate postinjection scintigram of the heels (**a**) showed left calcaneal hyperemia. Delayed views (**b**) showed increased left calcaneal tracer uptake corresponding to reparative bone activity at the site of osteomyelitis (*arrow*)

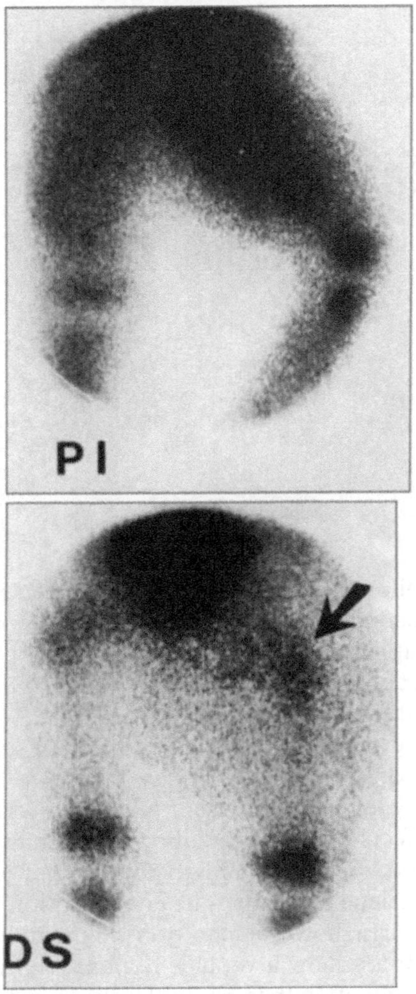

Fig. 6.36. A 1-year-old girl had a draining left-thigh pustule which her father attempted to drain vigorously, using an unsterile pin. Infection extended to involve the proximal left femur. The postinjection scintiphoto (*PI*) showed extreme left-thigh hyperemia while the delayed static view (*DS*) revealed an abnormal osseous localization of radionuclide (*arrow*)

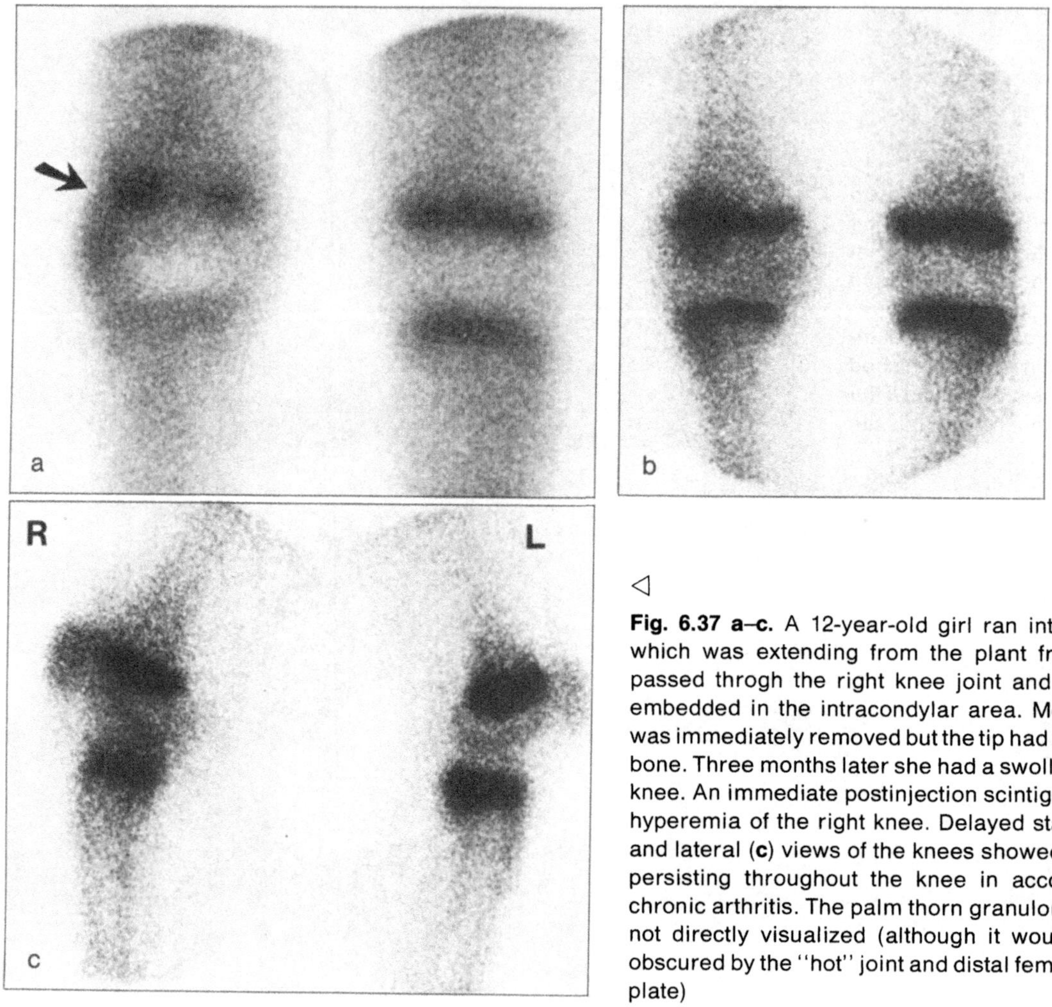

◁

Fig. 6.37 a–c. A 12-year-old girl ran into a palm thorn which was extending from the plant frond. The thorn passed throgh the right knee joint and its tip became embedded in the intracondylar area. Most of the thorn was immediately removed but the tip had broken off in the bone. Three months later she had a swollen, painful right knee. An immediate postinjection scintigram (**a**) showed hyperemia of the right knee. Delayed static anterior (**b**) and lateral (**c**) views of the knees showed diffuse uptake persisting throughout the knee in accordance with a chronic arthritis. The palm thorn granuloma, per se, was not directly visualized (although it would probably be obscured by the "hot" joint and distal femoral epiphyseal plate)

commonly follow such injuries where the tip of the thorn remains in bone. A lytic lesion is commonly seen radiographically.

Healing cephalohematomas may accumulate bone-seeking radiopharmaceuticals (Fig. 6.38). This probably corresponds to the calcific rim often seen with such lesions.

As is true with radiation therapy directed elsewhere, the effects of bone irradiation often include altered cellular metabolic activity, which can be detected by skeletal scanning. The configuration of the abnormal area, however, conforms to the radiation portal. Bones show a variable response during and immediately after therapeutic levels of radia-

▷

Fig. 6.38. Results of an old cephalohematoma seen as well delineated regions of right frontal uptake in an 8 month-old boy. The margins of radionuclide corresponded to the cephalohematoma boundaries

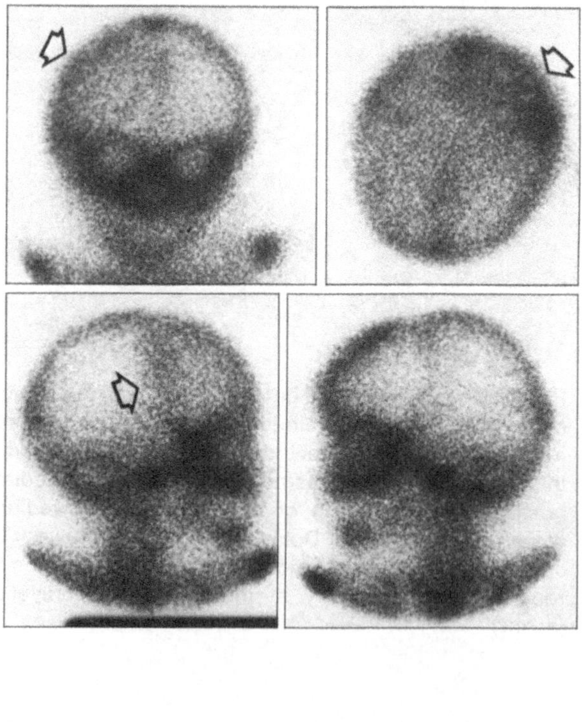

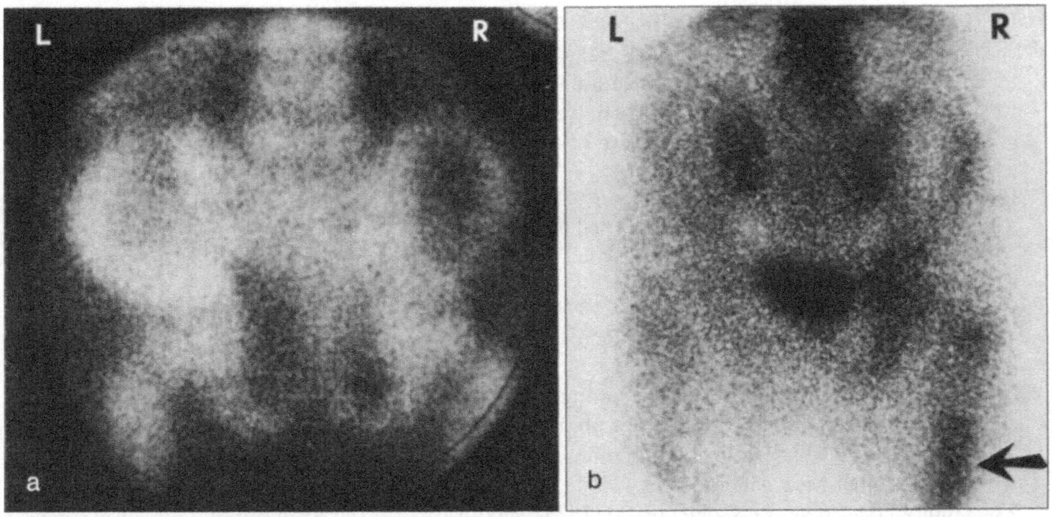

Fig. 6.39 a, b. An 8-year-old boy with a Ewing's tumor of the left ilium (**a**, posterior view) had supervoltage radiation therapy (over 5000 rad) to the left hemipelvis, including acetabulum and proximal femur. A repeat study $2^1/_2$ years later showed diminished tracer localization in the previously irradiated pelvis and proximal left femur (**b**, posterior view); however, a metastatic site in the right femur was evident (*arrow*)

tion, ranging from increased to decreased uptake, but the late effect is invariably one of sharply defined, diminished activity (Fig. 6.39).

6.6 Conclusion

Most standard radionuclide techniques can be utilized in assessing the traumatized child. The nuclear medicine examinations usually require a minimum (if any) patient cooperation and can be performed rapidly and safely in any modern hospital. Ultrasonography is a logical complementary test to include with nuclear imaging. The wide commercial availability of equipment and radiopharmaceuticals, plus increasing interest in pediatric nuclear medicine and ultrasound, will undoubtedly open new vistas of clinical scanning in traumatized children.

References

1. Alexander JM (1976) Radionuclide bone scanning in the diagnosis of lesions of the maxillofacial region. J Oral Surg 34:249–256
2. Apau RL, Saenz R, Siemsen JK (1972) Bloodless lung due to bronchial ostruction. J Nucl Med Allied Sci 13:561–562
3. Apfelbaum RI, Newman BA, Zingesser LH (1973) Dynamics of technetium scanning of subdural hematomas. Radiology 107:571–576
4. Ardran GM (1951) Bone destruction not demonstrable by radiography. Br J Radiol 24:107–109
5. Ash JH, Gilday DL (1977) Quantative analysis of pediatric renal function. 20th Annual Meeting of the Society for Pediatric Radiology, Boston, Massachusetts, September 25 1977
6. Berg BC Jr (1974) Radionuclide studies after urinary-tract injury. Semin Nucl Med 4:371–393
7. Bernard JD, McDonald RA, Verdon TA (1969) Brain scanning for subdural hematoma: Problems in interpretation. J. Nucl Med Allied Sci 10:322
8. Borak J (1942) Relationship between the clinical and roentgenological findings in bone metastases: Surg Gynecol Obstet 75:599–604
9. Buozas DJ, Barrett IR, Mishkin FS (1976) Diagnosis of epidural hematoma by brain scan and perfusion study. J Nucl Med Allied Sci 17:975–976
10. Caroll, CP, Cass KA, Whelan TJ (1973) Wounds of the liver in Vietnam: a critical analysis of 254 cases. Ann Surg 177:385–392
11. Conway JJ, Vollert JM (1972) The accuracy of radionuclide imaging in detecting pediatric dural fluid collection. Radiology 105:77–84
12. Conway JJ, Quinn JL III (1974) Brain imaging in pediatrics. In: (James AE, Wagner HN Jr, Cooke RE (eds) Pediatric nuclear medicine. Saunders, Philadelphia, pp 115–126
13. Cowan RJ, Maynard CD, Lassiter KR (1970) ^{99m}Tc technetium pertechnetate brain scan in detection of subdural hematoma. Study of age of lesion as related to development of a positive scan. J Neurosurg 32:30–34
14. Cowan RJ, Maynard CD (1974) Trauma to the brain and extracranial structures. Semin Nucl Med 4:319–338
15. De Nardo GL, Jacobson SJ, Raventos A (1972) ^{85}Sr bone scan in neoplastic disease. Semin Nucl Med 2:18–30

16. Edelystyn GA, Gillespie PJ, Grebbell FS (1967) The radiological demonstration of osseous metastasis: experimental observations. Clin Radiol 18:158–162
17. Faris IB, Dudley HAF (1973) Closed liver injury: an assessment of prognostic factors. Br J Surg 60:227–230
18. Fischer KC, Eraklis A. Rosello P et al (1978) Scintigraphy in the followup of pediatric splenic trauma treated without surgery. J Nucl Med Allied Sci 19:3–9
19. Fordham EW, Ramachandran PC (1974) Radionuclide imaging in osseous trauma. Semin Nucl Med 4:411–429
20. Gates GF (1974) Radionuclide scanning in cyanotic heart disease. Thomas, Springfield, pp 36–57
21. Gates GF (1978) Sepsis in children following splenectomy. J Nucl Med Allied Sci 19:113–115
22. Gilday DL, Coates G, Goldenber D (1973) Subdural hematoma – what is the role of brain scanning in its diagnosis. J Nucl Med Allied Sci 14:283–287
23. Gilday DL, Alderson PO (1974) Scintigraphic evaluation of liver and spleen injury. Semin Nucl Med 4:357–370
24. Gilday DL, Ash JM, Reilly BJ (1977) Radionuclide skeletal survey for pediatric neoplasms. Radiology 123:399–406
25. Gilson AJ, Gargano FP (1965) Correlation of brain scans and angiography in intracranial trauma. AJR 94:819–827
26. Goldman SM, Freeman LM, Ghossein NA et al (1969) Effects of thoracic irradiation on pulmonary arterial perfusion in man. Radiology 93:289–296
27. Handmaker H, Leonards R (1976) The bone scan in inflammatory osseous disease. Semin Nucl Med 6:95–105
28. Heiser WJ, Quinn JL III, Mollihan WV (1966) The crescent pattern of increased radioactivity in brain scanning. Radiology 87:483–488
29. Hellstrom G (1967) Traumatic liver injuries. In: Popper H, Schaffner F, (eds), Progress in liver disease. Grune & Stratton, New York p 432
30. Hopkins GB, Kristensen KAB (1973) Rapid sequential scintiphotography in the radionuclide detection of subdural hematoma. J Nucl Med Allied Sci 14:288–290
31. Johnson PM, Grossman FM, Atkins HL (1967) Radiation induced hepatic injury: its detection by scintillation scanning. AJR 99:453–462
32. Jones AG, Francis MD, Davis MA (1976) Bone scanning: radionuclide reaction mechanisms. Semin Nucl Med 6:3–18
33. Kassner EG, Solomon NA, Steiner P et al (1976) Persisting perfusion defects after bronchoscopic removal or spontaneous expulson of aspirated foreign objects. Radiology 121:139–142
34. Kerekes ES, Ewing J (1950) Traumatic liver cyst. Radiology 55:861–864
35. Kindling PH, Wilson RF, Walt AJ (1969) Hepatic trauma, with particular reference to blunt injury. J Trauma 9:17–26
36. Kurohara SS, Swensson L, Usselman JA et al (1967) Response and recovery of liver to radiation as determined by photoscans. Radiology 89:129–135
37. Lewin K, Millis RR (1973) Human radiation hepatitis. Arch Pathol Lab Med 96:21–26
38. Lewin W (1964) Cerebrospinal fluid rhinorrhea in nonmissile head injuries. Clin Neurosurg 12:237–252
39. Lin MS (1976) Diagnostic scintigraphic sign in epidural hematoma at the vertex. J Nucl Med Allied Sci 19:972–974
40. McCort JJ (1966) Radiologic examination in blunt abdominal trauma. Saunders, Philadelphia, pp 93–111
41. McKusick KA (1977) The diagnosis of traumatic cerebrospinal fluid rhinorrhea. J Nucl Med Allied Sci 18:1234–1235
42. Magmaes B, Solheim D Controlled over pressure cisternography to localize cerebrospinal fluid rhinorrhea. J Nucl Med Allied Sci 18:109–111
43. Marty R, Denny JD, McKame MR et al (1976) Bone trauma and related benign diseases. Semin Nucl Med 6: 107–120
44. Milstein D, Nusynowitz ML, Lull RJ (1974) Radionuclide diagnosis in chest disease resulting from trauma. Semin Nucl Med 4:339–355
45. Mishkin FS (1975) Central nervous system: brain. In: Handmaker H, Lowenstein JM, (eds) Nuclear medicine in clinical pediatrics Society of Nuclear Medicine, New York, pp 7–22
46. Richie JP, Fonkalstrud EW (1972) Subcapsular hematoma of the liver: non-operative management. Arch Surg 104:781–784
47. Ronai PM (1976) Epilogue on extradural hematoma. J Nucl Med Allied Sci 17:986–987
48. Rosenthall L (1974) Intravenous radionuclide angiography in the diagnosis of trauma. Semin Nucl Med 4:395–409
49. Schlegel JU, Hamway SA (1976) Individual renal plasma flow determinations in 2 minutes. J Urol 116:282–285
50. Siegel BA, Donovan RL, Alderson PO et al (1976) Skeletal uptake of ^{99m}Tc-diphosphonate in relation to local bone blood flow. Radiology 120:121–123
51. Stevenson JS, Bright RW, Dunson GL et al (1974) Technetium – ^{99m} phosphate bone imaging: a method for assessing bone graft healing. Radiology 110:391–394
52. Sugitani Y, Nakama M, Yamaguchi Y et al (1973) Neovascularization and increased uptake of ^{99m}Tc in experimentally produced cerebral hematoma. J Nucl Med Allied Sci 14:912–916
53. Tefft M, Mitus A, Das L et al (1970) Irradiation of the liver in children: review of experience in the acute and chronic phases, and in the intact normal and partially resected. AJR 108:365–385
54. Wendeberg B (1961) Mineral metabolism of fractures of the tibia in man: studies with external counting of Sr^{85}. Acta Orthop Scand [Suppl] 52:1–79
55. Willerson JT (1978) "Hot spot" scanning. Hosp Pract 13:82–88

56. Williams LF, Byrne JJ (1966) Trauma to the liver at Boston City Hospital from 1955 to 1965. Am J Surg 112:368–375
57. Woolf HB (ed) (1975) Websters New Collegiate Dictionary. Merriam, Springfield p 1243
58. Zilkha A, Irwin GAL (1976) The rim sign in epidural hematoma. J Nucl Med Allied Scie 17:977–979
59. Zingesser LH (1971) Scanning in diseases of the subdural space. Semin Nucl Med 1:41–47

7 Pancreatic and Adrenal Trauma

Philip Stanley and John L. Gwinn

7.1 Pancreatic Trauma

About 4% of children with blunt trauma to the abdomen have significant pancreatic injury [13] which is most frequently nonpenetrating. The pancreas is injured most frequently by automobile accidents and falling on bicycle handlebars [11]. Sporting injuries and child abuse are responsible for some cases [5]. The direction of force will determine to a certain degree the type and extent of the pancreatic injury [2, 10]. With the impact concentrated to the right of the spine, the head of the pancreas is crushed, along with possible avulsion of the common bile duct and gastroduodenal artery and also possible laceration of the superiorly placed liver. The duodenum and colon may also be damaged. With midline compression forces, classical compression damage to the pancreas occurs without associated injury. Injuries to the left of the spine can damage the tail of the pancreas and may be associated with splenic laceration.

Numerous classifications have been offered to define the extent and site of pancreatic trauma. The injuries may be classified as contusion, laceration, disruption, and complete transection, although other classifications have been offered [3, 8, 10]. As a result of trauma, there is hemorrhagic necrosis and enzymic exudation with subsequent pancreatic autodigestion [9]. A pseudocyst is a late complication [7, 11].

The symptoms, in the absence of injury to other organs, are typically slow to appear [1]. Upper or generalized abdominal pain appears after a few hours. There may be radiation of pain to the back or shoulders. Nausea and vomiting often occur later. Clinical examination reveals upper abdominal tenderness and guarding sometimes with a mass [9, 11]. The serum amylase is usually elevated [5].

The radiological features are variable. In severe cases, there may be pleural fluid at the bases. Plain abdominal films may show increased density in the left upper abdomen with sentinel loops (localized paralytic ileus of large or small bowel). There may be a colon cutoff sign (Fig. 7.1). There can be localized dilatation of the first and second portions of the duodenum. Increased spacing between the greater curvature of the stomach and adjacent jejunum or transverse colon may be present. If there is considerable retroperitoneal edema and/or hemorrhage, then obliteration of the psoas shadows will occur [14]. Abdominal calcification may be present (Fig. 7.1).

Contrast medium study may be normal initially, but later show a mass effect with forward displacement of the stomach, widening of the duodenal loop, elevation of the antrum, and displacement of the jejunum (Fig. 7.2). In addition to the mass effect, there may be coarsening of the duodenal folds with a "reversed 3" sign of Frostberg [14]. If the mass is in the tail of the pancreas, then there will be medial displacement of the greater curvature of the stomach (Fig. 7.3). A barium enema will show anterior/inferior displacement of the transverse colon. The mass may resolve spontaneously or continue, to become a pseudocyst. This is probably best demonstrated by ultrasound [14]. If there is associated duct damage, then fiber-optic endoscopic pancreatography may be helpful [4] although it is not a standard procedure in children.

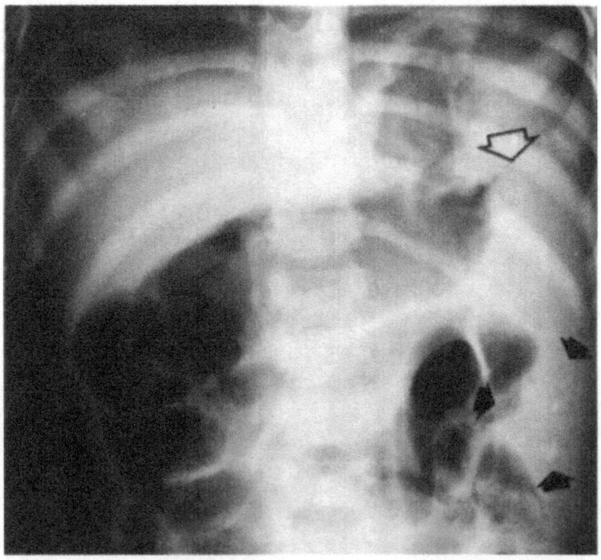

Fig. 7.1. Plain radiograph of the abdomen showing colon "cutoff" at the splenic flexure (*open arrow*). There is abdominal calcification (*solid arrows*)

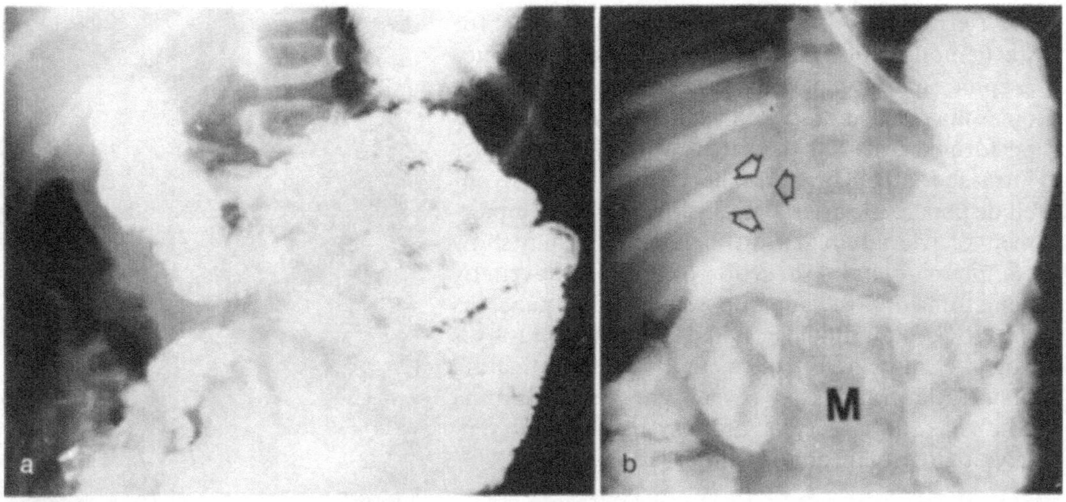

Fig. 7.2 a. Upper GI examination on 15 January showing no mass. **b** Repeat examination 4 days later demonstrating a mass in the region of the body of the pancreas (*M*) with upward displacement of the antrum and lateral displacement of loops of jejunum. There is right adrenal calcification (*open arrows*) due to old adrenal hemorrhage

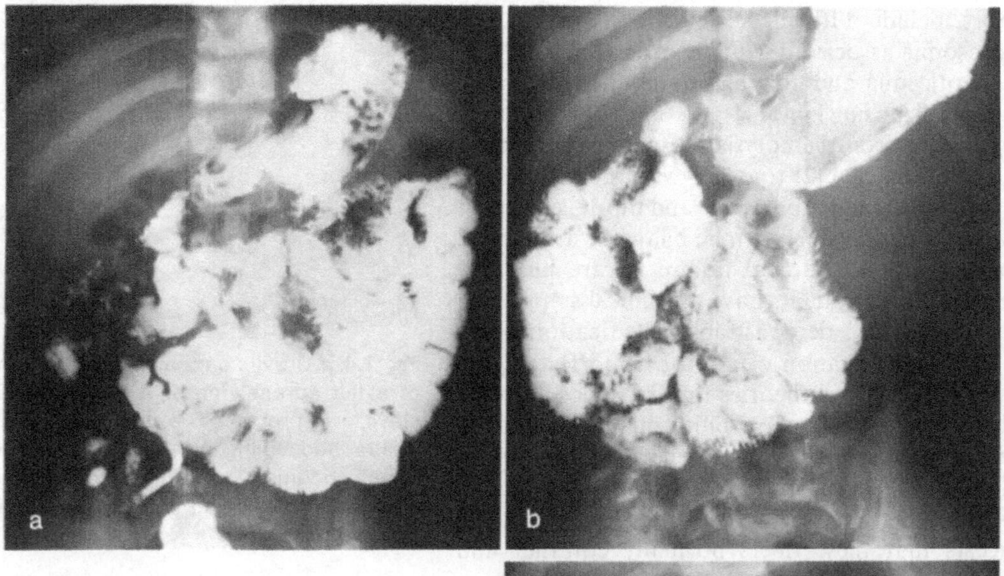

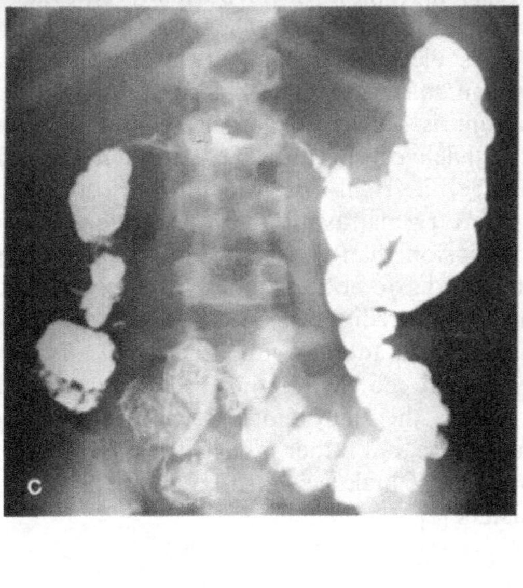

Fig. 7.3 a. Upper GI examination on day of trauma showing no abnormality **b** 5 days later, a mass in the region of the tail of the pancreas has appeared with displacement of the greater curvature of stomach and loops of jejunum. **c** 13 days later, the mass in no longer present

Arteriography is rarely performed primarily for the demonstration of pancreatic injuries but angiographic findings suggestive of trauma to the pancreas may be demonstrated when the examination is performed to assess the extent of damage to other intra-abdominal organs. The vascular changes include pancreatic arterial occlusion and local impairment of arterial circulation [6]. Later films may show compression and obstruction of the splenic vein by hematoma or posttraumatic swelling of the pancreas [6]. However, it should be noted that arteriography is not the most effective method of investigating pancreatic trauma as severe pancreatic trauma confirmed at surgery or autopsy may exhibit very few angiographic abnormalities [12].

7.2 Adrenal Trauma

Neonatal hemorrhagic necrosis of the adrenal is a well recognized clinical entity. The precipitating factors include difficult delivery, fetal anoxia, and macrosomia associated with maternal diabetes [1, 8, 10]. Septicemia and coagulation abnormalities are other predisposing factors [1, 4]. Signs of blood loss, [4] jaundice from hemolysis occurring in a closed space hemorrhage [2] together with an inability of the liver to conjugate bilirubin, and the development of a flank mass, which can be bilateral, are typical clinical features. Adrenal failure is rare but may occur [1]. Some patients have no clinical symptoms, radiographically, demonstrable calcification being the only manifestation of a prior hemorrhage [4].

Of the numerous theories that have been advanced to explain the susceptibility of the neonate to adrenal hemorrhage, the absence of bundles of longitudinal smooth muscle fibers in the neonatal adrenal veins is an attractive one. Heinivaara [5] suggests that these fibers normally contract and narrow the adrenal vein when the venous pressure becomes elevated. Their natural absence in the newborn makes the adrenal more susceptible to transient rises in venous pressure, especially during a difficult delivery. Because of the difference in venous drainage, the right side, which drains directly into the inferior vena cava, is more susceptible to venous hypertension than the left, which is partially protected by anastomotic channels. Most series report a right-sided predilection [1, 4, 6, 9]. In 10% of patients, both adrenals are affected.

Males are more commonly affected than females [1, 4, 6]; this may not be specific to adrenal hemorrhage, but rather reflects the generalized susceptibility of male newborn infants to a variety of disasters [1].

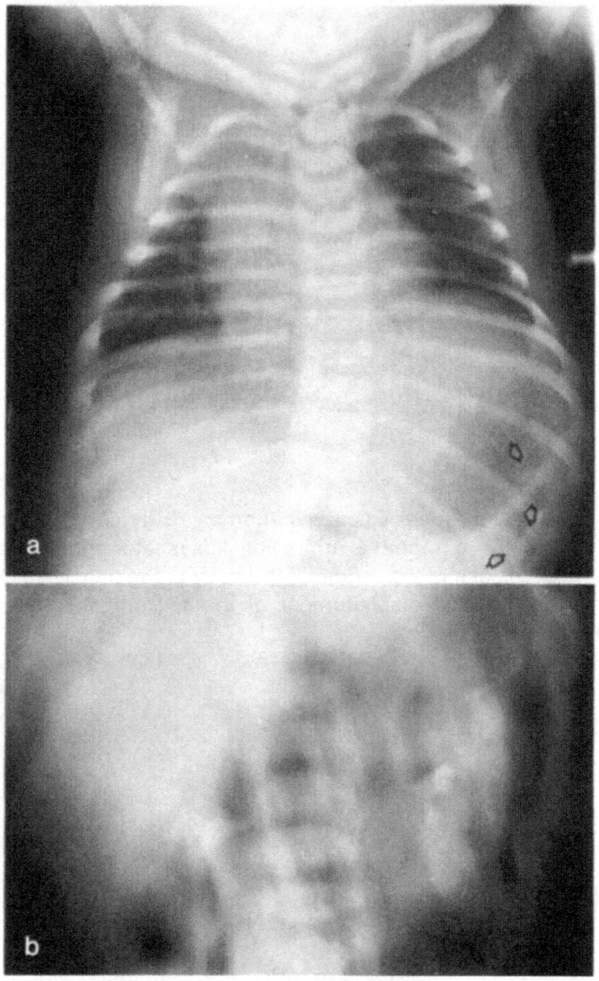

Fig. 7.4. a Curvilinear calcification around the periphery of a left adrenal mass. A healing fracture of the left clavicle is present. The infant, a product of a diabetic mother had a difficult delivery. **b** An AP tomogram of the upper abdomen following injection of contrast demonstrates the calcified adrenal hematoma displacing the left kidney downward

The most useful investigation is an intravenous urogram. On the preliminary film, there may be calcification, which may occur as early as 12 days [11] after the hemorrhage although usually it takes 3–4 weeks [1]. At first, the calcification is curvilinear around the periphery of the mass (Fig. 7.4) but as the hemorrhage is absorbed the calcification shrinks, becoming more dense and nodular and resembling the shape of the gland [1]. The calcification persists for life. Immediately following intravenous injection of contrast, a circumferential rim of adrenal tissue around a radiolucent center may be demonstrated in the total body opacification phase [2, 4]. The upper pole of the kidney is displaced inferiorly and may be rotated laterally (Figs. 7.5, 7.6). The upper pole of

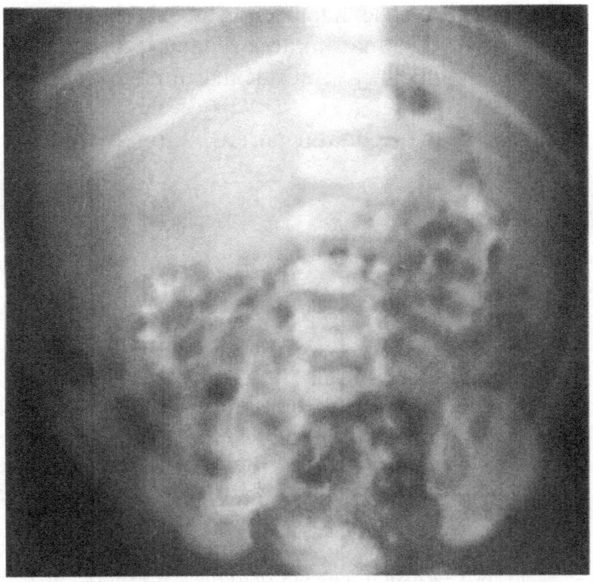

Fig. 7.5. Flatttening of the upper pole of the right kidney by an uncalcified adrenal hematoma

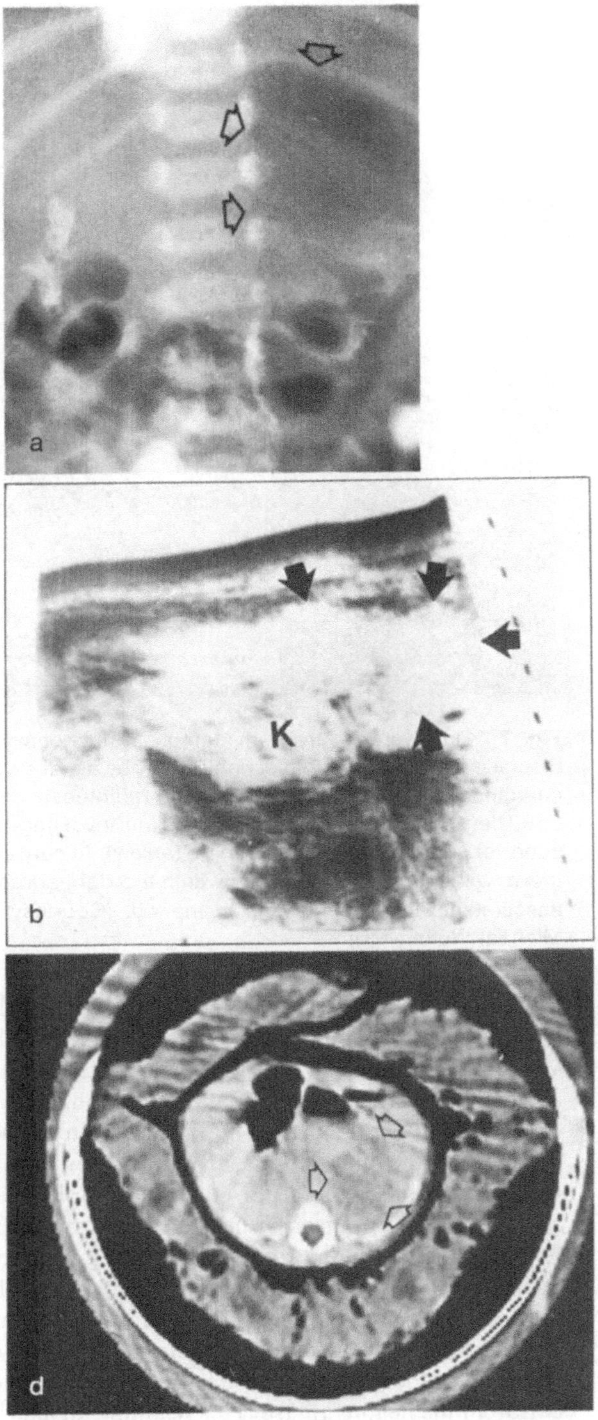

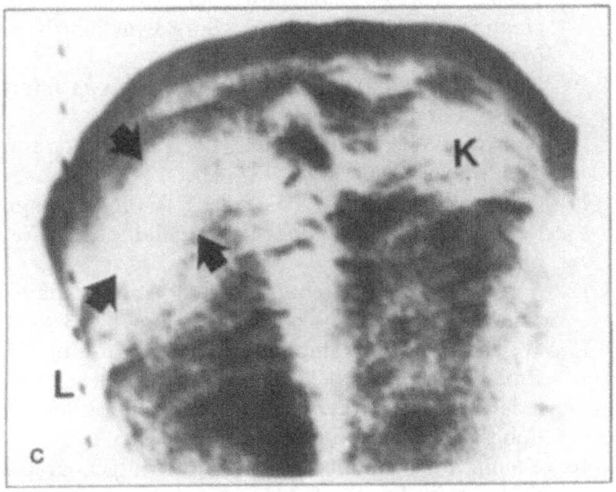

Fig. 7.6. a Intravenous urogram demonstrating a large adrenal hematoma displacing the left kidney downwards. **b** Longitudinal ultrasound scan showing a sonolucent mass above left kidney displacing the left kidney downwards. **c** Transverse scan demonstrating a sonolucent left adrenal mass. The opposite kidney is marked. **d** Computerized tomography of the upper abdomen following injection of contrast shows a mass of reduced attenuation in the region of the left adrenal

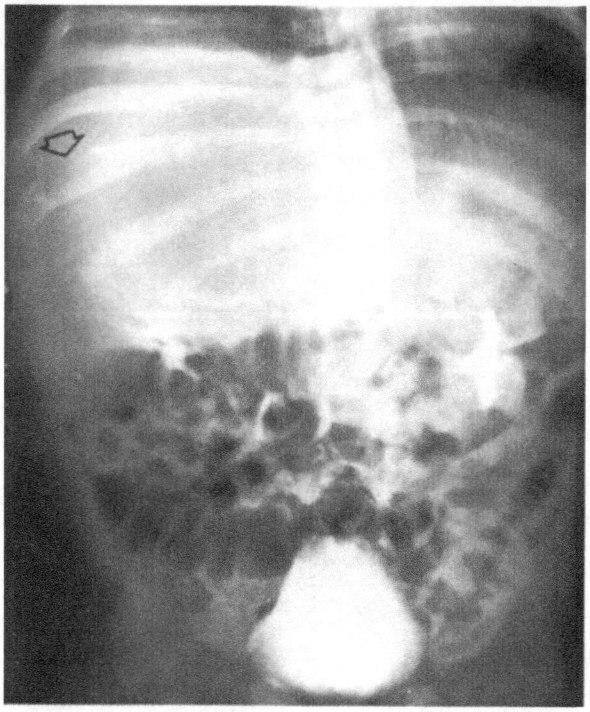

Fig. 7.7. Intravenous urogram demonstrating outward displacement of upper pole of right kidney by a mass with curvilinear peripheral calcification and radiolucent center. There is an area of bone destruction involving the superior surface of the right tenth rib (*arrow*). At surgery, there was a large abcess cavity within the right adrenal associated with osteomyelitis of the rib. (Courtesy of Michael Weller, MD)

the kidney is usually seen to be separate from the mass and a normal complement of calyces will be visualized. These last two features distinguish an adrenal hemorrhage from renal duplication with an obstructed upper polar moiety. If there is any doubt on the routine intravenous urogram, then tomography would be helpful. Ultrasonography will show a sonolucent mass without a solid component [9] and body computed tomography can give useful information, Fig. 7.6d although it will rarely be required with a good quality intravenous urogram. Serial intravenous urograms will show shrinkage of the mass and, possibly, the appearance of calcification in the healing phase. This healing can also be demonstrated by serial ultrasonography [9]. Normal levels of catecholamines in the urine should refute the possibility of a neuroblastoma causing adrenal enlargement.

Although arteriography is recommended for the correct diagnosis of adrenal hemorrhage by Iancu [7] it is not necessary in the majority of patients [4].

Unless there is life-threatening blood loss, which is rare, adrenal hematomas are treated conservatively once the diagnosis has been established. Occasionally, adrenal hematomata become secondarily infected in which case surgical drainage is usually required [3] (Fig. 7.7).

Outside the neonatal period, adrenal trauma is rare.

References

Pancreatic Trauma

1. Blandy JP, Hamblen DL, Kerr WF (1959) Isolation injury of pancreas from nonpenetrating abdominal trauma. Br J Surg 47:150–155
2. Donovan AJ, Turrill F, Berne CJ (1972) Injuries of the pancreas from blunt trauma. Surg Clin North Am 52:649–665
3. Freeark RJ, Corley RD, Norcross WJ, Baker RJ (1966) Unusual aspects of pancreatoduodenal trauma. J Trauma 6:482–492
4. Gougeon FW, Legros G, Archambault A, Bessette G, Bastein E (1976) Pancreatic trauma: a new diagnostic approach. Am J Surg 132:400–402
5. Grosfield JL, Cooney DR (1975) Pancreatic and gastrointestinal trauma in children. Pediatr Clin North Am 22:365–377
6. Haertel M, Fuchs WA (1974) Angiography in pancreatic trauma. Br J Radiol 47:641–645
7. Kilman JW, Kaiser GC, King RD, Shumacker HB (1964) Pancreatic pseudocysts in infancy and childhood. Surgery 55:455–461
8. Lucase CE (1977) Diagnosis and treatment of pancreatic and duodenal injury. Surg Clin North Am 57:49–65
9. Miller RE (1964) Pancreatic pseudocysts in infants and children. Arch Surg 89:517–521
10. Northrup WF, Simmons RL (1972) Pancreatic trauma: a review. Surgery 71:27–43
11. Otherson HG, Moore FT, Boles ET (1968) Traumatic pancreatitis and pseudocyst in childhood. J Trauma 8:535–545
12. Soroudi M, Bookstein JJ (1975) Angiography in acute pancreatic transection. Radiology 115:309–311
13. Welch KJ (1969) The pancreas. In: Mustard WT, Ravitch MM, Snyder WH, welch KJ, Benson CD (eds) Pediatric surgery 2nd edn. Year Book Medical Publishers, Chicago pp 750–767
14. Young LW, Adams JT (1967) Roentgenographic findings in localized trauma to the pancreas in children. AJR 101:639–648

Adrenal Trauma

1. Black J, Williams DI (1973) Natural history of adrenal hemorrhage in the newborn. Arch Dis Child 48:183–190
2. Brill PW, Krasna IH, Aaron H (1976) Early rim sign in neonatal adrenal hemorrhage. AJR 127:289–291

3. Carty A, Stanley P (1973) Bilateral adrenal abscesses in the newborn. Pediatr Radiol 1:63–64
4. Eklof O, Grotte G, Jorulf H, Lohr G, Ringertz H (1975) Perinatal hemorrhagic necrosis of the adrenal gland. Pediatr Radiol 4:31–36
5. Heinivaara O (1954) On the structure of the human suprarenal vein. Ann Med Internae Fenniae 43 Suppl 19
6. Hill EA, Williams JA (1959) Massive adrenal hemorrhage in the newborn. Arch Dis Child 34:178–182
7. Iancu T, Elian E, Lerner MA (1974) Angiography and the conservative management of neonatal adrenal hemorrhage. Pediatr Radiol 2:47–50
8. Kuhn J, Jewett T, Munschauer R (1971) The clinical and radiographic features of massive neonatal adrenal hemorrhage. Radiology 99:647–652
9. Pond GD, Haber K (1976) Echography: a new approach to the diagnosis of adrenal hemorrhage of the newborn. J Can Assoc Radiol 27:40–44
10. Schaffer AJ (1965) Diseases of the newborn, 2nd edn Saunders, Philadelphia p 502
11. Wagner AC (1961) Bilateral hemorrhagic pseudocysts of the adrenal glands in a newborn. AJR 86:540–544

8 Injuries to the Liver and Spleen

Philip Stanley and John L. Gwinn

8.1 Hepatic Trauma

Hepatic trauma is accompanied by high morbidity and mortality. The frequency is increasing, the majority of injuries being related to automobile accidents [6] although other accidents, child abuse [23], birth trauma [22], and liver biopsies are also responsible [28]. The injuries may be penetrating or blunt – the latter now forming the majority of injuries in children [20]. Many patients incurring severe hepatic injuries do not survive long enough to receive treatment. Among hospital patients, the overall mortality from two large series is around 13% [4, 26], although, for blunt trauma alone, the mortality rises to 32% [4] to 44.8% [3]. However, in one series, 74% of patients who arrived dead from blunt abdominal trauma had liver injuries [6]. The prinicpal causes of death are hemorrhage [26] and multiple injuries, including laceration of the heart and aorta [4]. Infection related to leakage of bile and sequestration of devitalized tissue [27], pulmonary insufficiency, and renal failure add to the mortality [4]. It is in the group of patients with severe blunt abdominal trauma that radiology is challenged to provide information regarding the nature and extent of the hepatic injury. This has become of increasing importance now that a more conservative approach to blunt trauma has been adopted, surgery being reserved for the more severe cases [4].

The spectrum of liver injury includes subcapsular hematoma, internal parenchymal rupture with hematoma formation, parenchymal and capsular laceration, parenchymal contusions, arteriovenous fistula, pseudoaneurysm with resultant hematobilia, laceration of vessels, and hepatic vein injury [4]. The intraparenchymal hematoma may undergo necrosis or cyst formation or become secondarily infected.

In addition to damage to intrahepatic structures, the injury may cause damage to the extrahepatic ducts [8, 17], the blunt force compressing the ducts against the spine. This may be accompanied by intrahepatic parenchymal trauma.

In most cases of hepatic injury, the patient is in shock with persistent right upper quadrant pain and the diagnosis of intra-abdominal bleeding is obvious [21]. A falling hematocrit and positive abdominal tap complete the clinical features. Even when the clinical features are typical, radiological investigations are most helpful if the patient's condition permits. Radiology is extremely useful if the clinical features are confusing. The range and type of investigations will depend on the patient's condition.

8.1.1 Plain Films

If the patient's condition permits, supine and erect films are taken together with appropriate views of the chest, skull, and limbs as dictated clinically.

Fractures of the lower right ribs indicate severe trauma in a child and are indicative of potential damage to the underlying liver and right kidney. A right pleural effusion may be present [15] (Fig. 8.1). In addition, contusion of the abdominal wall has been described [15]. This manifests itself as swelling of the muscles of the right lateral part of the abdomen with loss of normal muscle planes and properitoneal fat lines. This is present in just under half the patients with nonpenetrating trauma to the liver [15].

The soft tissue mass of the liver may be diffusely enlarged. There may be a localized swelling with an intact margin displacing the adjacent transverse colon due to a subcapsular hematoma. If there is localized bleeding into the subdiaphragmatic space, there may be elevation of the right dome of the diaphragm [15]. Signs of bleeding into the peritoneal cavity may be present, with blood in the flanks separating the colon from the properitoneal fat lines, and blood in the pelvis manifesting as symmetric densities on both sides of the bladder simulating dog's ears [16]. An adynamic ileus may be present [15].

8.1.2 Intravenous Urogram

Although obviously not performed primarily to demonstrate liver trauma, a urogram is usually undertaken in a patient with severe trauma to the right upper quadrant because of the possibility of renal damage. If sufficiently high dosage of contrast medium is given, laceration and hematomas will be

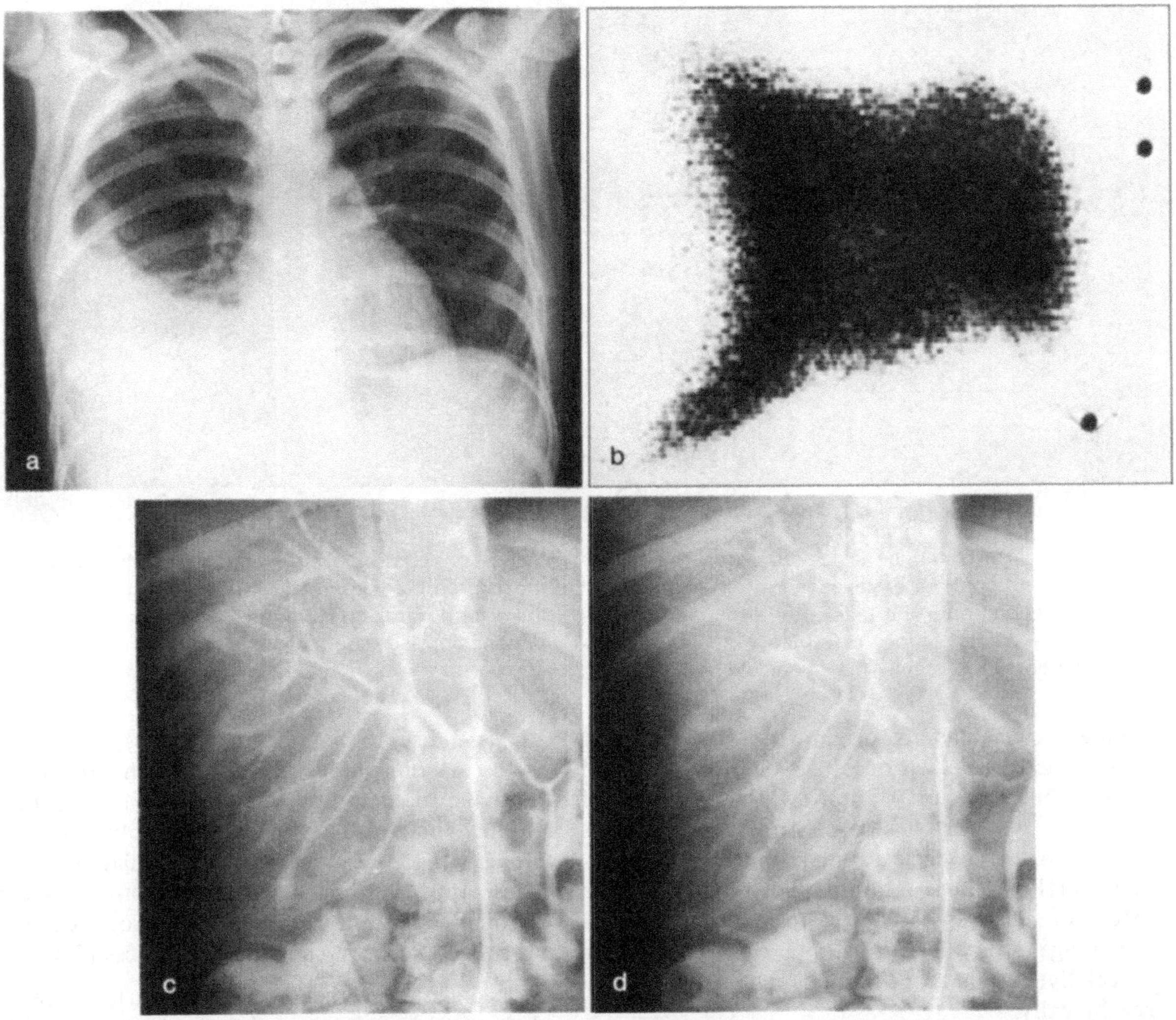

Fig. 8.1. a Frontal projections of the chest demonstrating a right pleural effusion. **b** Anterior scan showing a large void of radiocolloid accumulation in the region of the right lobe of theliver. **c** Arterial phase of hepatic arteriogram showing medial displacement of hepatic arterial branches. **d** Capillary phase of hepatic arteriogram demonstrating separation of the lateral edge of liver parenchyma from abdominal wall by subcapsular hematoma (proven by surgery)

seen as relative radiolucent defects in the total body opacification phase, particularly in neonates.

8.1.3 Isotopes and Ultrasound

If time and the patient's condition permit, then these investigations may be performed (see Chap. 6).

8.1.4 Arteriography

This investigation, although invasive, can be performed swiftly; it demonstrates better than any other imaging modality the extent and nature of the hepatic trauma. Provided the patient's condition permits, this is the investigation of choice in a severely ill patient, particularly if there is associated central nervous system damage, chest trauma, or multiple fractures. It is helpful when isotope scans and clinical findings are equivocal.

Preoperative angiography will demonstrate the nature and extent of the heaptic lesions, some of which may not be obvious on the external surface of the liver at surgery. Concealed and untreated intrahepatic injuries may lead to the late complications of infection, fistula formation, or infarction. The lobar and segmental anatomy will also be demonstrated along with the major arterial blood supply which can be variable. (In about 15% of patients, the right

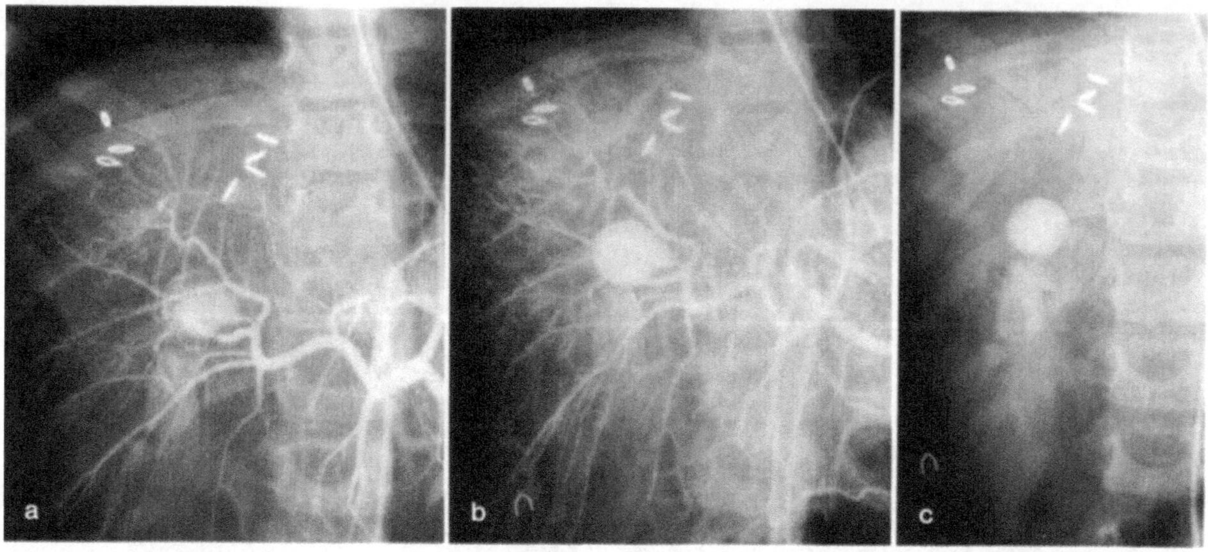

Fig. 8.2. a Arterial phase of celiac axis arteriogram demonstrating contrast extravasating from a branch of the right hepatic artery. **b** Late arterial phase showing progressive accumulation. **c** Capillary phase demonstrating a persistent stain. This 2-year-old had a hepatic laceration repaired at another hospital. Massive hematemesis prompted emergency arteriography. As a result of the arteriogram, the feeding vessels was ligated and the patient stopped bleeding

hepatic artery has its origin from the superior mesenteric.) Visualization of the blood supply and its variability is important now that ligation of hepatic artery branches to control hemorrhage is advocated to prevent exsanguination and hematobilia [26] (Fig. 8.2). In addition to demonstrating the extent of the liver damage, arteriography has the advantage of demonstrating injury to other organs, especiallythe right kidney which may not be suspected clinically.

Numerous arteriographic findings may be seen with hepatic trauma. Vessel narrowing or occlusion indicates severe trauma (Fig. 8.3) and it is often accompanied by other features indicative of liver damage [18], the most common being contrast accumulation (Fig. 8.4). This may be localized, representing active bleeding, which is often seen with hepatic laceration [2], or diffuse and variegated, suggestive of contusion [11, 13, 18]. An arteriographically demonstrable break in the liver parenchyma indicates a liver laceration. The viability of the liver margins adjacent to the tear is indicated by their staining quality [11]. The separation at the edge indicates the size of the interposed clot.

Pseudoaneurysm formation is another vascular manifestation of trauma and this may rupture into the portal or biliary system to give rise to a hepatoportal or hepatobiliary fistula [2]. Hepatoportal fistula can be responsible for portal hypertension later [7] and a hepatobiliary fistula can cause hematobilia.

Vessel displacement around a mass lesion is seen in the arterial phase, sometimes with slow arterial flow due to edema or compression [11, 22]. In the parenchymal phase there is a radiolucent center, often with a peripheral hypervascular zone [18]. These appearances usually indicate an intraparenchymal hematoma although a necrotic cavity or abscess could have similar appearances [18].

Medial displacement of the entire arterial tree and the presence of an external avascular space separating the liver from the abdominal wall in the parenchymal phase is characteristic of a subcapsular hematoma [18, 21] (Fig. 8.1).

Arteriography is useful in the postoperative patient in whom satisfactory progress is not being made following surgery for hepatic trauma [21]. Angiography will demonstrate the complications of hepatic artery fistulas between portal veins or biliary tract, unrecognized hematomas and areas of necrosis and abscess formation. Arteriography can also provide a route for embolization of hepatic artery-biliary tree fistulas although recent reports have recorded natural healing of the fistulas demonstrated by serial angiography [9].

There has been a report that hepatoportography via an umbilical vein cutdown should be the first contrast investigation in patients with liver trauma [1]. Truncated veins, pressure displacement and filling defects in the sinusoidal phase are all indicative of a hematoma. However, this technique, which

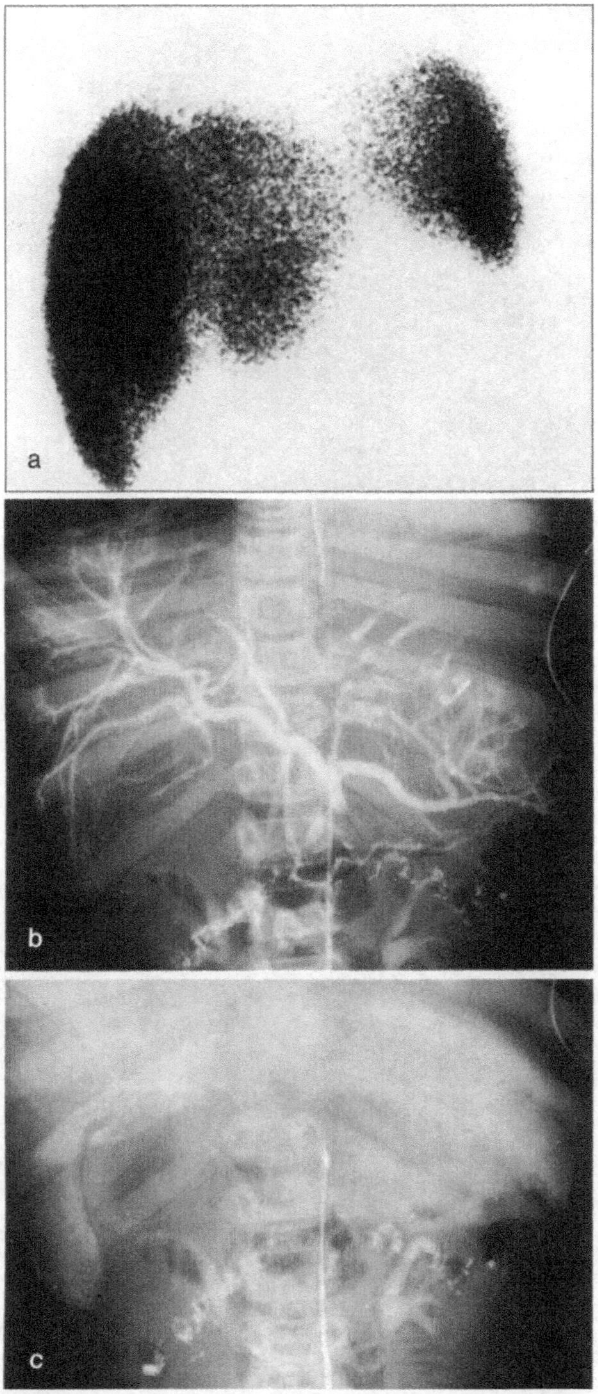

Fig. 8.3. a Anterior scan demonstrating a vertical cleft within the liver substance separating the right and left lobes. There is poor accumulation of the radiocolloid in the left lobe. **b** Arterial phase of hepatic arteriogram showing poor flow in the left hepatic artery. **c** Capillary phase of hepatic arteriogram showing homogeneous opacification of the right lobe with a lucency surrounding the gallbladder. The left lobe is poorly visualized. At surgery, there was a vertical fracture between the two lobes with contusion of the left lobe. There was a hematoma around the gallbladder

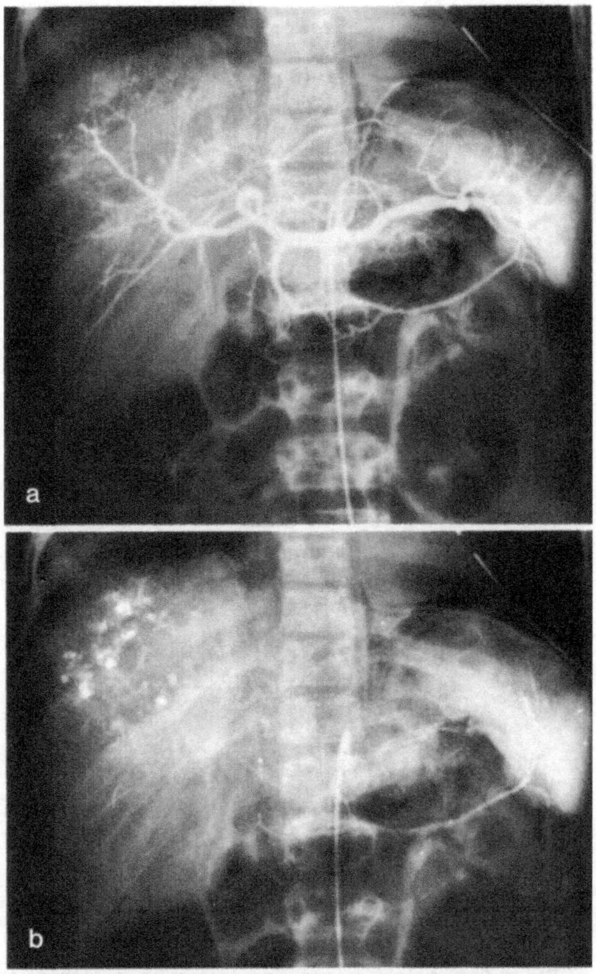

Fig. 8.4. a Celiac axis arteriogram in arterial phase. There is some separation of arterial branches in the right lobe with extravasation of contrast. **b** Capillary phase demonstrating a central lucency with peripheral collections of contrast compatible with severe contusion

involves surgical dissection, has not gained general acceptance.

Because of the association of hepatic vein injury with liver trauma and subsequent involvement of the inferior vena cava, it is recommended that patients have inferior vena cavography [12]. But it is not our routine.

8.1.5 Cholangiography

Intravenous cholangiography may be helpful in demonstrating duct trauma although, often, operative cholangiography is required [24]. If bile duct lacerations have been repaired over an indwelling catheter, follow-up T-tube cholangiograms are most helpful in determining healing, possible stricture formation, and in indicating for correct time for tube removal [14, 20] (Fig. 8.5).

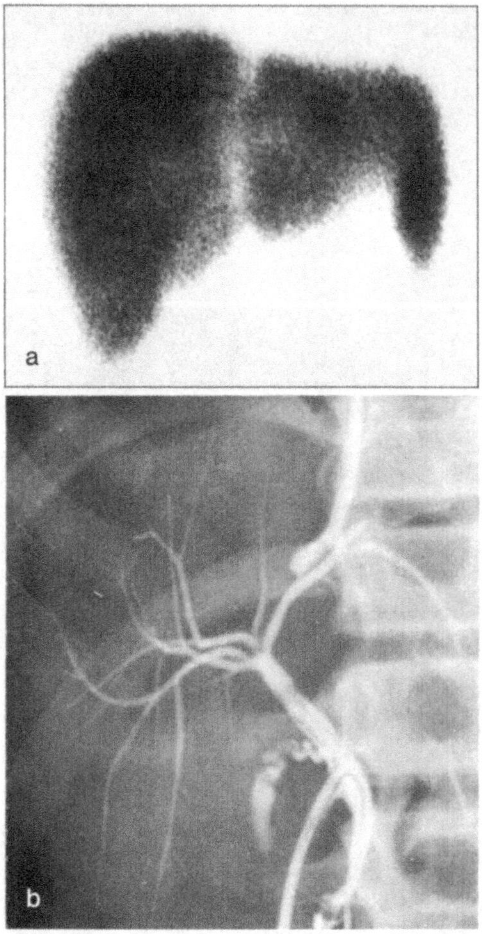

Fig. 8.5. a Anterior scan demonstrating a vertical cleft devoid of radiocolloid. Surgery demonstrated a vertical fracture. **b** T-tube cholangiogram showing extravasation of contrast from the left biliary duct system

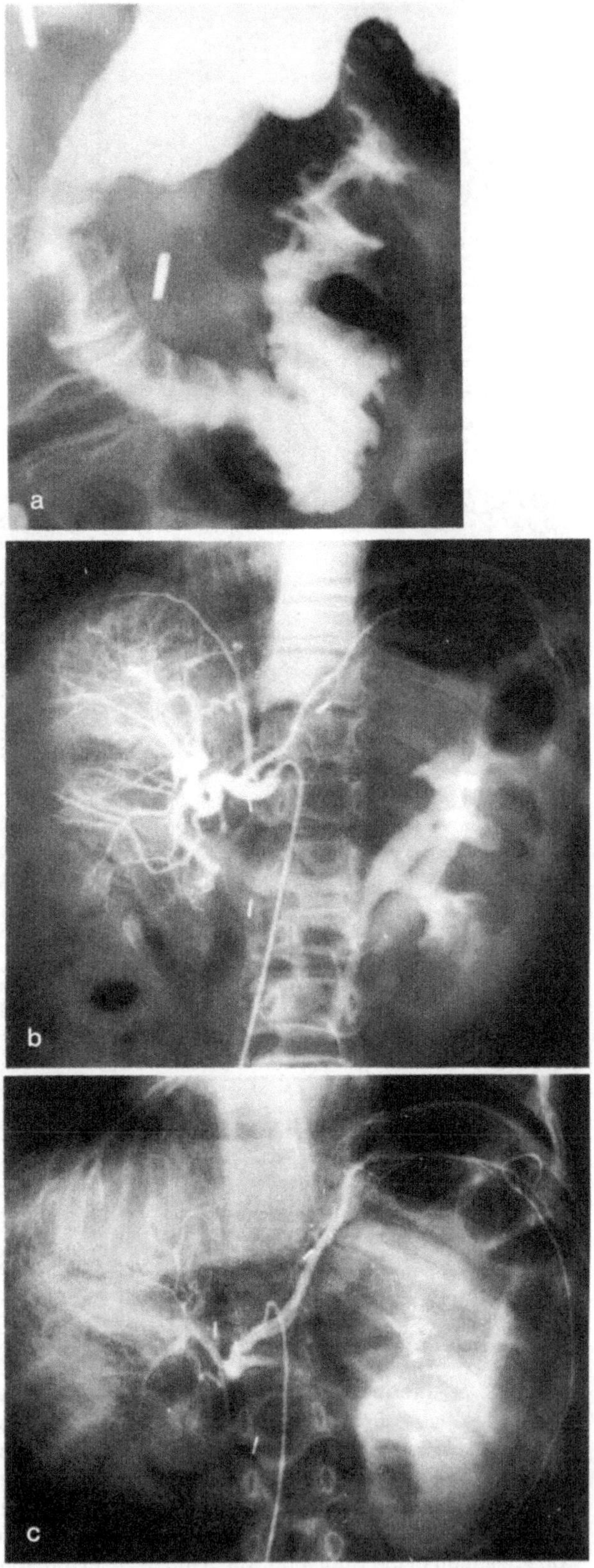

▷

Fig. 8.6. a Upper GI examination demonstrating narrowing of the duodenum with mucosal thickening and irregularity due to prior irradiation. There was a degree of obstruction to the flow of barium. **b** Celiac axis arteriogram in arterial phase. There is a small liver with vessel tortuosity and corkscrewing. (There has been a splenectomy.) **c** Celiac axis arteriogram in capillary phase. Shunting into pulmonary veins has been demonstrated. These changes are due to chronic irradiation injury to the liver. The patient had irradiation to the liver following surgical excision of Wilms' tumor

8.1.6 Computerized Tomography

This is a new diagnostic modality whose exact role in the diagnosis of abdominal trauma has yet to be fully assessed. However, contusions, lacerations, and hematomas in the liver should be easily demonstrable, as well as retroperitoneal hematomas. Fine vascular detail cannot be demonstrated.

8.1.7 Radiation-induced Injury

Initially it was thought that the liver was relatively resistant to radiation therapy. However, significant changes in hepatic morphology and function have been described following radiation therapy [5]. The injury usually manifests itself within a few weeks of the start of irradiation with an acute phase which may last a few months before progressing through a subacute stage to a chronic phase [5, 25]. These irradiation effects can be demonstrated by isotope scanning, showing decreased radioisotope uptake [5, 10], or with angiography [19]. In the acute phase there is arterial stretching and hepatofugal flow in the intrahepatic portal vein branches [19]. In the chronic phase there is corkscrewing of the hepatic arteries in the irradiated region [19] (Fig. 8.6). There may be irradiation changes in the underlying duodenum.

8.2 Injuries to the Spleen

In children, as in adults, the spleen is an organ most frequently injured by blunt trauma, motor vehicles being responsible for the majority of injuries [3, 25].

Injuries to the spleen are usually caused by acute bending or flexion of the relatively fixed spleen [25]. In children, the ribs are more resilient than in adults and usually spring back into position without fracturing [13] although, occasionally, broken ends of the ribs may pierce the spleen to cause a laceration and subcapsular hematoma. In children, due to the extreme elasticity of the ribs, force is easily and faithfully transmitted to the posterior abdominal wall, resulting in damage to the kidney and other neighboring structures. There is a significant incidence of trauma to the left kidney in children with splenic trauma [25].

Injuries to the spleen include intrasplenic and subcapsular hematomas, simple laceration, stellate laceration, and hilar rupture [3]. The late complications include posttraumatic splenic cyst, abdominal splenosis and delayed rupture, although the last appears to be uncommon in children [25]. The clinical features of splenic injury depend upon its severity. With moderate to severe injury, the child usually presents with abdominal pain and distension, left upper quadrant tenderness and a falling hematocrit. Although not always routinely performed, a peritoneal lavage may be positive [20]. Life-threatening hemorrhage from a splenic injury alone is unusual and so there is usually time for radiographic investigations to determine the extent of the injury and show involvement of other organs not suspected clinically [1]. Investigative techniques have become particularly important because of the tendency towards conservative treatment of splenic injuries (see later). In addition, radiographic techniques are very helpful when the clinical features are trivial or masked by more obvious skeletal, thoracic, and central nervous system injuries.

Plain radiographs of the abdomen may show fractures of the lower left rib cage [25]. There may be a soft tissue mass displacing the gastric air bubble towards the midline and depressing the splenic flexure [14]. There may be complete or partial loss of splenic outline [27]. A subsequent film showing a definite increase in the splenic soft tissue mass indicates active bleeding [25]. Thickening of the gastric rugae has been reported, along with elevation of the left dome of the diaphragm and a left pleural effusion [5, 17, 27]. There may be free fluid [21].

Splenic scintigraphy with ^{99m}Tc-sulphur colloid will demonstrate the site and extent of the laceration and surrounding hematoma [6, 16, 18, 26, 29] (see Chap. 6). Scintigraphy being noninvasive is the best investigation to demonstrate healing. This is particularly important in the diagnosis and follow-up of splenic trauma treated conservatively [9] (Fig. 8.7). Ultrasonography will also show the extent of the splenic trauma [28]. Arteriography may be performed, particularly if there are associated liver and renal injuries, or if the isotope scan and/or clinical features are equivocal. Arteriography has the advantage that there are no false negatives and very few false positives. The most reliable arteriographic signs of splenic rupture include extravasation, mottling of the parenchymal phase, and arteriovenous shunting [19, 11] (Fig. 8.8). With laceration and hematoma formation, there is vessel displacement by the hematoma which may be within the body of the spleen or subcapsular [19]. To the inexperience, gastric fundal arteries and parenchymal accumulation of contrast in the liver, stomach, colon, or pancreas may simulate splenic injury on arteriography [7]. An adherent omentum can cause a similar problem. Oblique views and gastric air insufflation or a selective splenic injection will usually provide

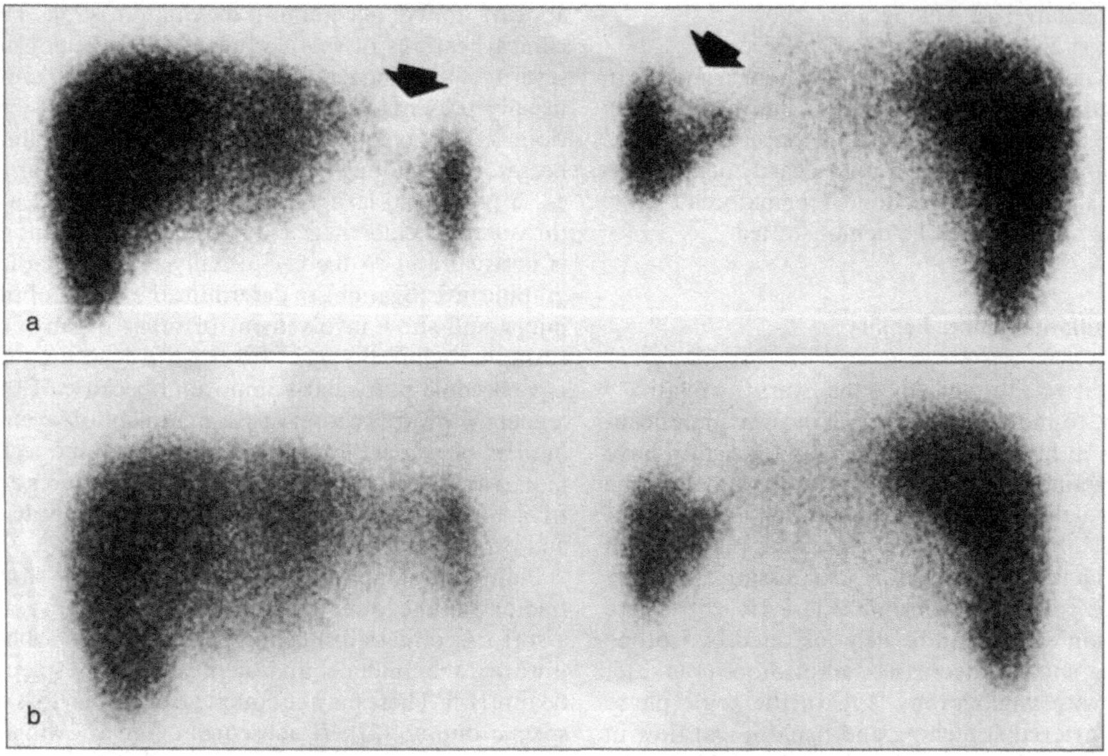

Fig. 8.7. Anterior (*left*) and posterior (*right*) scintiphotos showing a wedge-shaped defect in the posteromedial aspect of the spleen compatible with a fracture with a hematoma. (**a**) Repeat examination 47 days later shows some healing (**b**)

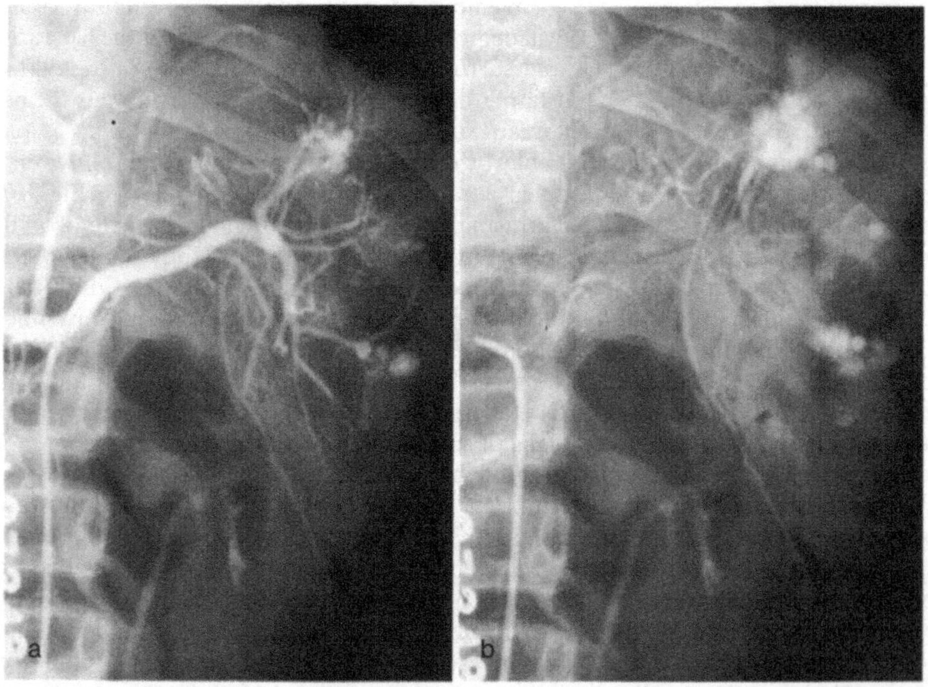

Fig. 8.8. Celiac axis arteriogram. **a** Arterial phase showing extravasation of contrast into the mid polar region with some separation of vessels. **b** Capillary phase contrast extravasation with a defect in the mid polar region. A splenic laceration in this area was found at surgery

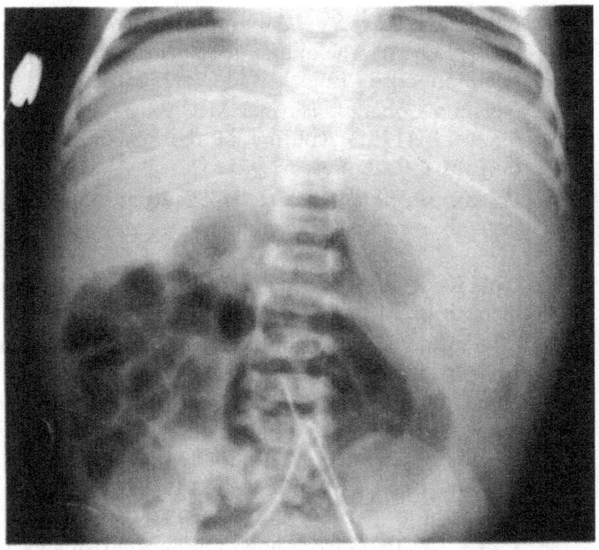

Fig. 8.9. Plain film of the abdomen showing soft tissue mass occupying the left upper quadrant. There is displacement of stomach and adjacement bowel loops

diagnostic distinction. Lobulation and a gap between the superior surface of the spleen and the diaphragm without other features of splenic injury may be considered normal. Sometimes following injury, intrasplenic aneurysms may be formed and these can be demonstrated only by arteriography [19].

Another late sequela is the development of intrasplenic cysts which show vascular displacement on arteriography but can be best identified by ultrasound [28].

Recent experience with CT scanning has demonstrated subcapsular splenic hematomas as a curvilinear low density mass between the spleen and left lateral part of the abdominal wall with a linear or concave outward border between the periphery of the spleen and the mass [10]. Immediately after trauma, the hematoma may be isodense with the normal spleen but later will be of lower attenuation value. Identification is usually easy after contrast because the normal spleen will increase in attenuation value while the surrounding hematoma remains essentially unchanged [10].

Although it has been denied by some authorities that there is an increased incidence of infections following splenectomy for trauma in children [4], more recent evidence suggests a significant incidence of fatal infections [23]. With this in mind, and provided the damage is not too severe, surgeons are pursuing reparative surgery [15] or a conservative nonoperative approach [25].

Rupture of the spleen may occur during birth, when it is usually associated with damage to other viscera, particularly the liver [8]. Pressure on the thorax during birth is an important factor, together with direct trauma, in producing these lesions, which are more common in large infants. A large spleen associated with erythroblastosis fetalis is apparently prone to trauma [22]. Clinical features include shock, falling hematocrit, and abdominal distension [24]. Plain radiographs reveal abdominal fluid with a vague soft tissues mass in the left upper quadrant (Fig. 8.9). Intravenous urography with immediate postinjection films for total body opacification will show a large zone of relative radiolucency in the left upper quadrant [12]. The high dose urogram not only demonstrates the splenic injury but has the advantage of showing trauma to other intra-abdominal organs. Laceration of the liver and suprarenal hemorrhage should always be considered with neonatal intraperitoneal hemorrhage [2].

References

Hepatic Trauma

1. Ayella RJ, Champion HR, Gill W, Hankins JR, Cowley RA (1974) Contrast roentgenolography in the management of major liver injury. Surg Gynecol Obstet 139:545–550
2. Boijsen E, Judkins MP, Simay A (1966) Angiographic diagnosis of hepatic rupture. AJR 86:66–72
3. Crosthwait RW, Allen JR, Murga F, Beall AC, De Bakey ME (1962) The surgical management of 640 consecutive liver injuries in civilian practice. Surg Gynecol Obstet 114:650–654
4. Defore WW, Mattox KL, Jordan GL, Beall AC (1976) Management of 1590 consecutive cases of liver trauma. Arch Surg 111:493–497
5. Fellows KE, Vawter GF, Tefft M (1968) Hepatic effects following abdominal irradiation in childhood: detection by Au 198 scan and confirmation by histologic examination AJR 103:422–431
6. Fitzgerald JB, Crawford ES, de Bakey ME (1960) Surgical considerations of non-penetrating abdominal injuries. Am J Surg 100:22–29
7. Foley WJ, Turcotte JG, Hoskins PA, Brant RL, Ause RG (1971) Intrahepatic arteriovenous fistulas between the hepatic artery and portal vein. Ann Surg 174:849–855
8. Hartman SW, Greaney EM (1964) Traumatic injuries to the biliary system in children. Am J Surg 108:150–156
9. Hendren WH, Warshaw AL, Fleischli DJ, Bartlett MK (1971) Traumatic hemobilia: non-operative management with healing documented by serial angiography. Ann Surg 174:991–993
10. Johnson PM, Grossman FM, Atkins HL (1967) Radiation induced hepatic injury: its detection by scintillation scanning. AJR 99:453–462

11. Lange EK (1976) The role of arteriography in trauma. Radiol Clin North Am 14:353–370
12. Levin DC, Watson RC, Sos TA, Baltaxe HA (1973) Angiography in blunt hepatic trauma. AJR 119:95–101
13. Love L (1975) Radiology of abdominal trauma. JAMA 231:1377–1380
14. Mays ET (1971) Complex penetrating hepatic wounds. Ann Surg 173:421–428
15. McCort JJ (1962) Rupture or laceration of the liver by non-penetrating trauma. Radiology 78:49–57
16. McCort JJ (1964) Radiological examination in blunt abdominal trauma. Radiol Clin North Am 2:121–143
17. Moyle WD, Karl RC (1969) Rupture of the extrahepatic biliary ducts by external blunt trauma. J Trauma 9:623–628
18. Nahum N, Levesque M (1973) Arteriography in hepatic trauma. Radiology 109:557–563
19. Nebesar RA, Tefft M, Vawter GF, Filler RM (1974) Angiography in radiation hepatitis. Br J Radiol 47:588–593
20. Noone RB, Mackie JA, Stoner R (1967) Liver and bile duct laceration from blunt abdominal trauma in children. Ann Surg 166:824–828
21. Osborn DJ, Glickman MG, Grnja V, Ramsby G (1973) The role of angiography in abdominal nonrenal trauma. Radiol Clin North Am 11:579–592
22. Smulewicz JJ, Tafreshi MM (1975) Hematoma of the liver due to birth trauma. J Natl. Med Assoc 67:214–215
23. Stone RK, Harawitz A, San Filippo JA, Gromisch DS (1976) Needle perforation of the liver in an abused infant. Clin Pediatr 15:958–959
24. Taylor B (1977) Newer aids in the diagnosis of blunt abdominal trauma. Can Med Assoc J 116:599–605
25. Tefft M, Mitus A, Das L, Vawter G, Filler RM (1970) Irradiation of the liver in children: review of experience in the acute and chronic phases, and in the intact normal and partially hepatectomised. AJR 108:365–385
26. Trunkey DD, Shires T, McClelland R (1974) Management of liver trauma in 811 Consecutive patients. Ann Surg 179:722–728
27. Turrill FL, Donovan AJ, Facey FL (1971) Traumatic hepatic sequestra. Am J Surg 122:175–182
28. Wallace S, Medellin H, Nelson RS (1972) Angiographic changes due to needle biopsy of the liver. Radiology 105:13–18

Injuries to the Spleen

1. Berk RN, Wholey MH, Stockdale R (1970) The angiographic diagnosis of splenic and hepatic trauma. J Can Assoc Radiol 21:230–234
2. Cywes S, Cremin BJ (1969) The roentgenologic features of hemoperitoneum in the newborn. AJR 106:193–199
3. Douglas GJ, Simpson JS (1971) The conservative management of splenic trauma. J Pediatr Surg 6:565–570
4. Eraklis AJ, Kevy SV, Diamond LK, Gross RE (1967) Hazard of overwhelming infection after splenectomy in childhood. N Engl J Med 276:1225–1229
5. Gershon-Cohen J, Hermel MB, Byrne RN, Bringhurst LS (1951) Rupture of the spleen: roentgen diagnosis. Radiology 57:521–527
6. Gilday DL, Alderson PO (1974) Scintigraphic evaluation of liver and spleen injury. Semin Nucl Med 4:357–370
7. Gold RE, Redman HC (1972) Splenic trauma: assessment of problems in diagnosis. AJR 116:413–418
8. Gruenwald P (1948) Rupture of liver and spleen in the newborn infant. J Pediatr 33:195–201
9. Howman-Giles R, Gilday DL, Venogopal S, Shandling B, Ash JM (1978) Splenic trauma – nonoperative management and long-term follow-up by scintiscan. J Pediatr Surg 13:121–126
10. Korobkin M, Moss AA, Callen PW, Demartini WJ, Kaiser JA (1978) Computed tomography of subcapsular splenic hematoma. Radiology 129:441–445
11. Lang EK (1976) The role of arteriography in trauma. Radiol Clin North Am 14:353–370
12. Marquis JR, Sun SC, Verasestakul S (1976) Rupture of the spleen in a newborn infant. Radiology 119:177–178
13. Mazel MS (1945) Traumatic rupture of the spleen. J Pediatr 26:82–88
14. McCort JJ (1964) Radiological examination in blunt abdominal trauma. Radiol Clin North Am 4:121–143
15. Mishalany H (1974) Repair of the ruptured spleen. J Pediatr Surg 9:175–178
16. Nebesar RA, Rabinov KR, Potsaid MS (1974) Radionuclide imaging of the spleen in suspected splenic injury. Radiology 110:609–614
17. Nelson JF (1966) The roentgenologic evaluation of abdominal trauma. Radiol Clin North Am 4:415–431
18. O'Marra RE, Hall RC, Dombroski DL (1970) Scintiscanning in the diagnosis of rupture of the spleen. Surg Gynecol Obstet 131:1077–1084
19. Osborn DJ, Glickman MG, Grnja V, Ramsby G (1973) The role of angiography in abdominal nonrenal trauma. Radiol Clin North Am 11:579–592
20. Root MD, Hauser CW, McKinley CR, Lafave JW, Mendiola RP (1965) Diagnostic peritoneal lavage. Surgery 57:633–637
21. Rosoff L, Cohen JL, Telfer N, Halpern M (1972) Injuries of the spleen. Surg Clin North Am 52:667–685
22. Simmons M, Burrington JD, Wayne ER, Hathaway WE (1973) Splenic rupture in neonates with erythroblastosis fetalis. Am J Dis Child 126:679–681
23. Singer DB (1973) Postsplenectomy sepsis. In: Rosenberg HS, Bolande RP (eds) Perspectives in pediatric pathology. Year Book Medical Publishers, Chicago, pp 289–290
24. Sokol DM, Tompkins D, Izant RJ (1974) Rupture of the spleen and liver in the newborn: a report of the first survivor and a review of the literature. J Pediatr Surg 9:227–229

25. Upadhyaya P, Simpson JS (1968) Splenic trauma in children. Surg Gynecol Obstet 126:781–790
26. Walsh JA, Ludrook J, Ronai PM (1974) Photoscanning – an aid to the early diagnosis of rupture of the spleen. Arch Surg 109:812–815
27. Wang CC, Robbins LL (1956) Roentgenologic diagnosis of ruptured spleen. N Engl J Med 10:455–449
28. Wilson RL, Rogers WF, Shaub MS, Birnbaum W (1978) Splenic subcapsular hematoma – ultrasonic diagnosis. West J Med 128:6–8
29. Witek JT, Spencer RP, Pearson HA, Touloukian RJ (1974) Diagnostic splenic scans in occult splenic injury. J Trauma 14:197–199

9 Gastrointestinal Trauma

John L. Gwinn and Philip Stanley

Abdominal trauma in children is not uncommon. Serious injury to the gastrointestinal tract is less frequent than to the other abdominal organs as the gastrointestinal tract, for the most part, is more mobile and compliant than the solid organs. This fact probably spares the bowel from injury. Blunt trauma to the gastrointestinal tract is seen much more frequently in childhood than is penetrating trauma [8, 9, 31]. Tunell [33], however, reported on 132 patients with 73 stab wounds and 59 gunshot injuries seen over a 10-year period. The involved abdominal organs were: liver 39, small bowel 23, stomach 18, colon 14, and duodenum 9.

Blunt injury to the gastrointestinal tract is usually produced by high velocity impact or sudden deceleration, as in a fall [9]. The bowel is often filled with fluid [9] and may be compressed against a solid structure such as the spine [23, 29, 35]. There may be a shearing or tearing of the bowel and mesentery at fixed points [9, 23].

In Grosfeld's [8] series of 40 children who suffered blunt gastrointestinal trauma, 82% of the patients were boys. One-half the cases were due to falls and one-thrid to vehicular accidents. Slightly over 37% had significant associated injury. These findings are true in other series [14, 28].

There are several radiological modalities available for assessing the type and extent of injury to the gastrointestinal tract. Even since the advent of nuclear medicine, ultrasonography, and CT scanning, the usual and very satisfactory studies of plain films, in various positions, and contrast studies of the gastrointestinal tract, remain as the most often used diagnostic procedures. If contrast studies are done, barium mixtures are usually the ones of choice. Water-soluble contrast medium is used for particular problems. Angiography is of value in cases of penetrating trauma and in evaluating injury to other abdominal organs but has little use in blunt trauma. The choice of the roentgenographic studies to be performed should be tailored to the individual patient [3, 6, 25].

9.1 Stomach

Rupture of the stomach in children is rare [2, 3, 10, 26, 34], but it occurs most often when the child is hit by a car or falls shortly after having eaten [1, 2, 34, 36]. The stomach is a mobile organ and is in a relatively protected position in relationship to the ribs [2, 8]. Rupture of the stomach may be seen in the battered child syndrome [3, 20, 26]. In this situation the nature of the blow and its vectors accounts for the paucity of splenic and hepatic injuries [26]. The rupture of the stomach is frequently linear, anteriorly located, and near the lesser curvature [2, 8].

Spontaneous rupture of the stomach in the newborn is thought to be due to: (1) distension of the stomach with or without obstruction, (2) mucosal trauma – feeding tubes, or (3) congenital absence or thinning of the musculature [25, 36] (Fig. 9.1).

9.1.1 Clinical

There is often a history of the child having had a recent meal that was followed by trauma to the abdomen. Usually, there is abdominal pain and distension. Vomiting is often present and there is peritoneal irritation. Respiratory distress may be secondary. Patients need airway support and their fluid volume carefully monitored.

9.1.2 Roentgenographic

Plain films of the abdomen in the supine, erect and/or left lateral decubitus positions, along with a chest film, should be obtained [22]. These may be the only studies needed. In selected cases, water-soluble contrast can be an aid in demonstrating the site of the perforation [32].

Most patients with rupture of the stomach will have free intraperitoneal air [2, 9, 20, 36] (Fig 9.2) and an air-fluid level. However, free air does not always occur [8, 12, 34]. Another finding may be the absence of the usual air-fluid level seen in the normal stomach. In the supine position, peritoneal fluid may be indicated by obliteration of the fat planes, displacement of the bowel, or the bowel floating in

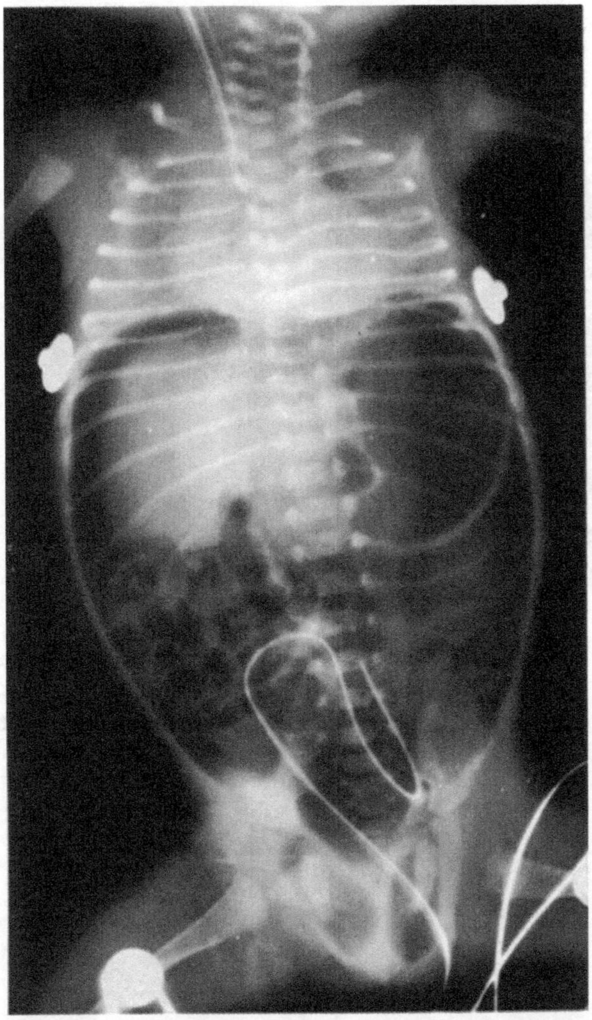

Fig. 9.1. Supine chest and abdomen of neonate. The changes in the lungs are those of hyaline membrane disease, and an endotracheal tube is in place. The patient also had esophageal atresia with tracheoesophageal fistula. With the infant on the respirator, oxygen was forced into the stomach resulting in perforation of the stomach and massive pneumoperitoneum even into the scrotum

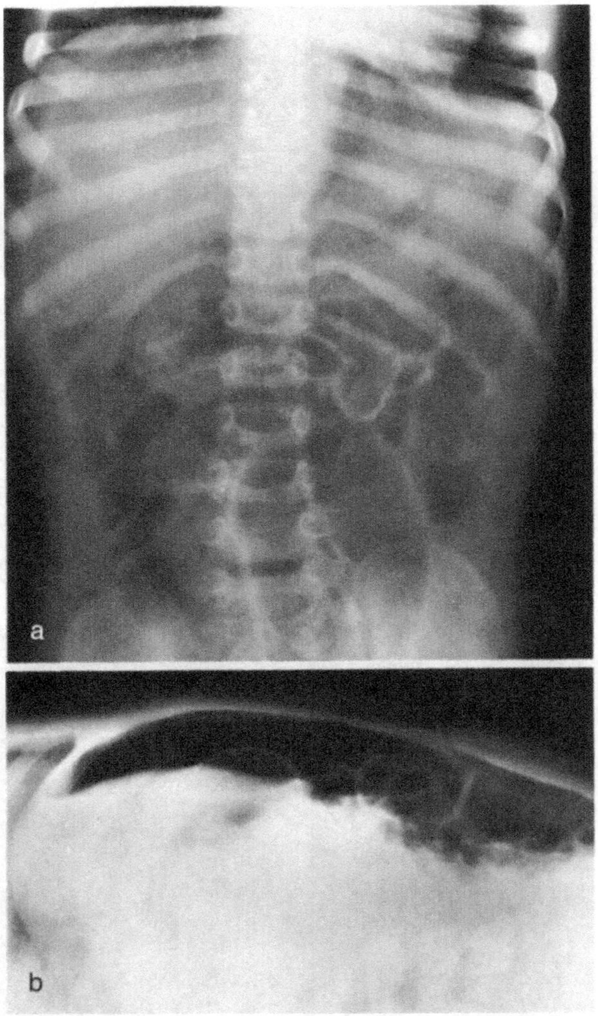

Fig. 9.2. a Supine abdomen with lucency in the abdomen, particularly noted over the liver and indicating free intraperitoneal air. **b** Cross-table lateral of the abdomen easily demonstrating free air. Both sides of the bowel are seen. This 3-year-old was struck in the abdomen by an automobile

the midabdomen. In the erect position, the so-called "dog ears" pattern in the pelvis may be present. Some of these features are not as readily perceived in a child as they are in adults.

Surgical intervention is necessary to repair the rupture of the stomach. Complications, consisting of abscess formation, general infection, and fistulization do occur.

9.2 Duodenum

Blunt trauma to the duodenum is more common than penetrating injury in childhood [7, 19, 29, 31], although Stone [30] reported on 27 penetrating injuries of the duodenum.

The second portion of the duodenum is in apposition to the hilum of the right kidney, and the third portion overlies the psoas muscle and the spine which are relatively fixed [32]. The third portion can easily be crushed against the spine [7, 14, 16, 29]. There is some evidence that the duodenojejunal

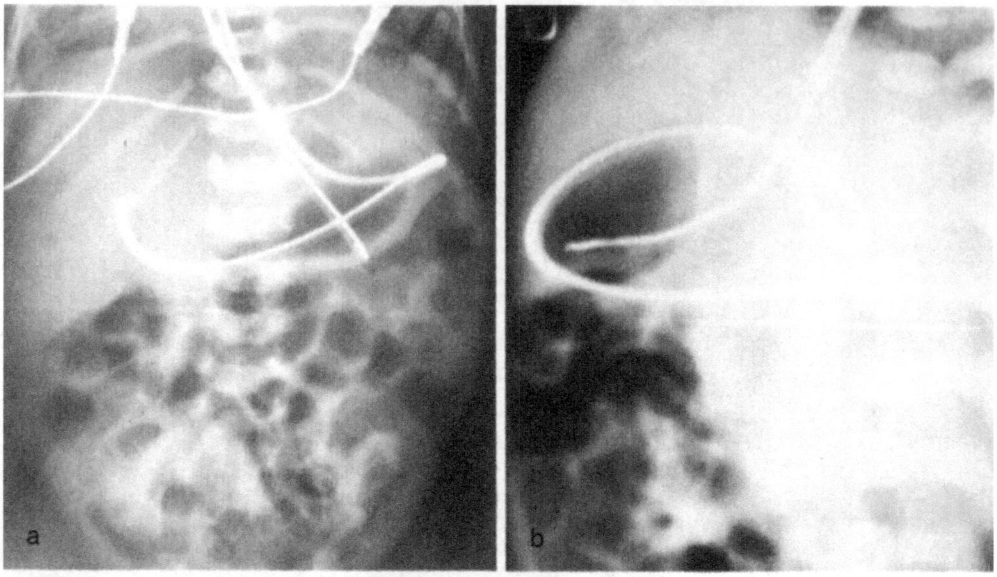

△
Fig. 9.3 a, b. Premature infant with duodenal tube in place. **a** Note abnormal position of the tip with relationship to normal duodenal position. **b** Lateral view of the abdomen with the duodenal tube much too far posterior to be in the duodenum. The tube had perforated the duodenum. (Courtesy of Hermann Grossmann, Durham, North Carolina)

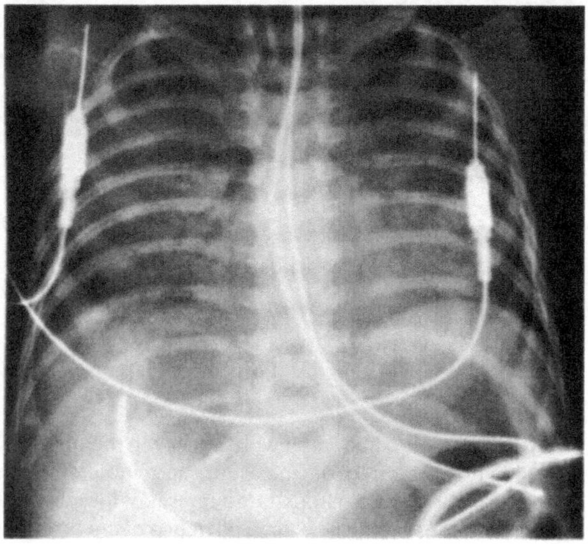

◁
Fig. 9.4. Same patient as in Fig. 9.3. Pulmonary changes of RDS. Note collection of air beneath right leaf of the diaphragm medially. (Courtesy of Herman Grossman, Durham, North Carolina)

junction in infants is mobile [Merten, personal communication].

Iatrogenic perforation of the duodenum is being reported with increasing frequency due to the increased use of nasojejunal feedings. Polyvinyl tubes apparently change consistency in as little as 6–12 h while within the bowel. Instead of remaining pliable they harden and become rigid [27]. Perforation can easily occur if the tube is manipulated after being in place for 12 h, hence repositioning of the tube is to be avoided [27]. Perforation of the duodenum by silicone rubber catheters has been reported [24] (Figs. 9.3, 9.4, 9.5).

Ingested material may injure the bowel at any level. Obviously, sharp, pointed, metallic substances can perforate the intestine but this is not common and surprisingly long, pointed objects may pass through the entire length of the bowel without damage.

Caustic materials and medications may also injure the intestine, causing scarring and stenosis (Fig. 9.6).

9.2.1 Clinical

Patients suffering blunt trauma to the duodenum may have immediate symptoms of pain and vomiting. These symptoms, however, are often delayed from one to several days [7, 13, 18, 19, 29]. Protracted vomiting in those with duodenal hematoma is found in almost all cases [19, 29]. The degree of trauma may appear to be mild [7, 13, 16]. Abdominal

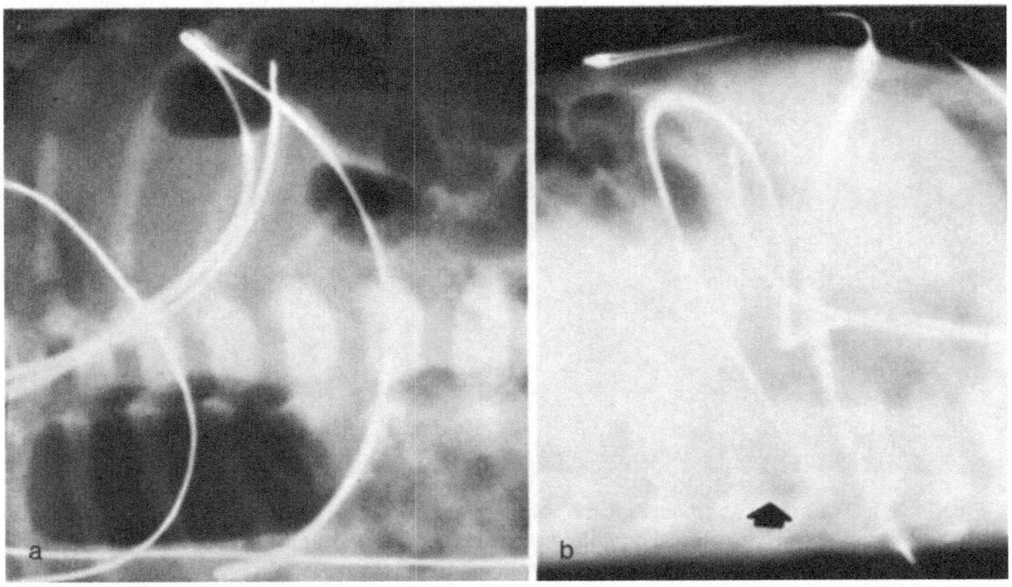

Fig. 9.5 a, b. Same patient, and on decubitus film (**a**) air-fluid level is present. **b** Cross-table lateral of abdomen showing air posteriorly (*arrow*) (Courtesy of Herman Grossman, Durham, North Carolina)

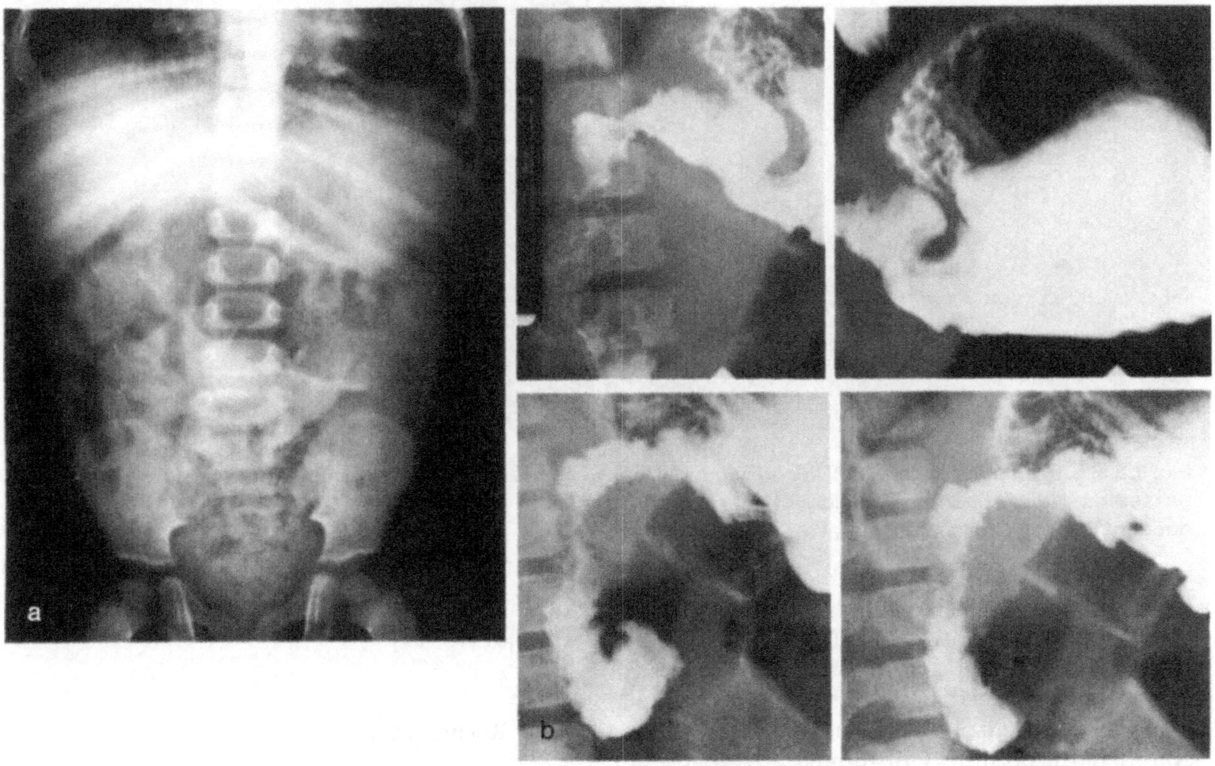

Fig. 9.6 a, b. Child had ingested iron tablets and continued to vomit. **a** Supine abdomen with nonspecific mild distension of bowel; **b** Gastrointestinal study – spot films of the duodenum with persistent narrowing of the duodenum and irregularity of the mucosa interpreted to be secondary to the iron ingestion

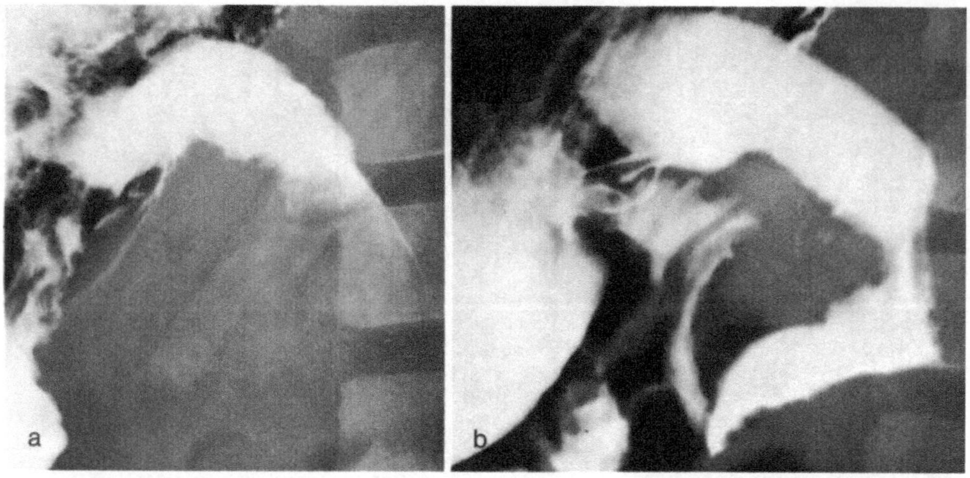

Fig. 9.7 a, b. Trauma to abdomen. **a** On original gastrointestinal series there was almost complete obstruction of the duodenum, thickening of the duodenal folds, and an intramural mass. **b** Repeat study 1 week later. There is still duodenal deformity but the duodenum is not obstructed and the mucosa has a much more normal appearance

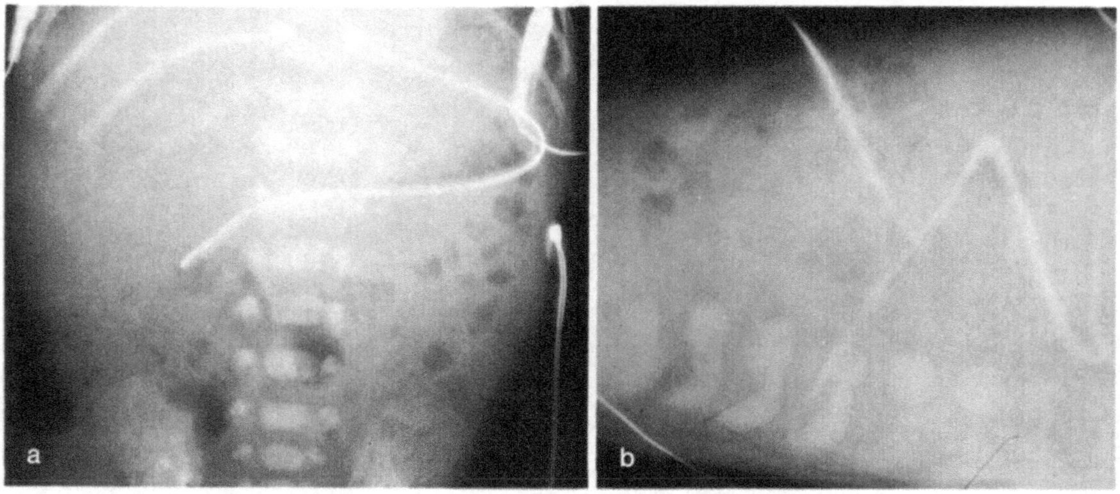

Fig. 9. 8 a, b. Premature child with RDS and duodenal tube passed. **a** Note abnormal position of the tip of the duodenal tube. **b** Cross-table lateral of the abdomen with marked posterior placement of the tip of the duodenal tube

tenderness is frequently elicited and may subside only to recur [18]. An abdominal mass may be palpated [19]. Besides trauma, other causes of intramural hemorrhage such as hemophilia, Henoch-Schönlein purpura, leukemia, etc., must be considered if no history of trauma is available [4].

Traumatic duodenal hematomas are located in the subserosal or intramural portion of the duodenal wall. There is a tearing of the small vessels in the wall without mucosal or serosal interruption [19, 29]. They may subside spontaneously [11] (Fig 9.7) or may increase in size due to accumulation of fluid secondary to the breakdown of hemoglobin which produces an increase in the osmotic pressure within the clot [13, 29].

9.2.2 Roentgenographic

Plain supine, erect, and/or left lateral decubitus films of the abdomen, along with a chest film, should be the first study. Technically excellent films are required for accuracy in diagnosis.

In perforation or rupture of the duodenum, free intraperitoneal air is rare [3, 10, 12, 18]. Nonspecific findings on the plain films include scoliosis, paralyt-

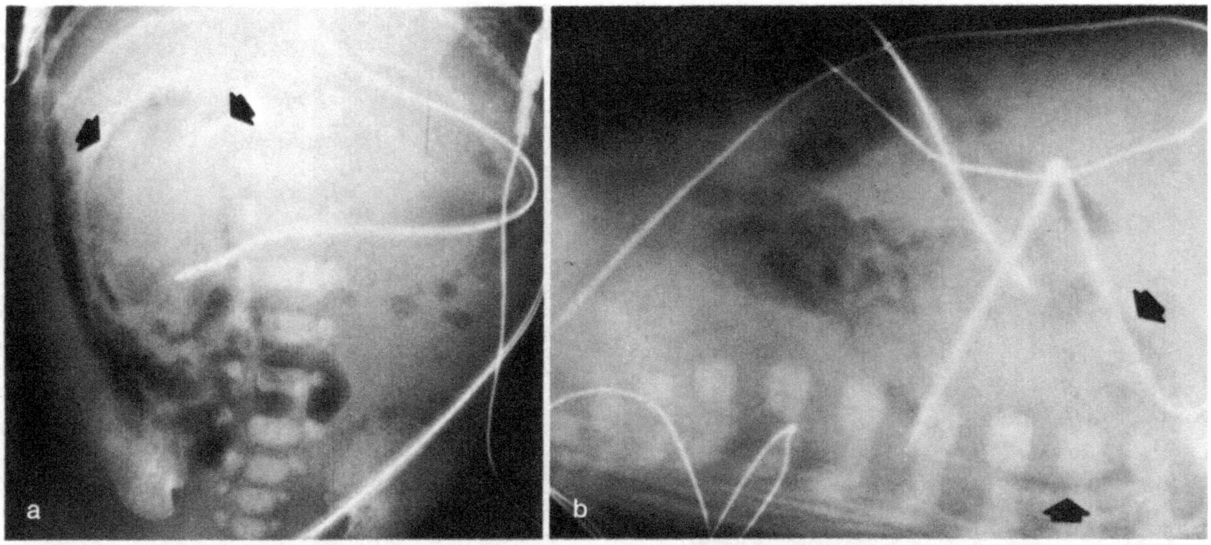

Fig. 9.9 a, b. Same patient as in fig. 9.8. **a** Supine abdomen with malplacement of the tube. Air is seen around the kidney and along the right flank due to perforation of the duodenum by the tube. **b** Cross-table lateral with air seen about the kidney (*arrows*)

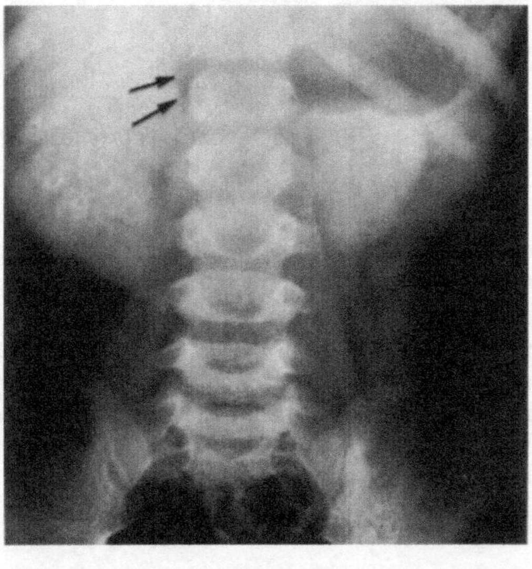

Fig. 9.10. Patient had trauma to abdomen followed by persistent vomiting. There is very little gas within the abdomen. *Arrows* mark a soft tissue mass partially obstructing the duodenum

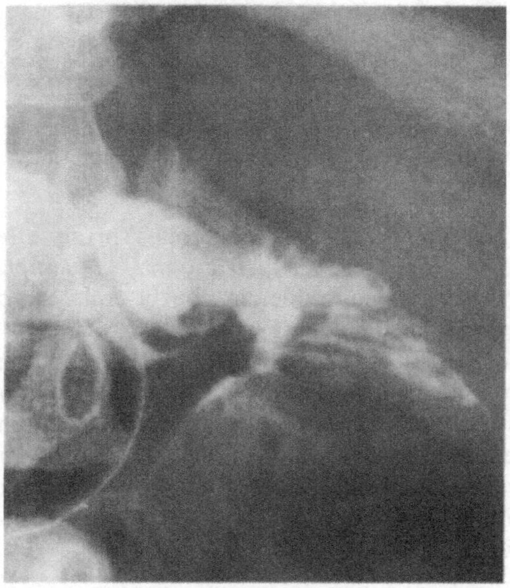

Fig. 9.11. Duodenal hematoma with mass effect, widening of the duodenum, and thickening of the mucosal folds

ic ileus and obliteration of the psoas margin [3, 10, 17, 32]. A more specific finding is retroperitoneal air usually around the right psoas muscle and the right kidney [3, 10, 17, 18, 32] (Figs 9.8, 9.9). This finding may be very subtle. Water-soluble contrast gastrointestinal study will usually show the site of rupture and contrast will flow into the retroperitoneal space [3, 10, 17, 32]. This type of duodenal injury is more commonly seen in adults than in children.

Duodenal hematoma due to blunt trauma is more common than perforation in children. In 1954, Felson and Levine [5] presented the classic roentgenographic findings in patients with duodenal hematoma. On plain films of the abdomen, the right psoas margin may be blurred. There may be gastroduodenal distension and a soft tissue mass may be seen [7] (Fig. 9.10). On the upper gastrointestinal study with barium as the contrast medium, the mucosal folds of the proximal area of the traumatized duodenum are thickened. More distally, there is an intramural mass widening the duodenum (Fig. 9.11). In this area the valvulae conniventes are

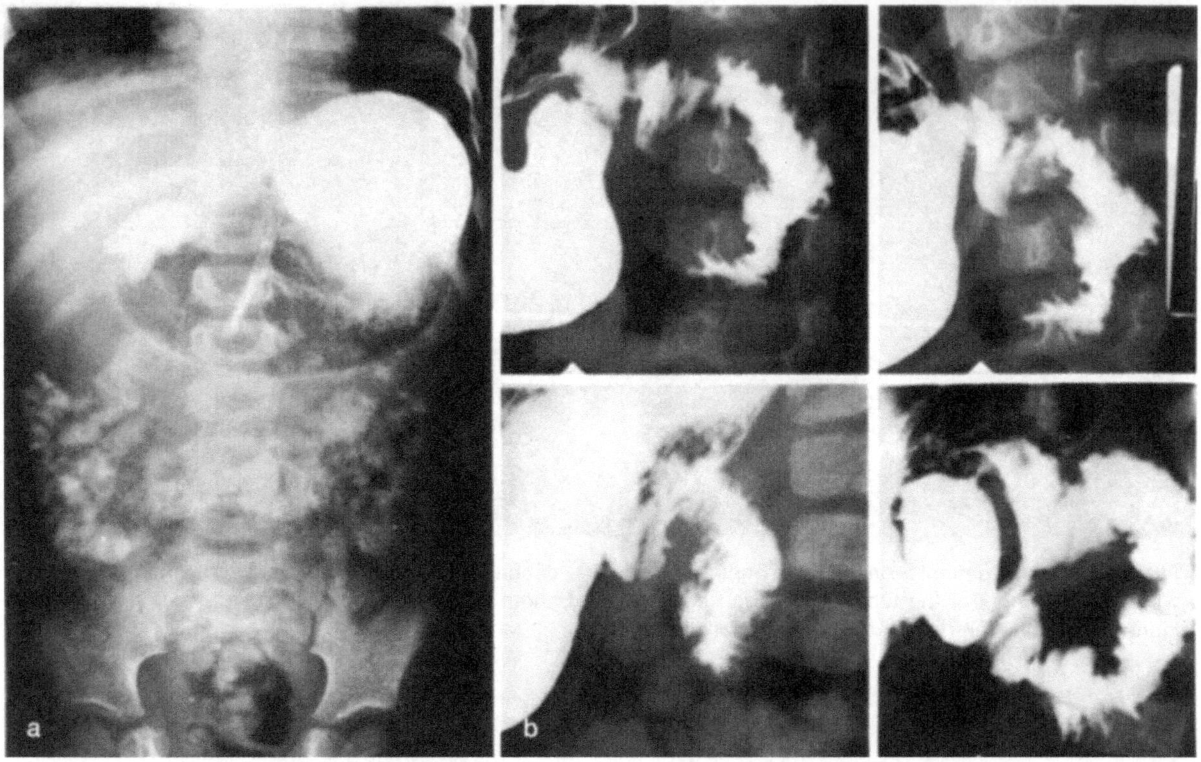

Fig. 9.12. a Incomplete obstruction of the duodenum due to duodenal hematoma. **b** Same patient 1 week after **a** with duodenum not obstructed. Some residual deformity

crowded together producing a "coiled spring" effect [3, 5, 6, 7, 10, 18, 19, 29]. There may be complete obstruction of the duodenum, but usually the obstruction is incomplete (Fig 9.12).

Most of the patients with duodenal hematoma can be managed conservatively [4, 11, 13, 19]. In our institution, the criteria for conservative management consist of no clinical, laboratory, or radiological evidence of associated injuries, no excessive continued blood loss, and subsidence of obstruction within 7–10 days.

9.3 Small Intestine

The small bowel is compressible and mobile, so injury by blunt trauma is less common than to other abdominal organs. When the small bowel is injured by blunt trauma, the usual sites of injury are at the area of the ligament of Treitz or the distal ileum where the bowel is relatively fixed [14]. There may be a shearing or tearing of the bowel and the mesentery at these fixed points [3, 8, 23]. This type of injury presents a complex diagnostic and therapeutic challenge [31]. The treatment is frequently hampered by delay in diagnosis [14].

Penetrating trauma to the small intestine probably occurs more frequently than blunt trauma. Retroperitoneal hematoma is often associated with penetrating injury of the small bowel [23]. Tunell et al. [33] in a series of 132 children who had penetrating abdominal injuries found that the small bowel was involved in 23 of them. In this type of injury, exploratory surgery is almost always done, usually with a minimum of roentgenographic studies [31].

9.3.1 Clinical

Abdominal pain is almost universally present and nausea and vomiting are frequent. There is generalized abdominal rigidity and tenderness. Peristalsis is diminished or absent. The leukocyte count is usually elevated [7, 8, 12]. There is a significant mortality (5%–20%) in these patients and a complication rate of up to 35% [8].

9.3.2 Roentgenographic

The basic roentgenographic series in evaluating a patient with abdominal trauma consists of plain films of the abdomen in the supine, erect, and/or left

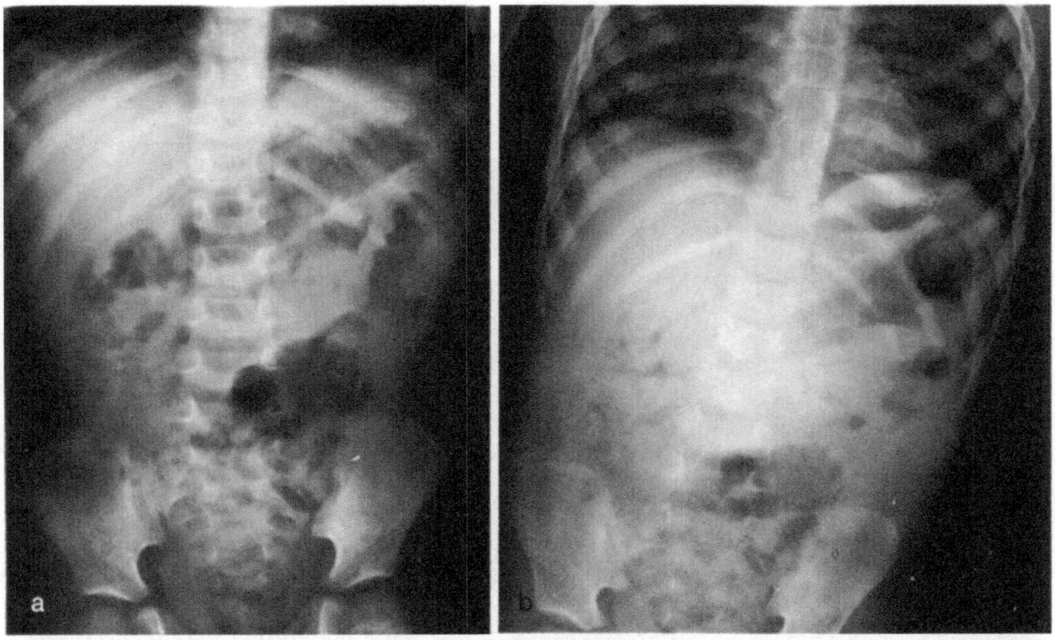

Fig. 9.13 a, b. Patient hit by a car. **a** Supine view of the abdomen with a mild adynamic ileus gas pattern; **b** erect abdomen with adynamic ileus. No free air

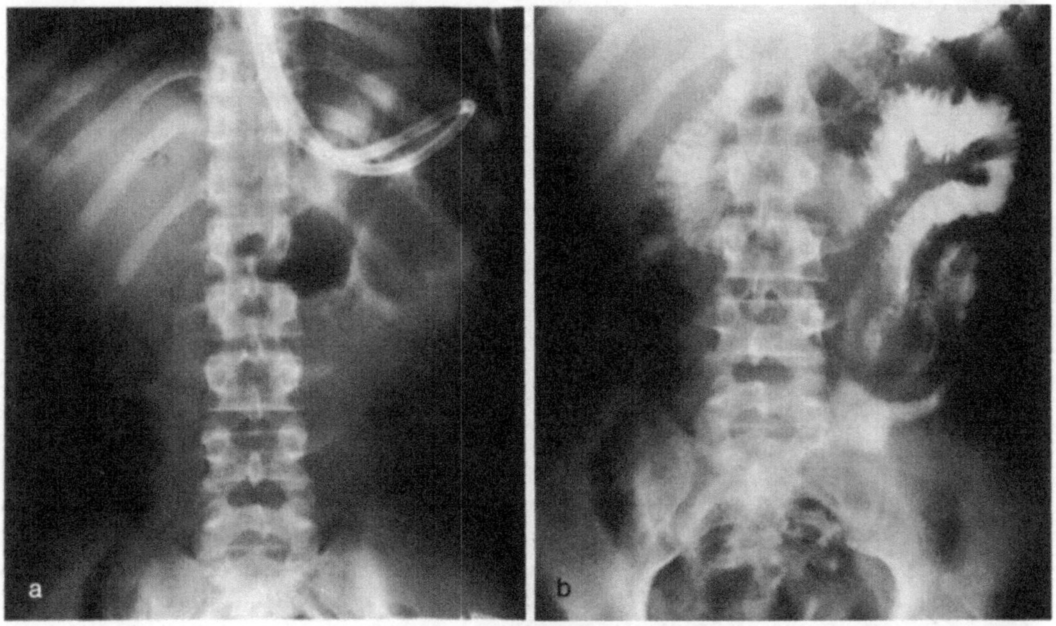

Fig. 9.14 a, b. Patient hit in abdomen with a bicycle handle. **a** Supine abdomen with nonspecific ileus pattern. Nasogastric tube in poor position. **b** Water-soluble contrast study demonstrating contrast outside of jejunal lumen due to perforation

lateral decubitus positions, along with a chest roentgenogram. The most prevalent finding in these studies is an adynamic ileus which is seen in most instances [6, 12, 22, 23] (Fig. 9.13). Free intraperitoneal air is seen in considerably less than 50% of the patients [6, 14, 23] and in some series free air is reported to be rare [3, 9, 12, 23].

The above studies are often all that are required for the management of the patient. However, in selected patients, water-soluble contrast studies of the

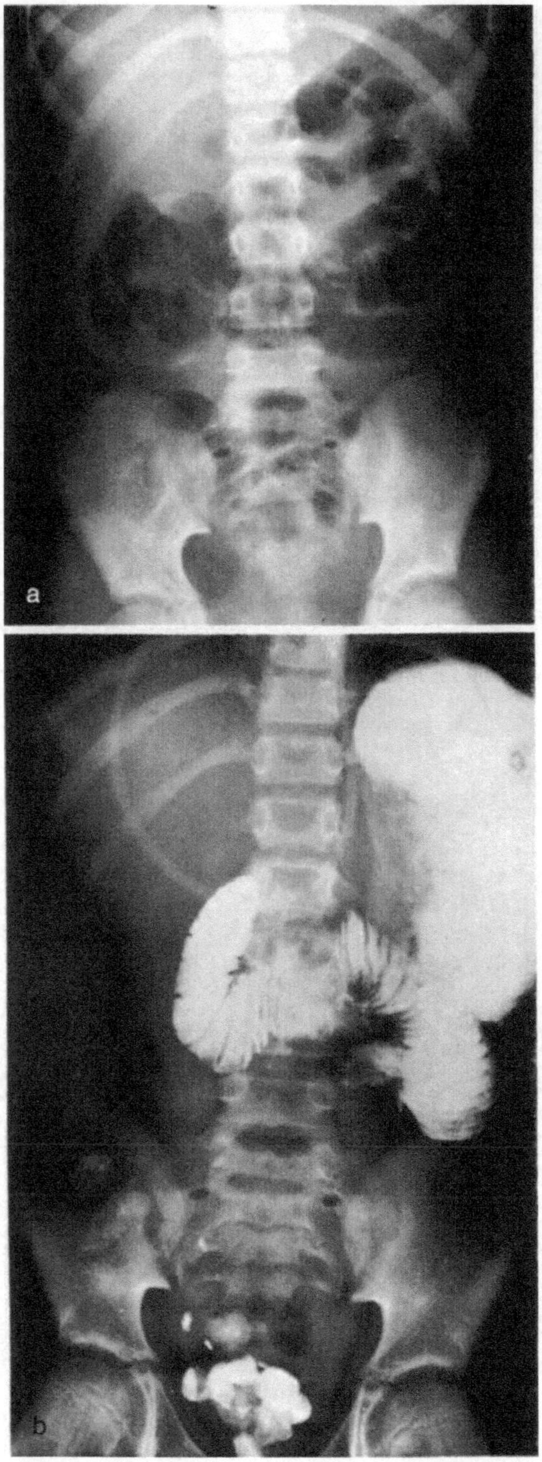

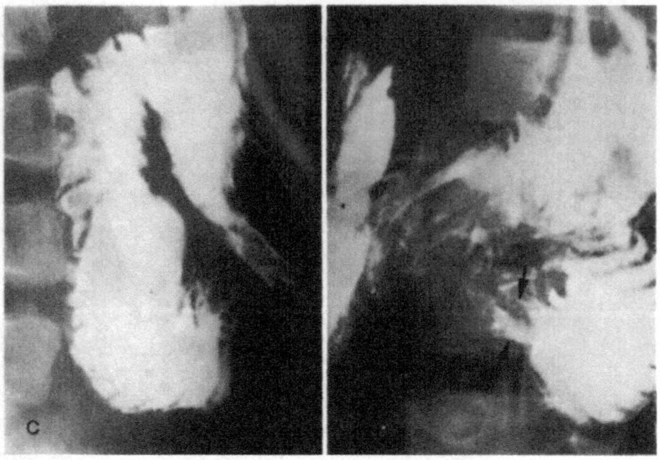

Fig. 9.15 a–c. Patient had suffered abdominal trauma. **a** Supine view of the abdomen with adynamic ileus pattern. No free air. Later, patient's clinical course deteriorated, and on a water-soluble gastrointestinal series **b** obstruction of the jejunum was found, and on a spot film **c** there is extravasation of contrast from the lumen of the bowel (*arrows*). (Courtesy of Lloyd Morris, MD, Adelaide, Australia)

small bowel are used to demonstrate the site of a leak or the area of hematoma [6, 22] (Figs. 9.14, 9.15). If significant intraperitoneal blood is present, abdominal angiography may be necessary to delineate the bleeding site.

9.4 Colon

Injuries to the colon in children are not common, and the majority are caused by penetrating trauma [15, 21]. In one series of 199 children, 99 of whom had blunt abdominal trauma and 100 penetrating trauma, the colon was not involved in any [28]. In a series of 132 children [33] with penetrating abdominal injury, the colon was involved in 14 patients. The force for injury from blunt trauma is severe and vehicular trauma is often involved. There is a high incidence of associated injury [15, 21].

Blunt abdominal trauma may produce immediate or delayed injury to the colon. The large bowel can be compressed against the spine, or even a seat belt, and then burst, particularly if the loop of compressed bowel is distended with gas. The mesentery may be avulsed, the colon may be lacerated, and there may be partial vascular disruption resulting in ischemia, hematoma formation, gangrene and perforation [3, 9, 15, 21].

In small children, in particular, perforation of the rectum may occur with the use of rectal thermometers [25] and may result from distension of the rectum by a Foley or Bardex balloon catheter.

The most common site of injury to the colon is in the descending colon and the rectum. Rectal injuries frequently have associated fractures of the pelvis. The ascending colon is the least often injured [15, 21].

9.4.1 Clinical

The clinical presentation will depend on the type and extent of the injury. There may be shock and peritoneal signs associated with colonic injury. In blunt trauma there is usually abdominal tenderness and mild distension. There may be bleeding from the rectum. The symptoms may be mild at first, only to progress later.

9.4.2 Roentgenographic

As in any abdominal trauma in children, plain films of the abdomen in the supine, erect, and/or left lateral decubitus positions should be obtained. Free intraperitoneal air is a common finding if the colon is lacerated or perforated [9, 17]. An adynamic ileus pattern is frequently observed [6, 22]. Fluid or blood may be suspected by displacement or floating of the bowel. Peritoneal lavage is often used as a diagnostic study in patients with colonic trauma so it is important to remember to obtain the roentgenograms prior to lavage since the lavage itself can produce free air [15].

Penetrating wounds of the colon, for all practical purposes, require exploration, and so the diagnosis of colon injury is established at surgery and probably no other roentgenographic studies beyond a plain film need be done. In blunt injury, a more selective approach can be taken. Careful contrast studies of the colon with water-soluble contrast medium will demonstrate the site of a perforation because of leakage from the bowel lumen. Hematomas, as an intramural mass, can also be identified in this manner.

9.5 Summary

With the possible exception of duodenal hematomas, trauma to the gastrointestinal tract in children is much less a problem than is trauma to other areas. The basic roentgenographic studies of plain films of the abdomen in various positions are the cornerstones for diagnosis of gastrointestinal injury. Contrast studies of the gastrointestinal tract are often useful, whereas the other imaging modalities play a lesser role than in solid organ injury.

References

1. Abrames JS (1975) Editorial comment. J Trauma 15:192
2. Asch MJ, Coran AG, Johnston PW (1975) Gastric perforation secondary to blunt trauma in children. J Trauma 15:187–189
3. Burrell M, Toffler R, Lowman R (1973) Blunt trauma to the abdomen and gastrointestinal tract: plain film and contrast study. Radiol Clin North Am 11:561–578
4. Eiland M, Sang YH, Hicks GM Jr (1978) Topics in radiology – intramural hemorrhage of the small intestine. JAMA 239:139–142
5. Felson B, Levin EJ (1954) Intramural hematoma of the duodenum: diagnostic roentgen sign. Radiology 63:823–830
6. Franken EA Jr, Smith JA (1975) Roentgenographic evaluation of infant and childhood trauma. Pediatr Clin North Am 22:301–315
7. Freeark RJ, Corley RD, Norcross WJ Strohl EL (1966) Intramural hematoma of the duodenum. Arch Surg 92:463
8. Grosfeld JL, Cooney DR (1975) Pancreatic and gastrointestinal trauma in children. Pediatr Clin North Am 22:365–377
9. Haller JA Jr (1966) Injuries of the gastrointestinal tract in children: notes on recognition and management. Clin Pediatr (Phila) 5:476–480
10. Harrison RC, Debas HT (1972) Injuries of the stomach and duodenum. Surg Clin North Am 52:635–648
11. Izant RJ, Drucker WR (1964) Duodenal obstruction due to intramural hematoma in children. J Trauma 4:797–813
12. Jacobson G, Carter RA (1951) Small intestine rupture due to nonpenetrating abdominal injury: roentgenologic study. AJR 66:52–64
13. Judd DR, Taybi H, King H (1964) Intramural hematoma of the small bowel. Arch Surg 89:527–535
14. Kakos GS, Grosfeld JL, Morse TE (1971) Small bowel injuries in children after blunt abdominal trauma. Ann Surg 174:238–241
15. Kirkpatrick JR (1977) Injuries of the colon. Surg Clin North Am 57:67–76
16. Kirkpatrick WE (1960) Submucosal hematoma of the duodenum: discussion and report of a case. AJR 83:857–860
17. Kurtzman RS (1977) Radiology of blunt abdominal trauma Surg Clin North Am 57:211–226
18. Lucas CE (1977) Diagnosis and treatment of pancreatic and duodenal injury. Surg Clin North Am 57:49–65
19. Mahour GH, Woolley MM, Gans SL, Payne VC (1971) Duodenal hematoma in infancy and childhood. J Pediatr Surg 6:153–160
20. McCort JJ, Vaudagna J (1964) Visceral injuries in battered children. Radiology 82:424–448

21. McKenzie AD, Bell GA (1972) Nonpenetrating injuries of the colon and rectum. Surg Clin North Am 52:735–746
22. Meyers HI (1968) Radiologic evaluation of patients with nonpenetrating abdominal trauma. Surg Clin North Am 48:1205–1219
23. Orloff MJ, Charters AC (1972) Injuries of the small bowel and mesentery and retroperitoneal hematoma. Surg Clin North Am 52:729–734
24. Perez-Rodrigues J, Quero J, Frias EG, Omenaca F (1978) Duodenorenal perforation in a neonate by tube of silicone rubber during transpyloric feeding. J Pediatr 92:113–114
25. Philippart AI (1977) Blunt abdominal trauma in childhood. Surg Clin North Am 57:151–162
26. Schechner SA, Ehrlich FE (1974) Gastric perforation and child abuse. J Trauma 14: 723–725
27. Siegel RL, Rabinowitz JG, Sarasohn C (1976) Intestinal perforation secondary to nasojejunal feeding tubes. AJR 126:1229–1232
28. Sinclair MC, Moore TC (1974) Major surgery for abdominal and thoracic trauma in childhood and adolescence. J Pediatr Surg 9:155–162
29. Stewart DR, Byrd CL, Schuster SR (1970) Intramural hematomas of the alimentary tract in children. Surgery 68:550–557
30. Stone HH (1972) Pancreatic and duodenal trauma in children. J Pediatr Surg 7:670–675
31. Touloukian RJ (1968) Abdominal trauma in childhood. Surg Gynecol Obstet 127:561–568
32. Toxopeus MD, Lucas CE, Krabbenhoft KL (1972) Roentgenographic diagnosis in blunt retroperitoneal duodenal rupture. AJR 115:281–282
33. Tunell WP, Knost J, Nance FC (1975) Penetrating abdominal injuries in children and adolescents. J Trauma 15:720–725
34. Vassey LE, Klecker RL, Koch E, Morse TS (1975) Traumatic gastric perforation in children from blunt abdominal trauma. J. Trauma 15:184–189
35. Williams RA, Sargent BA (1963) The mechanism of intestinal injury in trauma. J Trauma 3:288–294
36. Yajko RD, Seydel F, Trimble C (1975) Rupture of the stomach from blunt abdominal trauma. J Trauma 15:177–183

10 Chest Trauma

Philip Stanley and John L. Gwinn

Trauma to the chest in children may be minor, presenting no diagnostic or therapeutic difficulties, or it can be severe, jeopardizing the child's life.

Chest trauma is frequently due to vehicular accidents and these are an important cause of death and disability in children. Chest injuries are responsible for over 25% of fatal automobile accidents in the United States while in another 25% chest injuries were a major factor contributing to death [11]. It is likely, that with better transportation facilities to major centers equipped to deal with trauma in children, many of the patients who otherwise would die at the roadside or en route will arrive critically ill in the emergency room. Increasingly the radiology department will play an essential role in demonstrating the extent of the thoracic trauma and other associated injuries.

Chest radiographs are taken only after initial resuscitation and the establishment of an adequate airway and intravenous access. Occasionally, it is necessary to aspirate the chest in a patient with a suspected pneumothorax or massive hemothorax before initial chest radiographs have been taken. However, with X-ray facilities either within or in close proximity to the emergency room, a single anteroposterior (AP) view of the chest may be taken and processed within 5 min giving information essential for further management.

The ideal chest radiographic techniques of an upright posteroanterior (PA) film at 6 ft in full inspiration and a lateral projection are usually not possible and, with a critically ill child, a single AP film is taken. If the child is sufficiently stable clinically, then a regular upright PA projection is taken and, if abnormal, further views (lateral and lateral decubitus) may be taken as indicated.

The severely traumatized child with chest injuries will usually require skull, spine, abdominal, and limb radiographs because of the high incidence of associated trauma.

10.1 Soft Tissues

Injury to the chest wall may result in soft tissue swelling due to edema, which may be accompanied by hemorrhage, and this may be visible radiographically as a localized swelling with obliteration of the fascial planes. A penetrating wound may result in interstitial emphysema. Localized interstitial air and fluid, with an air-fluid level, may be confused with a lung abscess on a single erect view of the chest [52]. Interstitial air (frequently seen following chest surgery) may accompany lung trauma with fractures of the rib cage and penetration of the lung and pleura.

Interstitial emphysema in the soft tissues of the neck and supraclavicular region, discovered following trauma, may have tracked up from a pneumothorax or pneumomediastinum; such findings raise the possibility of damage to a major bronchus or its branches [52].

10.2 Fractures of the Rib Cage and Sternum

Unlike adults, rib fractures in children are usually obvious in a frontal projection of the chest without resort to oblique views (Fig. 10.1). The distribution of the fractures is important because of their relationship to underlying severe intrathoracic trauma.

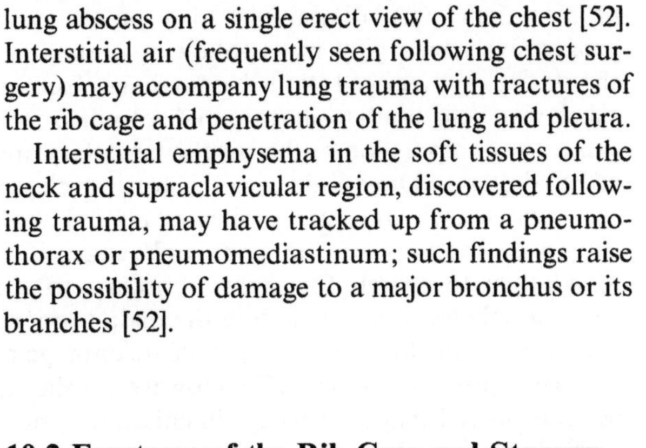

Fig. 10.1. Fractures of the posterior aspects of the left fourth and fifth ribs (*solid arrows*) and a fracture of the lateral aspect of the left fifth rib (*open arrow*). There is a hemothorax on left. Bilateral lung contusion is present with extensive alveolar consolidation and radiating air bronchograms. The tip of the endotracheal tube is a little too low, being down the right main bronchus. This 8-year-old boy was hit by a car

Chronic stress fractures apart, considerable force is required to cause a break in the first rib which is naturally well protected. In a large series that included adults, mortality in patients with first-rib fractures was high due to associated distant injuries to the head, heart, and abdomen [53]. Injury in the vicinity of the first rib included damage to the brachial plexus, subclavian artery, and lung [66]. Subclavian and related arterial thrombosis or hemorrhage may be present at the time of injury, but the development of a posttraumatic aneurysm may not be obvious until later. Arterial injuries are best demonstrated by arteriography, which is indicated in a patient with diminished arm pulses or a progressively enlarging mass following trauma. It should be appreciated that hemorrhage from a subclavian vein or adjacent fractured scapula or ribs can cause compression of the subclavian artery and brachial plexus. Direct injury to the aortic arch has been reported with fractures of the first rib [29]. With extensive fractures of the upper rib cage, it is mandatory to search for signs of injury to the mediastinal structures, including the main bronchi. Fractures of the lower ribs may indicate damage to the liver, spleen, or kidneys [52]. However, it should be remembered that the rib cage in children is more resilient than in adults and more force is required to fracture the rib [55]. It is possible to have severe intrathoracic or upper abdominal injury in a child with an intact rib cage.

Fractures of the posterior ribs in a young infant without a satisfactory history of accidental trauma always raises the possibility of child abuse. In this situation, the fractures are usually seen in a healing phase on the chest radiographs (Fig. 10.2). A violent squeeze is probably the underlying cause. Further fractures at various stages of healing, may be seen on a full skeletal survey.

Fracture of the clavicle in itself is not a serious injury [66]. In newborns, it results from a difficult delivery, particularly a breech. Abundant callus is seen within a few days of the injury. It is rare for there to be any associated complications, although in older patients subclavian artery damage has been reported. Clavicular fractures, although obvious in retrospect, can easily be missed on a routine chest film.

Traumatic retrosternal dislocation of the clavicle at the sternoclavicular joint may compress important structures at the root of the neck. If clinical examination shows asymmetry of the sternoclavicular joints following trauma, then special views, particularly the Heinig projection, are usually required to demonstrate the dislocation [38]. Superior dislocations at the sternoclavicular joint may be obvious on a routine chest film and not require any additional projections (Fig. 10.3).

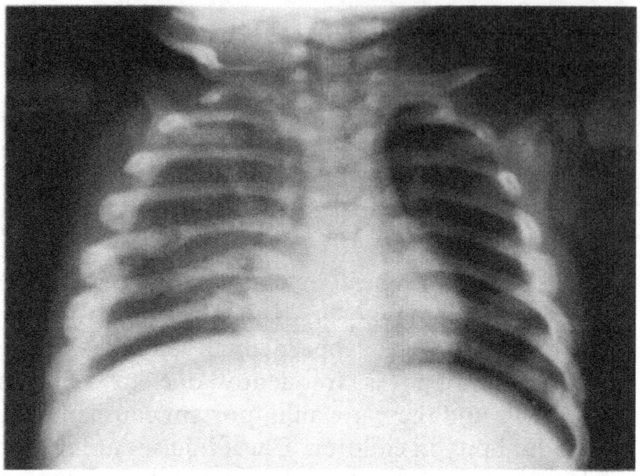

Fig. 10.2. Numerous rib fractures with excessive callus formation and in different stages of healing. A right-sides hemothorax is present. The parents admitted abusing the child

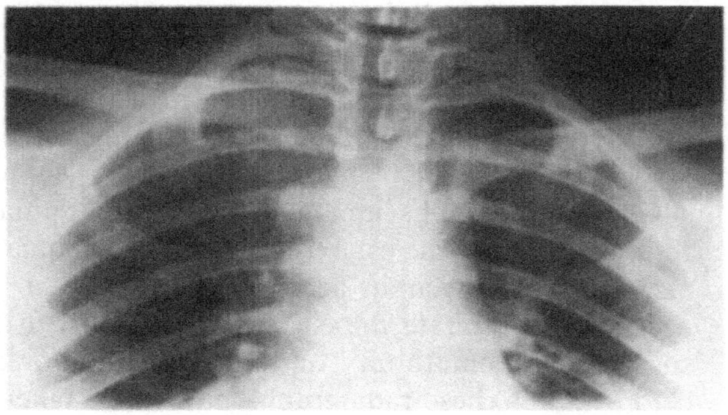

Fig. 10.3. Superior dislocation of the clavicle at the right sternoclavicular joint

Fractures of the sternum are almost always caused by nonpenetrating trauma and are usually associated with multiple fractures of the ribs and costal cartilages. True lateral projections (Fig. 10.4) and, occasionally, tomography are required to show the fracture and the deformity [66]. Cardiac contusion may accompany the injury [22].

10.3 Pneumothorax

A pneumothorax secondary to trauma is usually caused by a fractured rib puncturing the lung or by direct penetrating trauma. The pneumothorax will normally extend throughout the pleural space unless there are previous adhesions. On a routine projection, even the smallest pneumothorax is usually

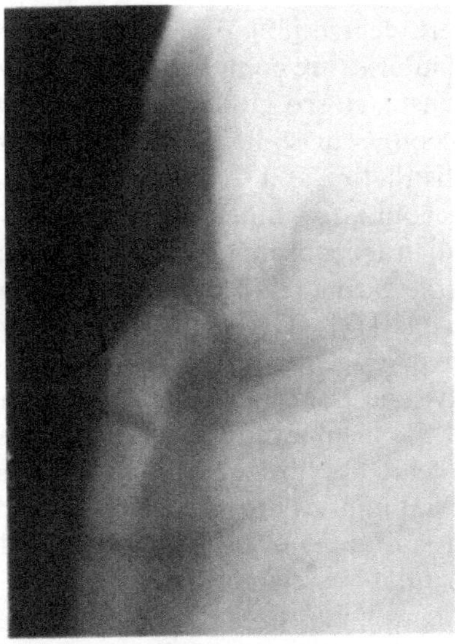

Fig. 10.4. Fracture of the sternum (*open arrow*) resulted when this infant was flung against the car's dashboard during a collision

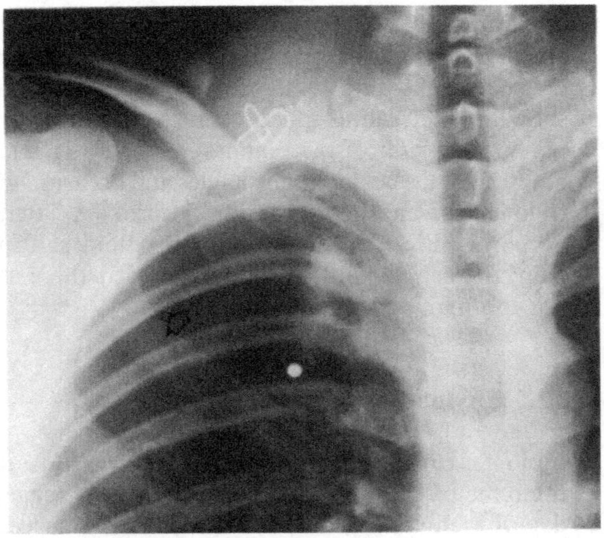

Fig. 10.5. Shallow pneumothorax is present (*open arrow*) following a pellet gun injury to the chest. A paper clip marks the entry site

visible as a lucency separating the lateral border of the lung from the chest wall (Fig. 10.5). In children, skin folds can occasionally simulate the lateral edge of the lung but close inspection reveals that the lung markings pass beyond the edge and that the edge extends beyond the thoracic boundaries (Fig. 10.6).

It is important to diagnose small pneumothoraxes because even these in the presence of severe intrathoracic damage can cause further strain on a critically embarrassed cardiorespiratory system. Medial extension of the pneumothorax can be confused with a pneumomediastinum although the latter usually extends more readily into the soft tissues of the neck and is usually seen on both sides of the mediastinum. In young patients, a pneumomediastinum will elevate the thymus, seen situated anteriorly on a lateral view of the chest. However, from the practical viewpoint, the distinction is immaterial as both indicate potential mediastinal damage following chest trauma.

A tension pneumothorax is obvious radiologically with collapse of the underlying lung and shift of the mediastinum to the opposite side.

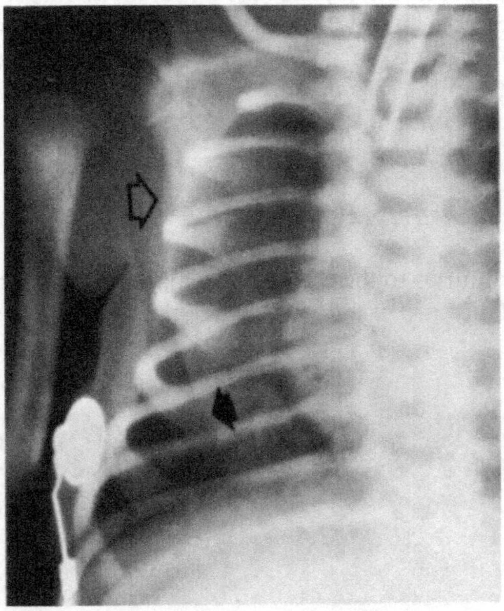

Fig. 10.6. A skin fold (*open arrow*) passing over the right hemithorax gives the spurious appearance of a pneumothorax (*closed arrow*)

10.4 Hemothorax

Blood in the pleural space following trauma results from lung laceration or disruption of vessels in the chest wall, diaphragm, or mediastinum [52, 67]. Although the exact site of bleeding is often difficult to determine, a progressing hemothorax seen on serial films usually indicates bleeding from sites other than the lung [52]. The blood in the pleural space, after initially clotting, liquefies and then moves freely in the pleural space. The fluid can usually be seen, on the routine chest PA projection, situated laterally and obscuring the costophrenic angle (Fig. 10.1). If there is air in the pleural space in addition to fluid, then an air-fluid level will be seen on an upright film. If the fluid is confined to the subpulmonic pleural space, then there will be apparent elevation of the diaphragm. There is often blunting of the costophrenic angles and occasionally fluid is present in the major fissures. A lateral decubitus film will usually show the fluid shifting from the subpulmonic position provided there are not too many adhesions.

10.5 Chylothorax

Fluid that contains a high proportion of fat and often recurs rapidly following aspiration is suggestive of a chylothorax. This usually follows surgery but can happen with other forms of penetrating trauma. The chylothorax does not become evident until several days after injury because, initially, the collection is mediastinal [67]. The site of leakage can be demonstrated with a positive contrast lymphangiogram [25] but it is usually apparent at surgery. No radiological criteria can distinguish chyle from any other fluid on a chest radiograph, although theoretically it would have a lower absorption coefficient on a CT scan of the thorax.

10.6 Tracheobronchial Injury

Major injuries to the trachea and major bronchi are rare. They are usually caused by a closed chest trauma of a severe degree [30]. The mechanics of tracheobronchial injuries are complex. Compressive forces acting against a closed glottis, with the lungs in inspiration, account for some of the injuries. A combination of distracting and shearing forces with some rotation account for other injuries [8, 66]. About 80% of all tracheobronchial injuries occur within 2.5 cm of the carina [8]. The rupture may be complete or partial [11]. The majority of large airway injuries involve the main stem bronchus and about 15% involve the trachea. In the trachea the tear is vertical in the membranous portion but just above the carina tears are horizontal [67]. Bilateral main stem bronchial injuries are rare. Survival with complete laceration of a major bronchus is possible only if the major hilar vessels are spared.

The chest radiograph may be surprisingly normal but with a complete tear there is usually a pneumomediastinum and a large pneumothroax, with the underlying collapsed lung falling away from the mediastinum on an upright film [45]. About 50% of patients with bronchial rupture have upper rib fractures [6, 8]. With an incomplete bronchial rupture, a bayonet deformity of the bronchus may be apparent on a penetrated chest film, and tomograms are often of assistance. Persistent collapse of the underlying lung following trauma suggests bronchial stenosis and this can be confirmed by bronchoscopy and bronchography [11] (Fig. 10.7). Good results following a late repair have been reported.

Acute injuries to the cervical trachea may follow blunt or penetrating trauma, a steering wheel blow to the trachea being a common form of injury. Views of

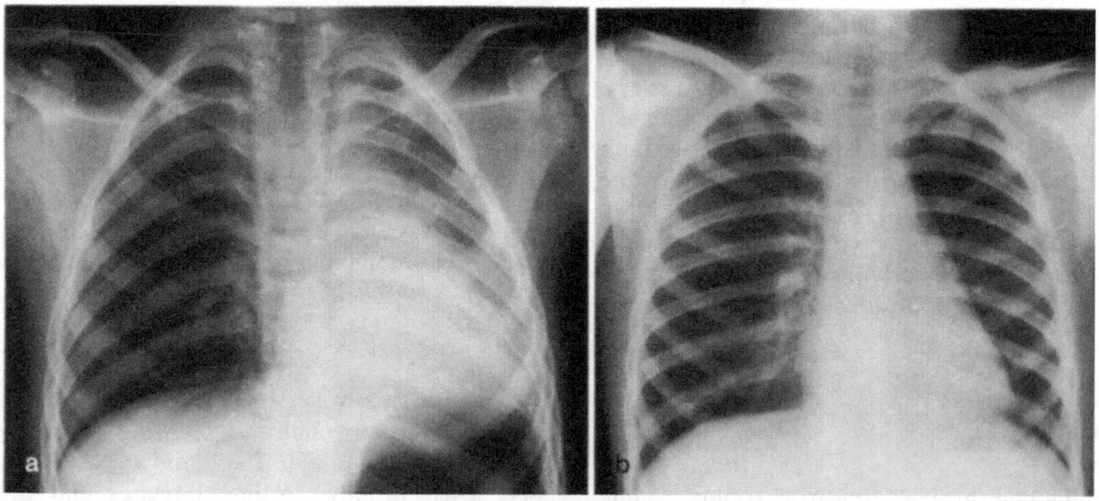

Fig. 10.7. a Chronic atelectasis of the left lower lobe 8 months after a vehicular accident. Bronchoscopy disclosed excessive granulation around an old left lower lobe bronchial rupture. **b** Complete expansion followed surgical repair

the neck will show subcutaneous emphysema, and actual tracheal laceration may be apparent on routine views or may require tomography or high kilovoltage lateral views.

10.7 Lung Contusion, Hematoma Formation, and Lung Cysts

Pulmonary contusion is the most common lesion resulting from closed chest trauma [65]. Within hours of the injury, a localized alveolar pattern, which may be patchy or confluent with radiating air bronchograms, is seen on the chest radiograph (Fig. 10.1). It should be emphasized that the chest radiograph may be normal on admission [34]. The contusion, unlike pneumonia, is not confined by lobar boundaries [11, 12, 28]. Aspiration and fluid overload and fat embolism are included in the differential diagnosis. However, the changes of fluid overload are usually more symmetrical when compared with contusion and the radiographic appearances of fat embolism usually do not appear until 1–2 days after injury. Resolution starts within 48–72 h. Failure to show progressive clearing within 72 h usually indicates continual parenchymal damage or development of pneumonia or atelectasis. There are often other injuries associated with lung contusion [1].

A cavitating pulmonary lesion may result from pulmonary laceration [12, 16, 48, 60]. The pulmonary injury leading to cavitation may be severe or relatively minor [10]. Within hours of the injury, single or multiple cavities, often containing airfluid levels surrounded by a variable amount of consolidation, will be apparent (Figs. 10.8, 10.9). The clinical course is usually benign. The presence of these cysts at the bases can make distinction from a ruptured diaphragm difficult on a plain film alone [10]. These cysts are usually present from the beginning although they may be obscured by surrounding consolidation. This distinguishes posttraumatic pneumatoceles from cavity-forming pulmonary hematomas where the cavity only appears as the hematoma resolves.

More severe blunt trauma, or injury by a fractured rib or weapon, may cause a pulmonary laceration and hematoma formation. Initially, there is radiological evidence of associated contusion which obscures the changes of pulmonary laceration and hematoma formation. When the initial changes have cleared, there is often a rounded well defined mass which may later be surrounded by an air meniscus as the hematoma resolves by solidifying and contracting over a period of days. A pneumatocele may be the end result of a hematoma. If the hematoma remains as a solid mass, then a history of trauma is of importance in reaching the correct diagnosis. However, most hematomas resolve within 5 weeks.

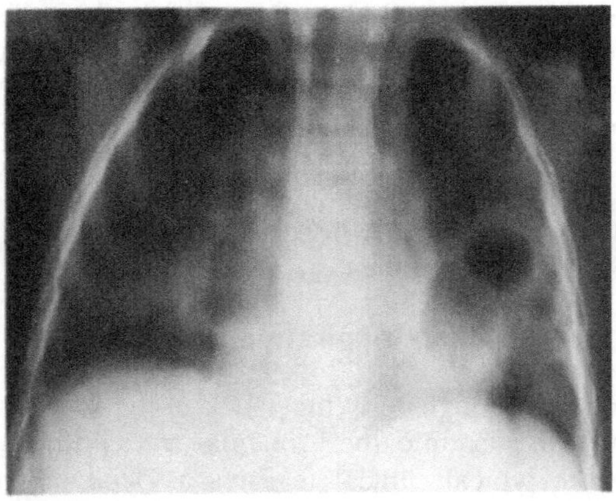

Fig. 10.8. AP tomogram revealing numerous pneumatoceles with surrounding contusion in 18-month-old child who had been savaged by a great dane

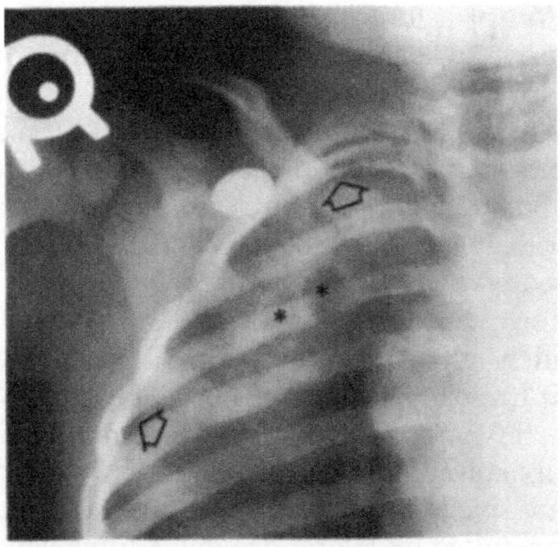

Fig. 10.9. Shallow pneumothorax with pneumatoceles and contusion in the underlying lung. Fractures of the posterior aspects of the first and second ribs are present. The patient was struck by a car

10.8 Postshock Lung

Following severe trauma, respiratory difficulties may later become apparent. The etiology is controversial and several factors acting either alone or in combination have been implicated. The precipitating agents include fat embolism, oxygen toxicity, fluid overload, infection, aspiration, and hyperconsumptive coagulopathy [50]. After a few hours, the initial clear lung will show interstitial edema followed by progressive alveolar consolidation, often symmetrical, and in a bat's wing distribution. The heart remains normal in size and there is usually no pleural effusion. Pathologically, there is loss of lung surfactant, decreased pulmonary compliance, damage to alveoli, and hyaline membrane formation.

10.9 Foreign Body Aspiration

An inhaled foreign body may stick in the larynx or trachea or pass into the bronchial tree. Although there are typical clinical features associated with laryngeal foreign bodies, AP and lateral views and sometimes fluoroscopy are necessary to demonstrate the foreign body for certainty. A radiopaque foreign body in the trachea is usually obvious on routine AP/lateral views of the neck (Fig. 10.10).

Inhalation of a foreign body into the bronchial tree can prove to be a diagnostic dilemma for both pediatrician and radiologist, particularly with chronic cases. In this situation the initial event may not be remembered, and the child presents with recurrent pneumonia resistant to therapy. The consolidation is often lobar or segmental in distribution. Bronchoscopy, and occasionally bronchography, is required for the correct diagnosis.

The acutely inhaled body may act as a check valve, causing air trapping distal to the partial obstruction. In adults, this is usually best demonstrated by an inspiration/expiration films. However, in children who are not so cooperative, selective air trapping is best demonstrated by lateral decubitus films which will demonstrate selective air trapping in the lowermost lung.

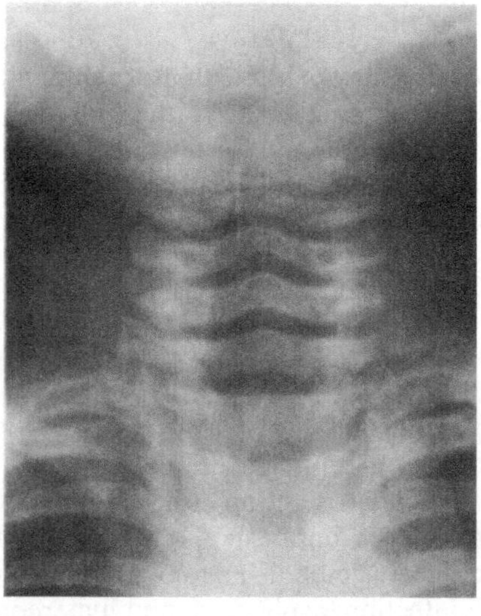

Fig. 10.10. Radiopaque foreign body in the upper trachea

10.10 Toxic Inhalation Pneumonitis

The most common group of inhaled toxins are the hydrocarbons. These include gasolene, lighter fuels, kerosene, cleaning fluids, and liquid polishes and waxes [14]. These hydrocarbons have decreased surface tension and viscosity and increased volatility all of which increase the risk of lung damage and aspiration [18]. The lower the surface tension the more likely aspiration is to occur, with the hydrocarbon "creeping" into the lungs [13]. There is considerable evidence to show that absorption from the gastrointestinal tract does not play a significant part in producing pulmonary lesions [5, 14].

Significant involvement of the respiratory tract occurs in 25%–40% of patients [14]. Symptoms of respiratory involvement (dyspnea with nonproductive cough) usually progress for 24 h and then plateau before subsiding between the 2nd and 5th days [14]. Pathological examinations of fatal cases have shown formation of hyaline membranes together with a necrotizing bronchopneumonia and polymorphonuclear exudate [14].

The radiological changes may vary from a normal chest or slight lung hyperexpansion to alveolar infiltrates, atelectasis, pneumothorax, pneumomediastinum, and pneumopericardium [2]. Pneumatoceles have recently been described [2, 24] (Fig. 10.11). They usually appear within a discrete area of consolidation during the 2nd or 3rd week of the illness and may not be discovered if radiographs are not taken because the disease appears to be resolving satisfactorily on clinical findings. The pneumatoceles are probably due to a check valve mechanism. They usually resolve with no sequelae.

Inhalation of barium will occur if excessive contrast is injected into the upper pouch of a patient with esophageal atresia (Fig. 10.12) and in patients with paryngeal incoordination. A lipoid inhalation pneumonia can occur in infants given oral oily solutions over a long period of time. Patchy asymmetric consolidation that often involves the upper lobes is seen radiologically. A barium esophagram should be performed to look for reflux or obstruction which could be responsible for the inhalation pneumonia.

Another form of lipoid pneumonia may follow lymphangiography [20]. Within hours, the patient develops fever, cough, and dyspnea. A chest radiograph shows diffuse ground-glass appearance, but in severe cases there may be more confluent consolidation which usually resolves within 36–48 h.

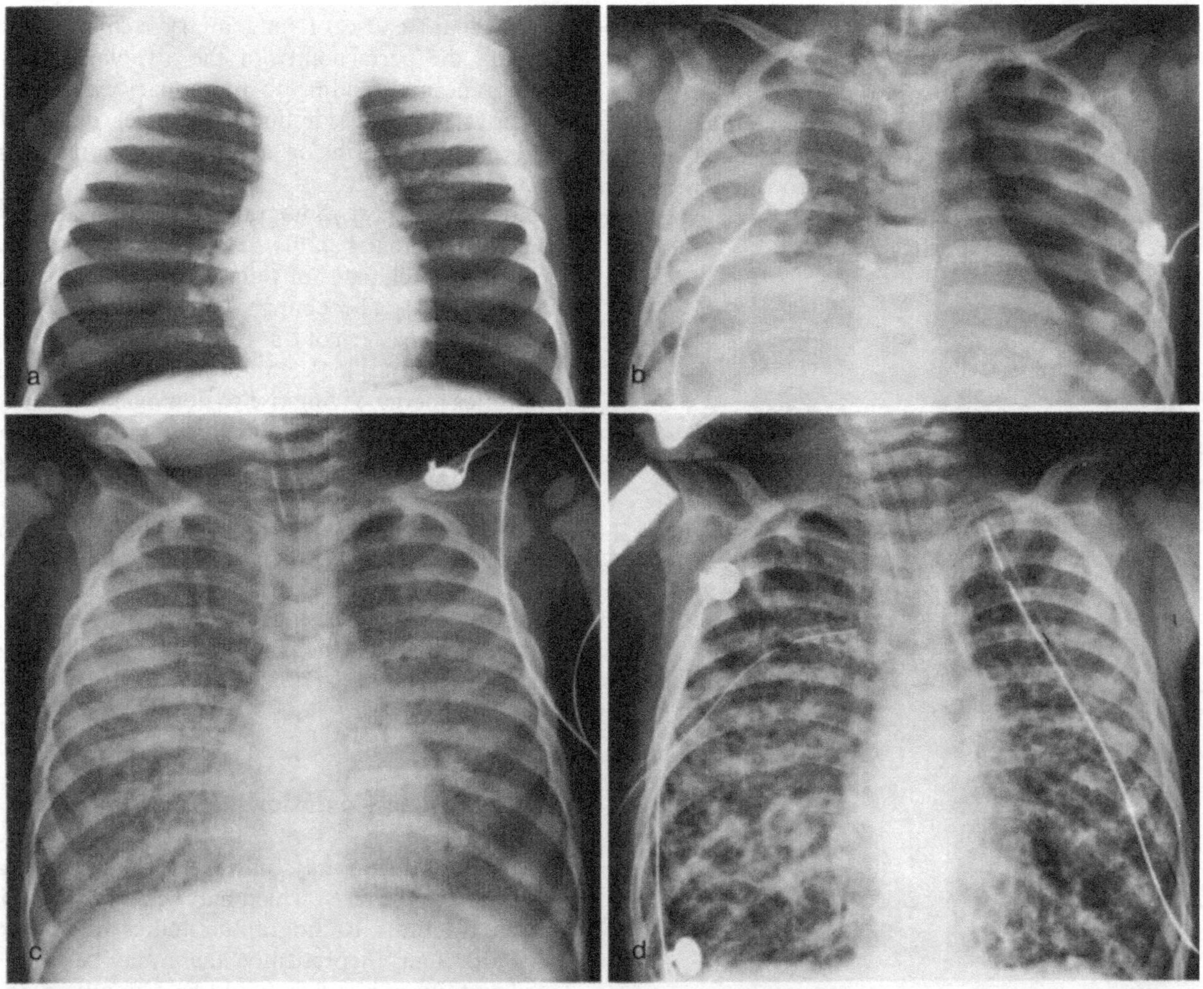

△

Fig. 10.11. a Admission chest film immediately after inhalation of *Old English* furniture polish shows hyperexpansion. **b** Three days later there is a pneumomediastinum with extensive lung consolidation especially on the right. **c** Twelve days later: symmetrical alveolar infiltrates with early cyst formation are present. **d** 24 days later: extensive honeycombing of the lungs has occurred with bilateral pneumothoraxes. The patient died the following day

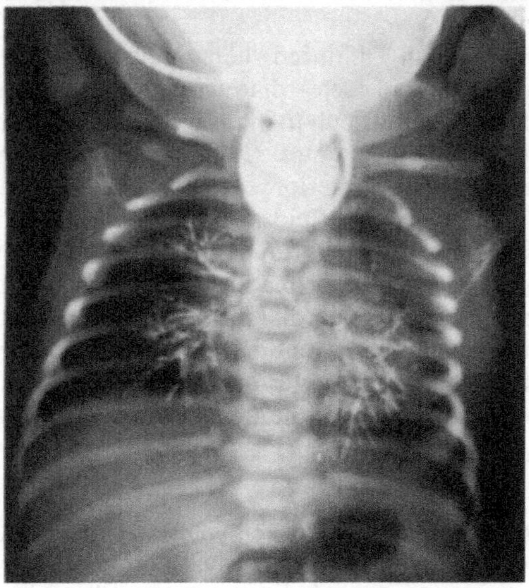

◁ **Fig. 10.12.** Excessive barium introduced into the upper pouch with overflow into the lungs. This is preventable with caution and fluoroscopy

10.11 Near Drowning

In the United States, particularly in California, drowning is a common cause of accidental death in children. Many children who are rescued in time exhibit the syndrome of near drowning in which hypoxia, pulmonary edema, acidosis, and aspiration are the prime composites [51].

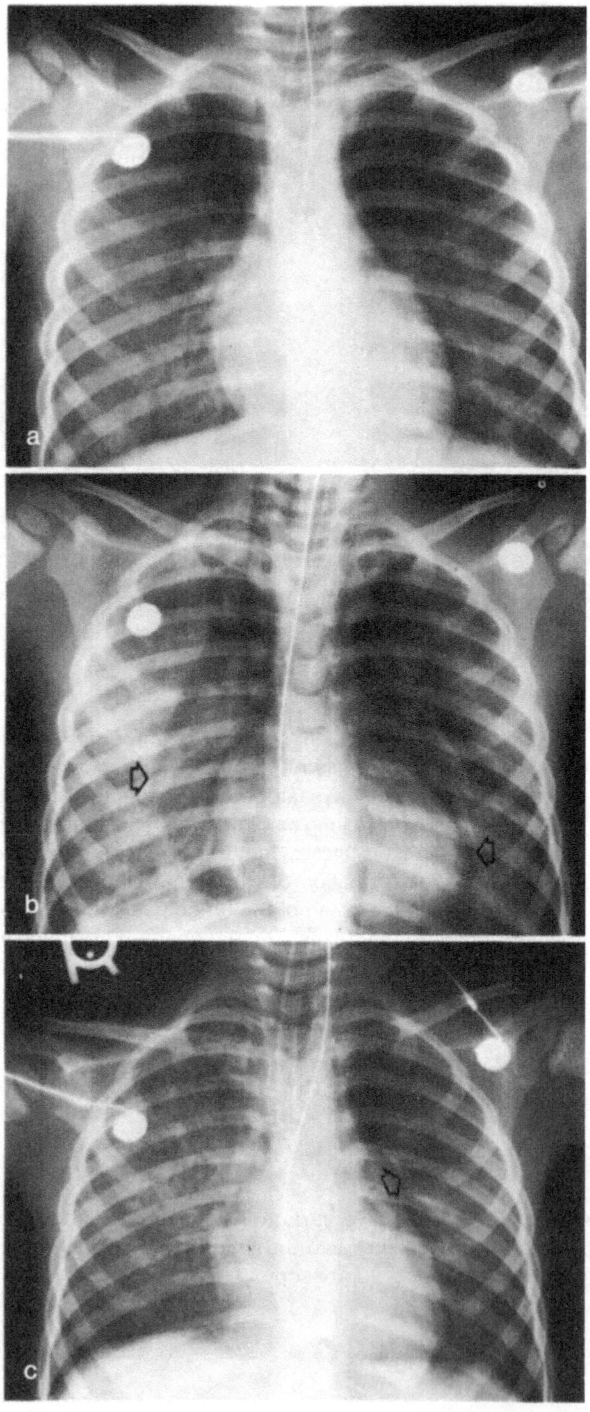

The main cause of lung injury is hypoxia [31] altering the permeability of the alveolar/capillary membrane and leading to pulmonary edema [51], which is also caused, but to a lesser degree, by aspiration of chlorine or salt/fresh water and gastric juices [31].

The initial chest radiograph bears little relationship to the clinical status. A delay of 24–48 h may occur before changes of pulmonary edema become apparent [51]. The changes may be mild, with a symmetrical pattern of fine alveolar infiltrates in the perihilar regions [51]. In more severe cases, the infiltrates merge, giving rise to homogeneous opacification of both lungs on air bronchograms. There is a degree of air block and there is always the danger of barotrauma if a respirator is required (Fig. 10.13).

There is usually clearing of the lung in 3–5 days, some taking up to 10 days. Superimposed pneumonia will prolong the clearing [31]. The radiological features appear to be independent of the composition of the fluid in which the child has been immersed [51].

10.12 Cardiac Contusion

Cardiac contusion may follow severe nonpenetrating injury to the chest which may be associated with sternal fractures. Radiographic studies are unnecessary although, theoretically, there may be signs of cardiac failure, but this would be difficult to diagnose in the presence of other severe intrathoracic injury.

Traumatically induced hemopericardium may show widening of the cardiac silhouette (Fig. 10.14) but this may be difficult to interpret on a AP film at a short film-focus distance. On a lateral projection, there may be fluid anterior to the epicardial fat stripe although pericardial fluid is best assessed by echocardiography if there is doubt clinically. If there is a penetrating wound, air may be introduced into the pericardiac sac. Pericardial air can be differentiated from a pneumomediastinum because a pneumopericardium is limited anteriorly by the pericardial reflection at the root of the great vessels and will pass

◁

Fig. 10.13. a Initial chest radiograph showing faint alveolar infiltrates. The patient was found floating head down in a swimming pool. **b** Following day, there is an extensive pneumomediastinum (*arrows*) with extensive consolidation on the right side. **c** Two days later, there has been considerable resolution although a small pneumomediastinum is still present

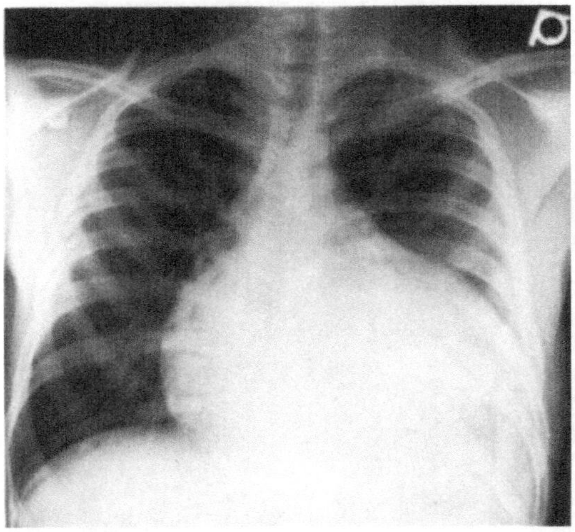

Fig. 10.14. This 18-year-old boy was stabbed in the chest. The cardiac silhouette is widened. At surgery, a hemopericardium was drained. Old shotgun pellets to the left chest wall are noted

under the base of the heart, whereas a pneumomediastinum will not.

10.13 Aortic Laceration/Rupture

Severe deceleration forces to the chest can impose such a severe shearing stress that the aortic wall can be disrupted [41]. This usually occurs at the aortic isthmus where the relatively fixed arch joins the more mobile descending aorta [41]. A less common site is just above the aortic valve [61]. The tear, which is usually anterior, starts at the intima and may involve the media and adventitia [17]. Even with disruption of the adventitia, fatal hemorrhage may be prevented by the restraining action of the mediastinal structures. With an incomplete tear, a false aneurysm may result and this may not manifest itself clinically for some time. Rarely a dissection will occur [66]. To a certain extent, patients with aortic tears are self-selective, 80%–90% dying immediately following the accident [17, 37]. Of the survivors, many are critically ill on arrival in the emergency room while a small group is deceptively well. Clinical findings include retrosternal pain, upper arm hypertension, and diminished or absent femoral pulses. There may be an interscapular bruit [17]. Associated severe injuries are not uncommon [17], including cardiac injury [47]. A chest radiograph will often show rib fractures. There is usually widening of the upper mediastinum, but this may be difficult to interpret with an AP film that has a relatively short film-tube distance. If at all possible, a 6-ft PA film should be taken. In addition to the mediastinal widening, there may be blurring of the left lateral border of the aortic arch and downward depression of the left main bronchus [17, 66]. The trachea is usually displaced to the right along with the esophagus as shown by the position of the nasogastric tube. There may be an associated pneumothorax with an apical component [17]. Left-sided hemothorax, pneumothorax, pneumomediastinum and intrapulmonary hemorrhage, reflecting severe trauma, are often present [36]. If there is doubt clinically and the patient's condition permits, a repeat AP film will often show progressive widening with obliteration of the aortopulmonary window. A lateral projection will also confirm these finding.

The exact site and number of tears of the aorta can only be demonstrated by arteriography. The catheter is usually introduced through the right brachial artery, particularly if there are poor femoral pulses, to avoid passing the catheter through the tear. However, the femoral route has been used in many patients in which event the catheter should be preceded by a soft-tip J-shaped guide wire [17]. Filming in the left anterior oblique projection is useful. The tear is usually in the anterior wall of the aorta at the site of the isthmus. Angiographic findings are variable [17]. A thin radiolucent line of rolled-up edge indicates an intimal flap [36] whereas filling of an aneurysm means a more severe disruption. The aorta is often narrowed at the site of disruption, partly by the tear and also by the surrounding hematoma. Extravasation from the aorta is rare although leakage of contrast has been recorded from tears in smaller vessels (e. g., internal mammary) which can clinically mimic aortic rupture [64]. Documentation of a double-barred lumen or intimal septa establishes the diagnosis of a dissecting aneurysm. Multiple aortic tears which can only be revealed by arteriography have been reported [17]. Aortography has the additional advantage that injuries to other intrathoracic vessels may be demonstrated [17, 37].

A periaortic hematoma due to thoracic injuries other than aortic laceration can best be diagnosed by aortography (Fig. 10.15).

10.14 Esophagus

In children, rupture of the esophagus is usually due to blunt trauma to the chest or neck. This is often complicated by mediastinitis. Chest pain, dysphagia, and crepitation in the soft tissues of the neck are usually present. A chest radiograph usually reveals

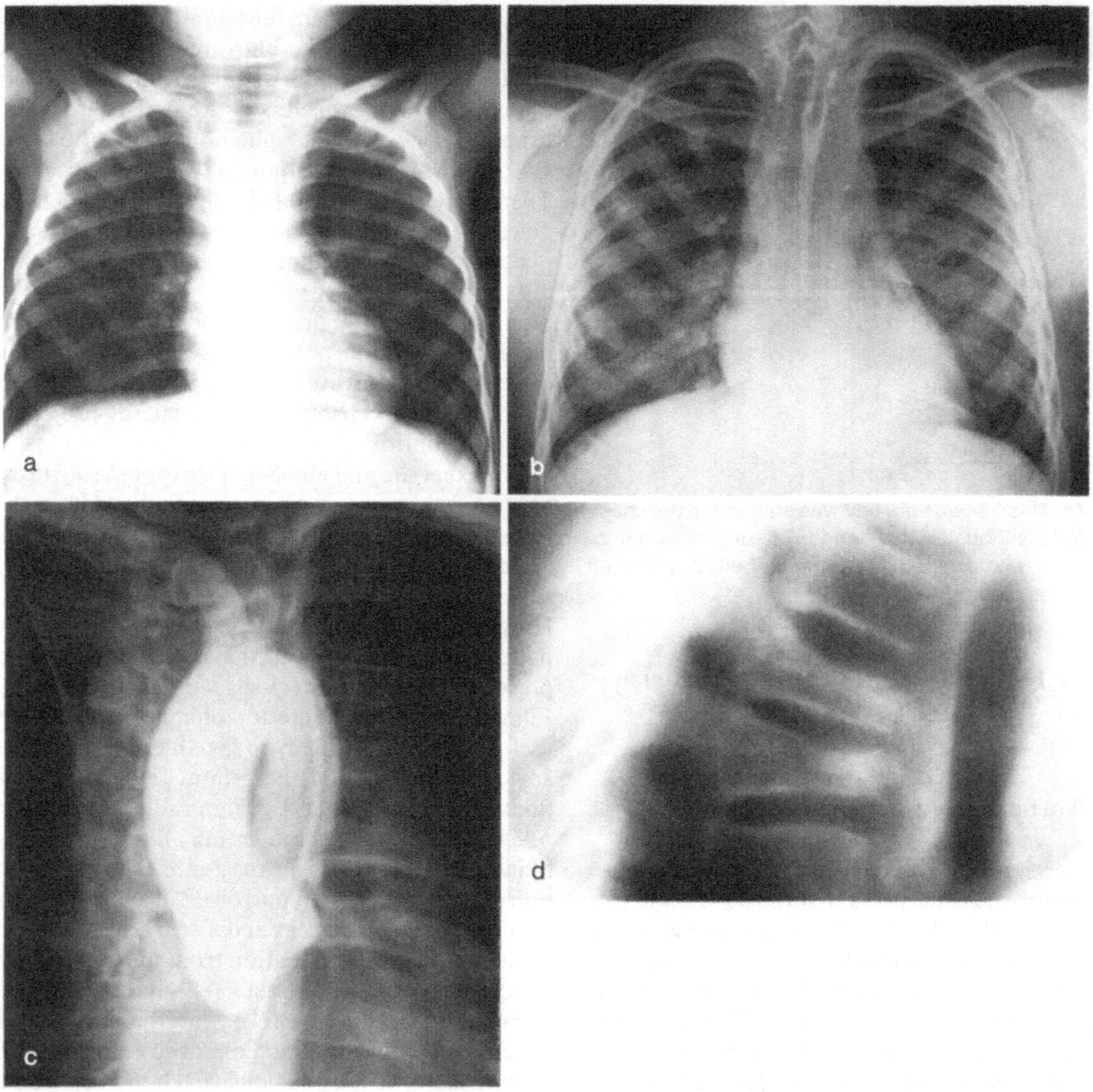

Fig. 10.15. a Initial chest film of a 10-year-old boy revealed widening of the mediastinum following an automobile accident. **b** No significant deviation of the esophagus was demonstrated. **c** Aortogram shows no dissection or extravasation. **d** Lateral *tomogram* demonstrates traumatic wedging of two consecutive thoracic vertebrae which were responsible for the mediastinal hematoma

subcutaneous emphysema and pneumomediastinum with pleural fluid. A pneumothorax may also be present. The site and extent of the rupture can best be demonstrated by water-soluble contrast medium (Fig. 10.16). A high or mid-esophageal tear may communicate with the trachea. The prognosis is usually better if this does occur. Later complications include esophageal stenosis and posttraumatic tracheoesophageal fistula [22].

The most common cause of esophageal trauma in children is ingestion of lye. Initially, there is spasm, edema, and ulceration which may resolve but is usually followed by a fibrous stricture. The stricture is often of some length and may not be obvious clinically until the child swallows a large poorly masticated bolus of food. This also applies to other strictures as a result of reflux esophagitis or secondary to repair of a congenital tracheoesophageal fistula. With the latter group there may, in addition, be esophageal dyskinesia and a lower stricture, either of unknown etiology or secondary to reflux esophagitis, which is often present in these children.

Swallowed foreign bodies may ulcerate the esophagus, and the subsequent periesophageal inflammatory tissue encases the trachea, causing stridor. A tracheoesophageal fistula may occur. Sometimes,

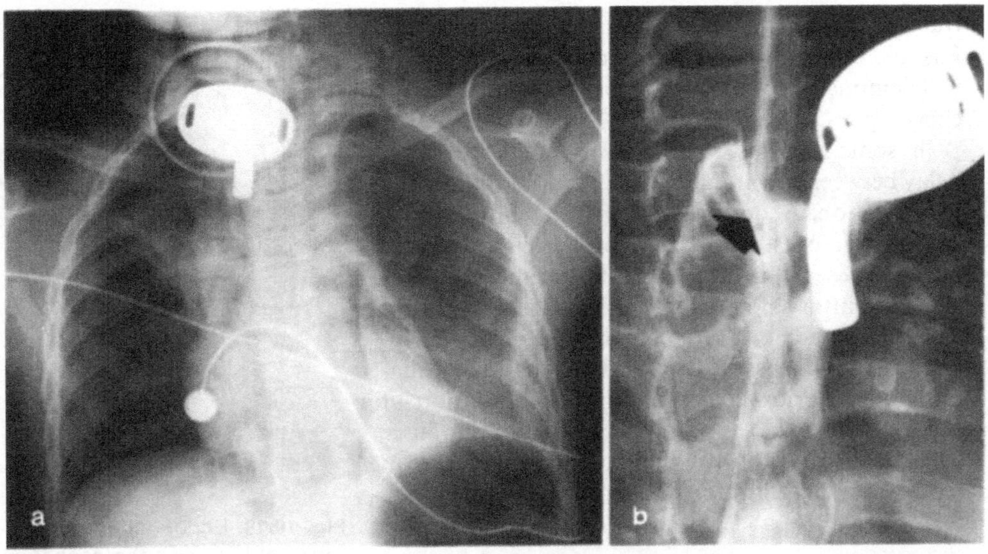

Fig. 10.16. a Chest film of teenager who was struck in the neck by a shopping cart shows mediastinal air (present before the emergency tracheostomy). Consolidation at the left base and a left pleural effusion are also present. **b** Water-soluble contrast esophagram showing extravasation of contrast from a tear (*arrow*)

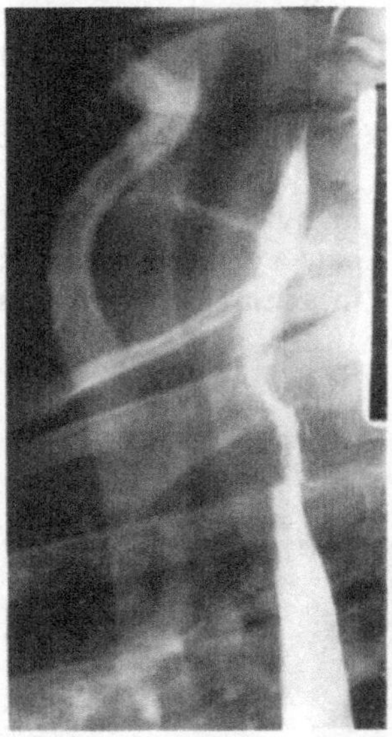

Fig. 10.17. A barium esophagram showing mucosal irregularity with some narrowing of the lumen due to an ingested can "pop top." Note narrowing of the adjacent trachea

because of its shape and limited radiopacity, a foreign body may not be visible in a single projection [43]. If there is a definite history of an ingested foreign body, then films in multiple projections and a barium esophagram are required. Newman [43] draws attention to the variety of respiratory symptoms that can be associated with an esophageal foreign body. The symptoms are related to the surrounding edema and inflammatory tissue, usually located just below the cricopharyngeal constriction or the thoracic inlet [32] which is the most common site for impaction for esophageal foreign bodies (Fig. 10.17).

10.15 Diaphragmatic Injury

The diaphragm is not infrequently injured by penetrating wounds or blunt trauma to the lower thorax and upper abdomen. In *blunt* trauma, the left diaphragm, particularly the dome, is most frequently injured, the right being protected by the liver [3, 27, 68].

If all types of injury, including penetrating wounds, are considered, then there is no predilection to either side [68]. Associated injuries to the liver and stomach accompany penetrating trauma, and fractured ribs and splenic rupture are often seen with blunt trauma [62, 68]. Bilateral diaphragmatic rupture [42] and multiple defects within a single diaphragmatic leaf have been reported [3].

Usually, diagnostic difficulties are not encountered with penetrating trauma. With blunt trauma, radiology has a more important role. The chest radiograph may show hemothorax, elevation of the diaphragm, or herniation of a hollow organ, usually the stomach, into the chest. In one series, every patient with diaphragmatic rupture had some abnormality on the admission chest radiograph [62] although in another review of patients with blunt trauma, only 37% had abnormal radiographs [68]. Passage of a nasogastric tube and instillation of air will demonstrate if the stomach is herniated into the chest.

In some patients there may be an appreciable delay between the moment of injury and the start of investigation. Abdominal symptoms relating to incarceration of strangulation of herniated viscera may be present. In these patients, barium examinations and intravenous urograms may be helpful. The barium will demonstrate constriction of the herniated gut as it passes through the rent in the diaphragm. Arteriographic findings of herniation of the liver through a ruptured right diaphragm have been described [15] although a radionuclide scan would give similar information and is noninvasive.

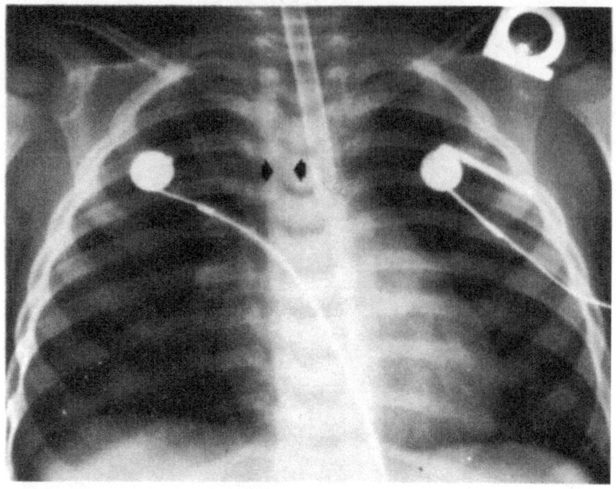

Fig. 10.18. Endotracheal tube is not within the trachea (*arrows*) but down the esophagus

10.16 Trauma Related to Artificial Support Systems and Resuscitation

10.16.1 Endotracheal Intubation

Overzealous insertion of an endotracheal tube is usually manifested radiographically with the tip down a main bronchus, usually the right. Depending upon the size of the tube and exact position of its tip, there may be a combination of atelectasis and hyperexpansion (Fig. 10.17). In a large series, which includes children, intubation of the right main bronchus was associated with decreased survival [69].

If the tube appears to project beyond the radiographically visible walls of the trachea, then it may well have been inadvertently introduced into the esophagus (Fig. 10.18). Clinical inspection or a lateral projection will usually resolve the doubt.

A pneumomediastinum and subcutaneous emphysema is occasionally seen when there have been many attempts by inexperienced personnel to intubate a child. Presumably the attempts have resulted in a tear in the mucosa of the hypopharynx (Fig. 10.19).

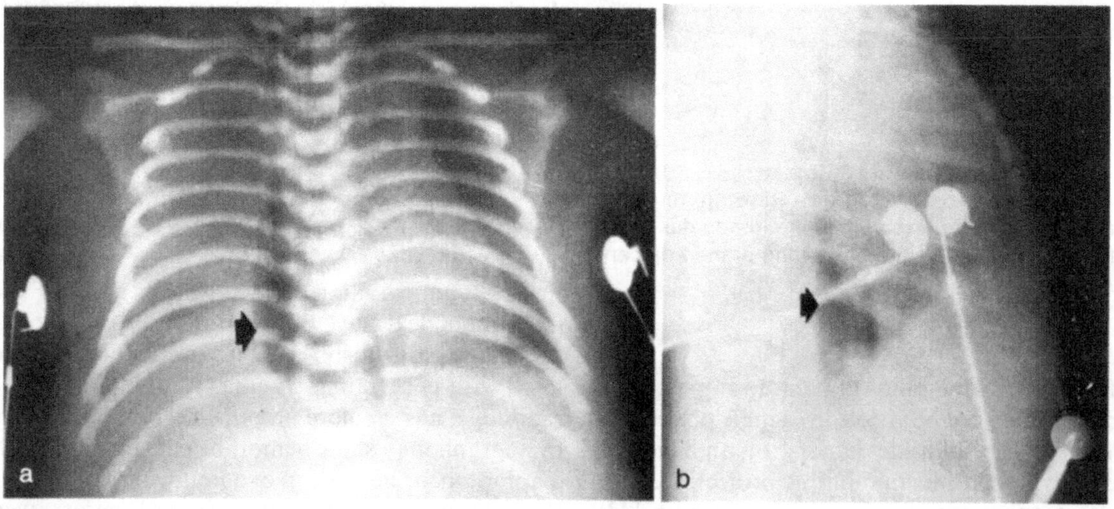

Fig. 10.19. a Numerous attempts were made to intubate this newborn infant. There was a collection of posterior mediastinal air (*solid arrow*) presumably secondary to a breech in the pharyngeal mucosa. **b** Lateral projection confirming the posterior distribution of the mediastinal air

10.16.2 Vascular Catheters

Intravenous access catheters are introduced either for measurement of central venous pressure or for long-term intravenous therapy. The tip of the catheter should, ideally, be within the body of the right atrium or immediate superior vena cava where there is a high flow rate to dilute the thrombogenic hyperosmolar solutions [35]. Progressive widening of the mediastinum with pleural effusions suggests that the catheter has perforated the heart or superior vena cava resulting in extravasation of intravenous fluid [35]. If confirmation is required, then the injection of 2–3 ml dilute water-soluble contrast agent and a single film taken at the end of injection will show the leakage (Fig. 10.20). Other complications associated with the intravascular catheter include septicemia, thrombosis of major vessels, and catheter emboli [26, 35].

10.16.3 Esophageal Pseudodiverticula in the Newborn

Overenthusiastic probing with a suction catheter or finger at delivery can tear the mucosa of the posterior wall of the pharynx, causing a dissection [19, 39]. The breach is always just above the level of the cricopharyngeus. A nasogastric tube often passes preferentially into the pseudodiverticulum and can cause further dissection (Fig. 10.21). A barium esophagram will outline a variable-length diverticulum that is situated posteriorly. There may be a re-entry into the esophagus at a lower level. There is usually filling of the true esophagus although it is often compressed by the diverticulum. However, at esophagoscopy, the true esophageal opening can sometimes be difficult to see. Although having a similar appearance to a traumatic diverticulum on barium swallow, a true diverticulum can be differentiated by esophagoscopy. A pseudodiverticulum usually contains purulent material and has a rough dull appearance, and an irregular tear is always visible [39]. Congenital diverticula are lined with stratified squamous epithelium and have both mucosa and submucosa. Duplications of the esophagus lie anteriorly [59] as opposed to traumatic pseudodiverticula which lie posteriorly. Infants with traumatic pseudodiverticula are usually treated conservatively with spontaneous healing of the diverticula.

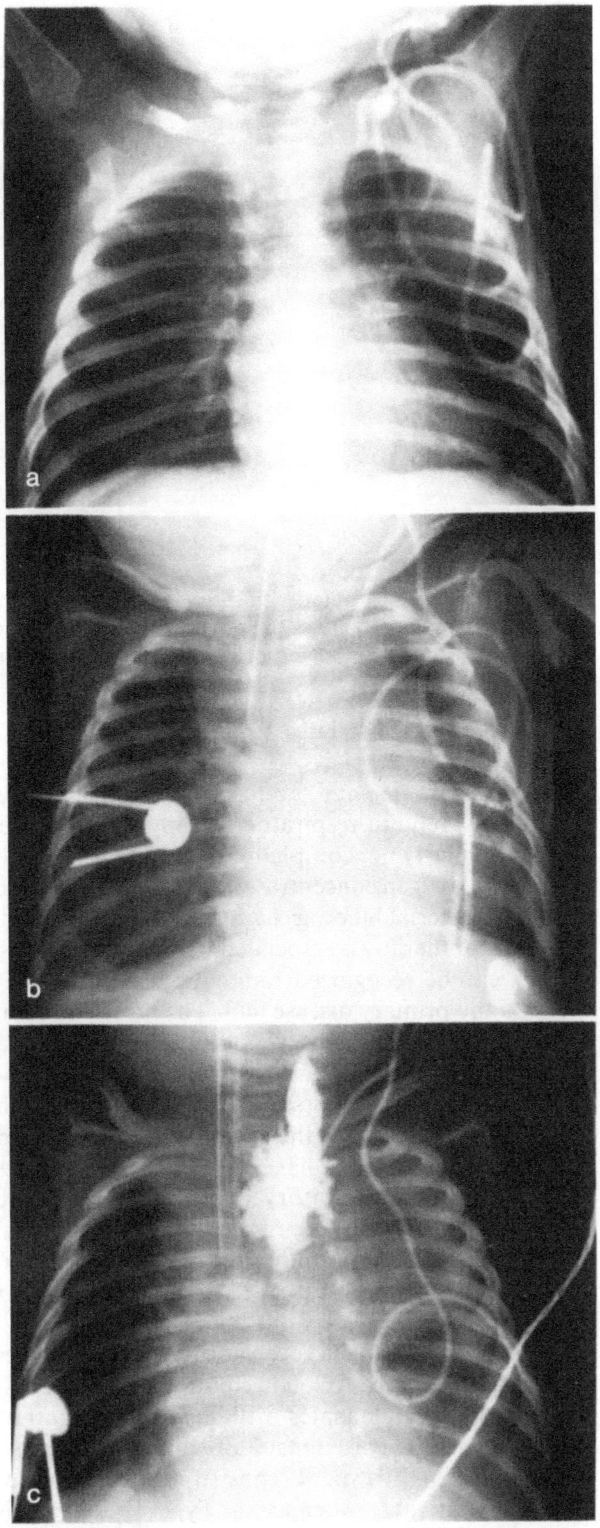

Fig. 10.20. a No important abnormality is seen on this chest radiograph of the child with hyperalimentation. **b** Five days later, there is widening of the mediastinum. **c** Injection of contrast shows extravasation of contrast from the hyperalimentation catheter

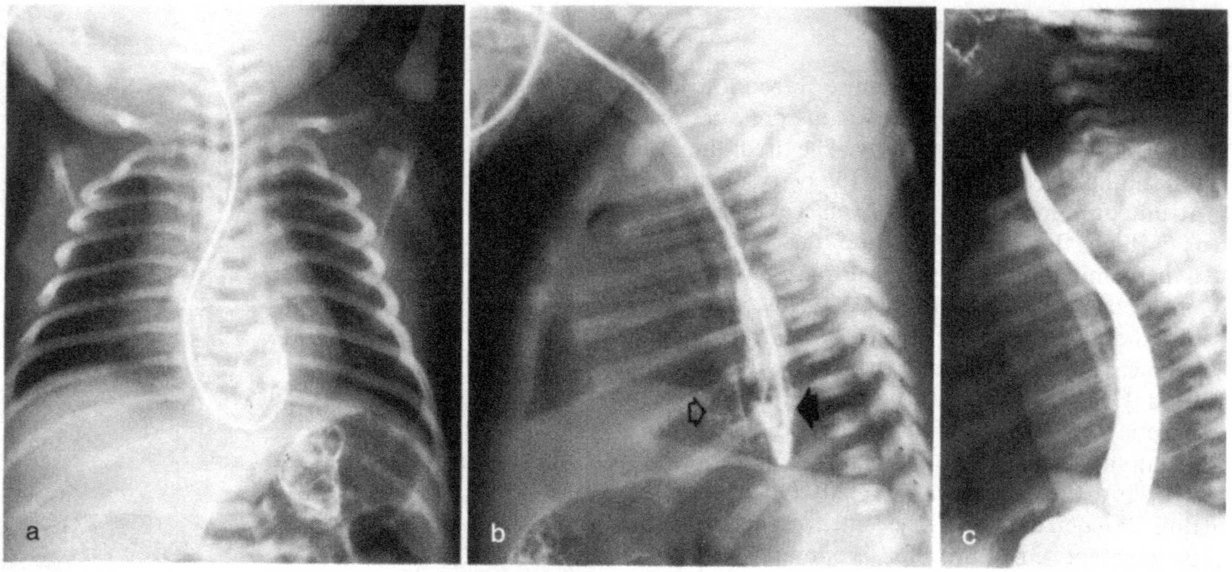

Fig. 10.21. a Initial radiograph after introduction of an esophageal catheter shows the catheter curled up in the lower end of the pseudodiverticulum. **b** Lateral projection confirms the posterior position of the diverticulum. **c** Nine days later, there has been complete healing

10.16.4 Respirator-related Problems

Newborn infants with severe respiratory problems frequently require respirator therapy. If the lungs are particularly noncompliant, then increasing pressures and oxygen concentrations may be required to keep the arterial blood gases at a satisfactory level. Respirator therapy is associated with complications, which can be recognized radiographically in addition to the primary disease [40]. The most common complication of assisted ventilation is barotrauma (pneumothorax, pneumomediastinum, pneumopericardium, and interstitial emphysema) which adds significantly to the overall morbidity and mortality. Barotrauma has been noted when infants with idiopathic respiratory distress syndrome are improving, probably because as the parenchymal disease improves, continuous use of pressures necessary earlier in the disease will now cause alveolar overdistension [23].

In a radiological survey, Swischuk [63] describes three different types of bubble pattern seen on chest radiographs of neonates with hyaline membrane disease which may be a result of respirator therapy. The bubbles in Type I consist of dilatation of terminal airways, whereas in Type II the air is located in the pulmonary interstitium, and Type III is seen in the reparative stage of hyaline membrane disease with underlying bronchopulmonary dysplasia. Air that is interstitial (Type II) will track along the bronchovascular pathways to the hilum to collect as a pneumothorax or pneumomediastinum.

Intravascular air embolism is a rare but well recognized complication of positive pressure ventilation in hyaline membrane disease. Air escaping from a ruptured alveolus passes into a pulmonary venule and then into the arterial circulation [4, 21, 58]. Gas dissecting into the subadventitial plane of the pulmonary veins may not dissect further into the veins but may pass centrifugally to cause a pneumopericardium or hilar compression of pulmonary veins by subadventitial air [4]. However, Gregory and Tooley [21] offer the alternative theory of air being sucked into the umbilical vein around the catheter, and air may also enter the circulation this way via the umbilical artery. Research in rats has shown that the use of high inspiratory and expiratory pressures increases the incidence of air embolism, and conditions associated with pulmonary edema decrease the probability of its occurrence [33].

Intermittent positive pressure ventilation via an endotracheal tube together with high oxygen toxicity over a period of time has been implicated as a contributing factor to the origin of bronchopulmonary dysplasia [44, 49].

Gastric distension and perforation, which can be seen radiographically, are other important complications accompanying positive pressure ventilation in infants and children [40].

Oh [46] found certain radiological patterns in children who were on continuous positive pressure breathing. The lungs are usually hyperinflated. As a result, a paralyzed diaphragm may be depressed to a normal level and not detected on the chest radiograph. There is rapid clearing of pulmonary edema and focal atelectasis and also exaggerated shift of the mediastinum with continuing lobar atelectasis.

10.17 Trauma Related to Therapy

10.17.1 Radiation- and Chemotherapy-induced Pneumonitis

Radiation therapy may result in acute radiation pneumonitis or chronic interstitial fibrosis. The acute reaction occurs from 2 weeks to 6 months following completion of therapy [56]. Cough, dyspnea, and fever are characteristic features. The chest radiograph shows alveolar consolidation within the irradiated field (Fig. 10.22) which may either resolve or progress to the chronic fibrotic form of the disease. In the latter case, the fibrotic changes are clearly delineated and reflect the field limited by the port aperture.

Natural progression of the malignant disease, superimposed infections and drug-related pulmonary disease have to be considered in the differential diagnosis of acute radiation pneumonitis [56]. *Pneumocystis carinii* pneumonia can resemble acute radiation pneumonia radiographically; both have diffuse perihilar alveolar infiltrates. A biopsy may be necessary to differentiate between the two.

Three drugs used in the therapy of malignant disease have been implicated in causing diffuse pulmonary disease. Busulfan and bleomycin can cause progressive dyspnea accompanied by diffuse interstitial infiltrates [56]. Methotrexate may manifest itself acutely with cough, fever, and dyspnea, with bilateral confluent alveolar and interstitial infiltrates [9]. There is a chronic form manifested by dyspnea and diffuse interstitial infiltrates similar to busulfan, bleomycin, and chronic irradiation [7]. It should be noted that prior irradiation predisposes to bleomycin-related pulmonary toxicity and can be of a fulminating nature [54].

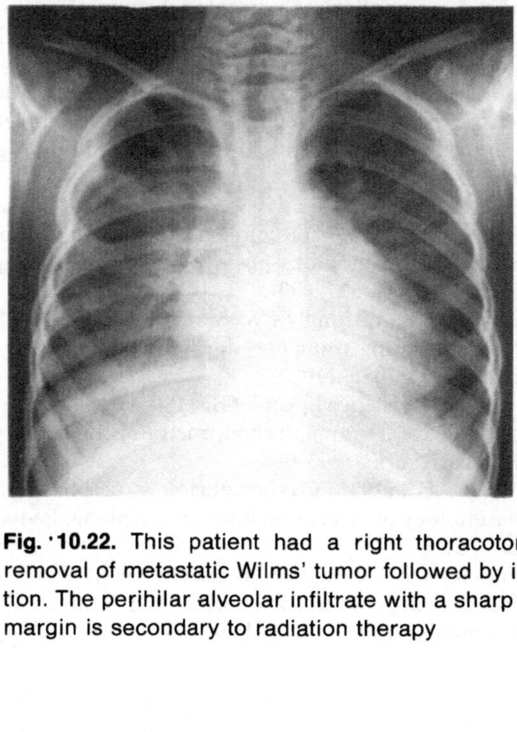

Fig. 10.22. This patient had a right thoracotomy for removal of metastatic Wilms' tumor followed by irradiation. The perihilar alveolar infiltrate with a sharp lateral margin is secondary to radiation therapy

10.17.2 Tracheostomy Complications

Tracheostomy is an important surgical procedure in infants with congenital and inflammatory disorders of the airway. In the majority of patients decannulation proceeds without incident and the tracheostomy heals normally, leaving an uncompromised airway. However, because the complications of tracheostomy can be so devastating and those patients at risk can be difficult to identify, some authorities [57] recommend that all infants with tracheostomies have radiographic studies at the time of decannulation. By using conventional radiographs or xeroradiographs, problems with persistent tracheal narrowing or granuloma formation can be anticipated and appropriate action taken.

References

1. Barnes RW, Merendino KA (1972) Post traumatic pulmonary insufficiency syndrome. Surg Clin North Am 52:625–633
2. Bergeson PS, Hales SW, Lustgarten MD, Lipow HW (1975) Pneumatoceles following hydrocarbon ingestion. Am J Dis Child 129:49–54
3. Bernatz PE, Burnside AF, Clagett OT (1958) Problem of the ruptured diaphragm. JAMA 168:877–881
4. Bowen FW, Chandra R, Avery GB (1973) Pulmonary interstitial emphysema with gas embolism in hyaline membrane disease. Am J Dis Child 126:117–118
5. Bratton L, Haddow JE (1975) Ingestion of charcoal lighter fluid. J Pediatr 87:633–636
6. Burke JF (1962) Early diagnosis of traumatic rupture of the bronchus. JAMA 181:682–686
7. Burns WA, McFarland W, Matthews MJ (1970) Busulfan induced pulmonarv disease. Am Rev Res Dis 101:408–413
8. Chesterman JT, Satsangi PN (1966) Rupture of the trachea and bronchi by closed injury. Thorax 21: 21–27
9. Clarysse AM, Cathey WJ, Cartwright GE, Wintrobe MM (1969) Pulmonary disease complicating intermittent therapy with methotrexate. JAMA 209:1861–1864

10. Cochlin DLl, Shaw MRP (1978) Traumatic lung cysts following minor blunt chest trauma. Clin Radiol 29:151–154
11. Cohn R (1972) Nonpenetrating wounds of the lungs and bronchi. Surg Clin North Am 52:585–595
12. Crawford WO (1973) Pulmonary injury in thoracic and nonthoracic trauma. Rad Clin North Am 11:527–541
13. Done AK (1974) The fuel shortage: a dangerous spinoff. Emerg Med 6:289–296
14. Eade NR, Taussig LM, Marks MI (1974) Hydrocarbon pneumonitis. Pediatrics 54:351–356
15. Enge I Forysaker T (1969) Rupture of the right hemidiaphragm with herniation of the liver. Radiology 92:1273–1274
16. Fagan CJ, Swischuk LE (1976) Traumatic lung and paramediastinal pneumatoceles. Radiology 120: 11–18
17. Fishbone G, Robbins DI, Osborn DJ, Grnja V (1973) Trauma to the thoracic aorta and great vessels. Radiol Clin North Am 11:543–554
18. Gerarde HW (1963) Toxicological studies on hydrocarbons. The aspiration hazard and toxicity of hydrocarbons and hydrocarbon mixtures. Arch Environ Health 6:329–341
19. Girdany BR, Sieber WK, Osman MZ (1969) Traumatic pseudodiverticulums of the pharynx in newborn infants. N Eng J Med 280:237–240
20. Gough JH, Gough MA, Thomas ML (1964) Pulmonary complications occurring after lymphangiography. Br J Radiol 37:416–421
21. Gregory GA, Tooley WH (1970) Gas embolism in hyaline membrane disease. N Eng J Med 282:1141–1142
22. Grimes OF (1972) Nonpenetrating injuries to the chest wall and esophagus. Surg Clin North Am 52:597–609
23. Hall RT, Rhodes PG (1975) Pneumothorax and pneumomediastinum in infants with idiopathic respiratory distress syndrome receiving continuous positive airway pressure. Pediatrics 55:493–496
24. Harris VJ, Brown R (1975) Pneumatoceles as complication of chemical pneumonia after hydrocarbon ingestion. AJR 125:531–537
25. Heilman RD, Collins VP (1963) Identification of laceration of the thoracic duct by lymphangiography. Radiology 81:470–472
26. Heird WC, Driscoll JM, Schullinger JN, Grebin B, Winters RW (1972) Intravenous alimentation in pediatric patients. J Pediatrics 80:351–372
27. Hill LD (1972) Injuries of the diaphragm following blunt trauma. Surg Clin North Am 52:611–624
28. Hirsch M, Banzini J (1969) Blast injury of the chest. Clin Radiology 20:362–370
29. Holmes TW, Netterville RE (1956) Complications of first rib fracture including one case each of tracheoesophageal fistula and aortic arch aneurysm. J Thor Surg 32:74–91
30. Hood RM, Sloan HE (1959) Injuries of the trachea and major bronchi. J Thor Cardiovascular Surg 38:458–480
31. Hunter TB, Whitehouse WM (1974) Fresh-water near-drowning: radiological aspects. Radiology 112:51–56
32. Jackson C, Jackson CL (1950) Bronchoesophagoscopy. Saunders, Philadelphia, p. 13
33. Kao DK, Tierney DF (1977) Air embolism with positive pressure ventilation of rats. J Appl Physiol 42:368–371
34. Kilman JW, Charnock E (1969) Thoracic trauma in infancy and childhood. J Trauma 9:863–873
35. Knight L, Tobin J, L'Heureux P (1974) Hydrothorax – a complication of hyperalimentation with radiologic manifestations. Radiology 111:693–695
36. Lang EK (1976) The role of arteriography in trauma. Radiol Clin North Am 14:353–370
37. Le Cudonnec B, Vasile N, Ferrane J (1978) Les ruptures traumatiques de l'aorte isthmique.A propos de dix cas. Ann Radiol 21:9–18
38. Lee FA, Gwinn JL (1974) Retrosternal dislocation of the clavicle. Radiology 110:631–634
39. Lynch FP, Coran AG, Cohen SR, Lee FA (1974) Traumatic esophageal pseudodiverticula in the newborn. J Pediatr Surg 9:675–681
40. MacPherson RI, Chernick V, Reed M (1973) The complications of respirator therapy in the newborn. J Can Assoc Radiol 23:91–102
41. Molnar W, Page WG (1966) Traumatic rupture of the thoracic aorta. Radiol Clin North Am 2:403–414
42. Manlove CH, Baronofsky ID (1955) Traumatic rupture of both leaves of the diaphragm. Surgery 37:461–462
43. Newman DE (1978) The radiolucent esophageal foreign body: an often forgotten cause of respiratory symptoms. J Pediatr 92:60–63
44. Northway WH, Rosan RC, Porter DY (1967) Pulmonary disease following respirator therapy of hyaline membrane disease – bronchopulmonary dysplasia. N Eng J Med 276:357–368
45. Oh KS, Fleishner FG, Wyman SM (1969) Characteristic pulmonary finding in traumatic complete transection of a main-stem bronchus. Radiology 92:371–372
46. Oh SK, Stitik FP, Galvis AG, Bearman SB, Heller RM, Dorst JP (1974) Radiological manifestations in patients on continuous positive-pressure breathing. Radiology 110:627–630
47. Parmley LF, Mattingly TW, Manion WC et al (1958) Nonpenetrating traumatic injury of the aorta. Circulation 17:1086–1101
48. Pearl M, Milstein M, Rook GD (1973) Pseudocyst of the lung due to traumatic nonpenetrating lung injury. J Pediatr Surg 8:967–968
49. Philip AGS (1975) Oxygen plus pressure plus time: the etiology of bronchopulmonary dysplasia. Pediatrics 55:44–51
50. Putnam CE, Minagi H, Blaisdell FW (1973) The roentgen appearance of disseminated intravascular coagulation (DIC). Radiology 109–13–18

51. Putnam CE, Tummillo AM, Myerson DA, Myerson PJ (1975) Drowning: another plunge. AJR 125:543–548
52. Reynolds J, Davis JT (1966) Injuries of the chest wall, pleura, pericardium, lungs, bronchi and esophagus. Radiol Clin North Am IV:383–401
53. Richardson JD, McElvein RB, Trinkle JK (1975) First rib fracture: a hallmark of severe trauma. Ann Surg 181:251–254
54. Samuels ML, Johnson DE, Holoye PY, Lanzotti VJ (1976) Large-dose bleomycin therapy and pulmonary toxicity – a possible role of prior radiotherapy. JAMA 235:1117–1120
55. Schralmel R, Kellum H, Creech O (1961) Analysis of factors affecting survival after chest injuries. J Trauma 1:600–607
56. Schwarz MI, Whitcomb ME, Goldman AL (1973) The spectrum of diffuse pulmonary infiltration in malignant disease. Chest 64:88–93
57. Scott JR, Kramer SS (1978) Pediatric tracheostomy II: radiographic features of difficult decannulations. AJR 130:393–398
58. Shook DR, Cram KB, Williams HJ (1975) Pulmonary venous air embolism in hyaline membrane disease. AJR 125:538–542
59. Sidaway MD (1964) Duplication of oesophagus. Ann Radiol 7:400–405
60. Sorsdahl OA, Powell JW (1965) Cavitary pulmonary lesions following nonpenetrating chest trauma in children. AJR 95:118–124
61. Strassman G (1947) Traumatic rupture of the aorta. Am Heart J 33:508–515
62. Strug B, Noon GP, Beall AC (1974) Traumatic diaphragmatic hernia. Ann Thorac Surg 17:444–449
63. Swischuck LE (1977) Bubbles in hyaline membrane disease. Radiology 122:417–426
64. Weiss JM (1975) Widened mediastinum after a penetrating injury of the chest. JAMA 233:366
65. Williams JR, Stembridge VA (1964) Pulmonary contusions secondary to nonpenetrating chest trauma. AJR 91:284–290
66. Wilson RF, Murray C, Antonenko DR (1977) Nonpenetrating thoracic injuries. Surg Clin North Am 57:17–36
67. Wiot JF (1975) The radiologic manifestations of blunt chest trauma. JAMA 231:500–503
68. Wise L, Connors J, Hwang YH, Anderson C (1973) Traumatic injuries to the diaphragm. J Trauma 13:946–950
69. Zwillich CW, Pierson DJ, Creagh CE, Sutton FD, Schatz E, Petty TL (1974) Complications of assisted ventilation. Am J Med 57:161–170

11 Skeletal Trauma

Fred A. Lee

The skeleton provides the framework for support and locomotion of the body and acts as a protective barrier for the vital internal organs. It bears the brunt of traumatic forces which may disrupt the integrity of the individual bones and the normal articulation between bones. This occurs more frequently in children than in adults because of their more exuberant and carefree activities and because their bones are slender and weaker. Fortunately, a child's skeleton heals rapidly and with a great capacity for remodeling. The rate of bone healing is greater in the younger age. As an illustration, Salter cites the fact that a femoral shaft fracture will unite in 3 weeks in a neonate, in 8 weeks in an 8-year-old child, and in 12 weeks at the age of 12 years; whereas it will take approximately 20 weeks in adults [31]. A remarkable amount of callus can be deposited in a matter of days in a neonate (Fig. 11.1).

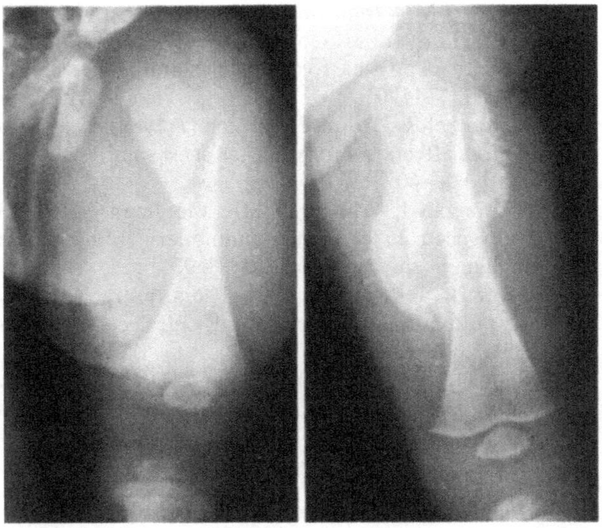

Fig. 11.1. Fracture healing is rapid in neonates. A large amount of bony callus has formed in 1 week in this 2-month-old girl with a fractured femur. *Left:* Shortly after fracture; *right:* one week later

Angulation and displacement deformities are usually spontaneously corrected if there are at least two more years of bone growth ahead for the child. Correction of angulation is more likely if the deformity is near a joint rather than in mid shaft and if the angulation is in the same plane as the usual motion at the contiguous joint. If the angulation is perpendicular to the joint motion, remodeling is less likely to occur.

Side-by-side displacement (bayonet deformity) and even slight override of the fracture segments will heal and remodel with surprisingly little residual deformity in young children (Fig. 11.2). With femoral shaft fractures in particular, the regional hyperemia to the epiphysis subsequent to the fracture can result in overgrowth of the bone if the fracture segments are reduced anatomically; in these instances, healing of a side-by-side displacement is preferred.

Rotational deformity, however, cannot be spontaneously remodeled and must be recognized and corrected during reduction and casting of the acute fracture.

In young children, ligaments and tendons and, to a lesser extent, fibrous capsular structures are relatively stronger than the contiguous bones to which they attach. These bony attachments are usually torn before the tendons rupture. Joint sprains or strains are therefore much less common in children, and subtle fractures of the adjacent bones and epiphyseal injuries must be carefully ruled out before these diagnoses are considered.

11.1 Diagnosis

The diagnosis of fracture or dislocation is frequently quite obvious on clinical inspection. Subtle fractures, however, can be recognized only on radiographs. Radiographs are also required to assess the presence of comminution, the degree of angulation and rotation, and the amount of displacement, override, or distraction of clinically apparent fractures. Radiographs of the injured part should routinely be exposed in at least two projections perpendicular to each other. Even widely displaced fractures may be missed on a single projection (Fig. 11.3). The examination should include the entire bone plus the proximal and distal joints. The films should be evaluated immediately and additional views obtained ad lib if there is inconclusive evidence of a fracture (Fig. 11.4). Occasionally, when a fracture cannot be definitely demonstrated, a repeat

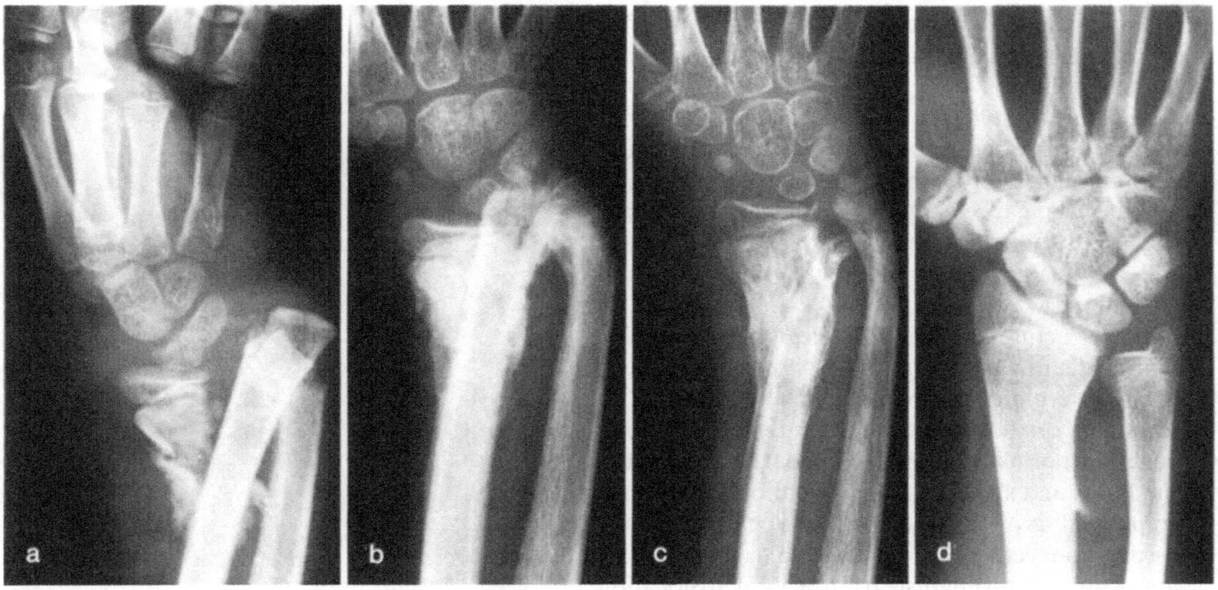

Fig. 11.2 a–d. A growing child has a remarkable capacity for spontaneous correction and remodeling of significant postfracture deformities. This 6-year-old girl suffered severe fracture-dislocation of the wrist which was not initially reduced because of more urgent serious head injuries. **a** Persistent deformity and early callus formation are present 2 weeks following trauma. **b** There are progressive healing and persistent deformities 3 weeks later. **c** Good healing and remodeling have occurred 4 months after trauma. **d** Nearly normal appearance of wrist 6 years later

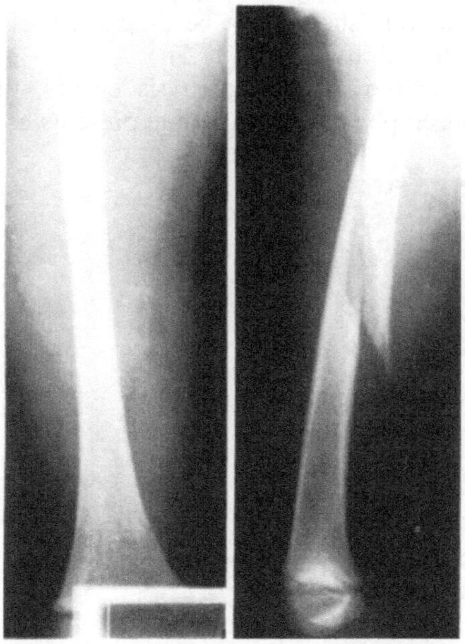

Fig. 11.3. Displaced spiral fracture of femoral midshaft in a 5-year-old boy is clearly seen on lateral view but not on frontal view

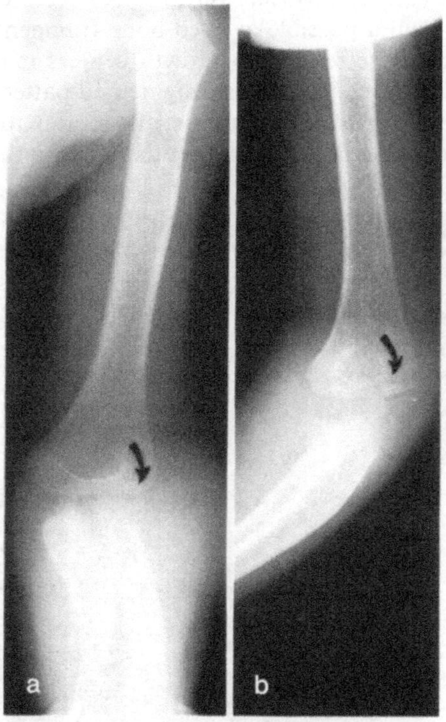

Fig. 11.4 a, b. Lateral condylar fracture of distal humerus in a 3-year-old girl is barely detectable on routine frontal view (**a**), but is clearly demonstrated on an oblique projection (**b**)

examination in a week will clearly show it. The injured part should be protected by a splint or cast in the meantime.

The films should be of good technical quality but this should not be achieved at the cost of patient comfort and safety. Obtaining diagnostic films in severely traumatized patients should await stabilization of the patient's clinical course and frequently will tax the ingenuity of the physician and the technologist.

Most fractures are easily detected on radiographs. Normal features of the growing skeleton should not be misinterpreted as pathologic alterations. The secondary ossification centers at the ends of the long bones are normally not mineralized at birth except at the knees and shoulders, and fractures through the epiphyseal growth plate with dislocation of the ossification center are difficult to recognize and impossible to distinguish from a joint dislocation until healing occurs. The long axis of the long bone should always be carefully evaluated to detect any malalignment of the bone in relation to the contiguous joint socket. The times of ossification of the various growth centers differ and tables listing the normal times should be consulted in standard textbooks such as Caffey [7], Keats [18], or Kohler [20] to differentiate early epiphyseal ossification or accessory ossicles from a possible avulsed bone fragment. Ossification of the secondary growth centers may occur in a very irregular almost fragmented pattern which should not be misinterpreted for traumatic comminution. This is particularly bothersome at the elbow. Ossification may also arise from two or more foci producing a multipartite appearance to an epiphysis and this should not be diagnosed as a fracture of the epiphysis (Fig. 11.5).

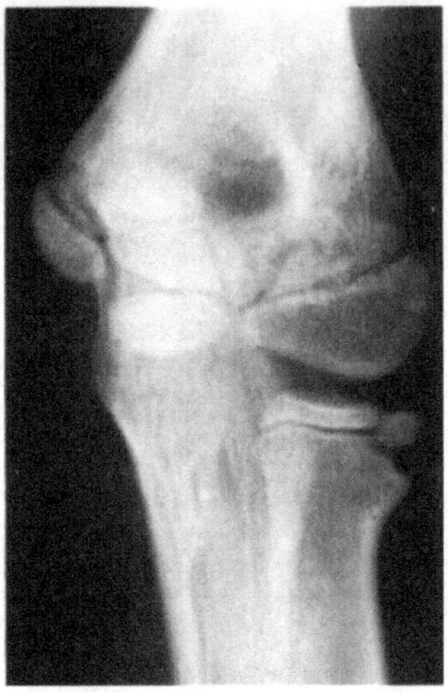

Fig. 11.5. Frontal projection of normal elbow in a 12-year-old boy demonstrates separate ossification centers of the medial condyle, trochlea, and capitellum of the distal humerus. The radial head epiphysis is bipartite and the proximal radial metaphysis has a notched appearance. These normal findings should not be considered pathological

Once ossification of the epiphysis occurs, the cartilaginous epiphyseal growth plate presents as a

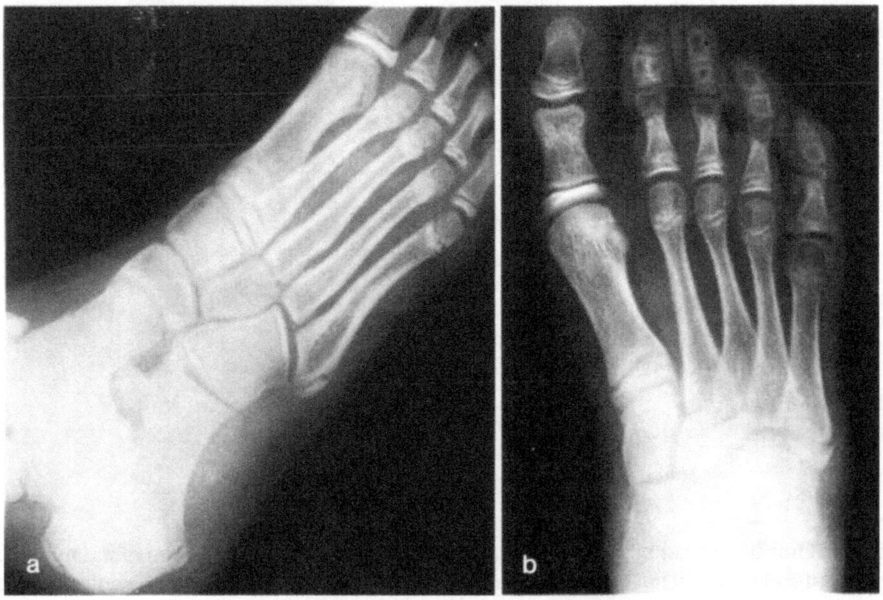

Fig. 11.6 a, b. The apophysis at the proximal 5th metatarsal is normally obliquely positioned and may appear quite fragmented (**a**). Fracture through the base of the 5th metatarsal is usually transverse in position (**b**)

transverse radiolucent strip at the ends of the bones which normally would not be confused for a fracture except by the very inexperienced neophyte. Occasionally, if a radiograph is exposed obliquely to a plane of the growth plate, the projection of the growth plate in two different planes could mimic a fracture, but attention to the positioning of the X-ray beam and the part examined should avoid this.

The cartilage growth plate of an apophysis (traction epiphysis) is usually more obliquely placed in relation to the long axis of the bone and should not be misconstrued as a fracture. This mistake occurs most often in the base of the fifth metatarsal bone (Fig. 11.6).

Partial fusion of the epiphysis to the shaft (Fig. 11.7) and pseudoepiphyses present as cleftlike defects at the ends of long and short tubular bones and may mimic a fracture. The more prominent nutrient foramen in children may also simulate a fracture line. Sesamoid and accessory bones should not be confused for traumatic lesions (Fig. 11.8).

If there is a finding which is unfamiliar or equivocal, the radiologist should personally examine the patient. If no swelling or tenderness is present in the region in question, fracture is highly unlikely.

Also, in these tentative situations, radiographs of the opposite normal limb for comparison may be useful, but one should recognize that normal variants need not be present symmetrically. Comparison views are frequently useful as a guide for the orthopedic surgeon in planning treatment. While comparison views are not obtained routinely in most large pediatric centers [26] and are not needed most of the time for accurate diagnosis [24], there should be no hesitation in obtaining them if there is any uncertainty on the part of the physician who must initially interpret the films or who is providing the primary care for the patient.

In most instances, routine radiographs will provide all the information needed. Special procedures are seldom necessary. Tomography is helpful in

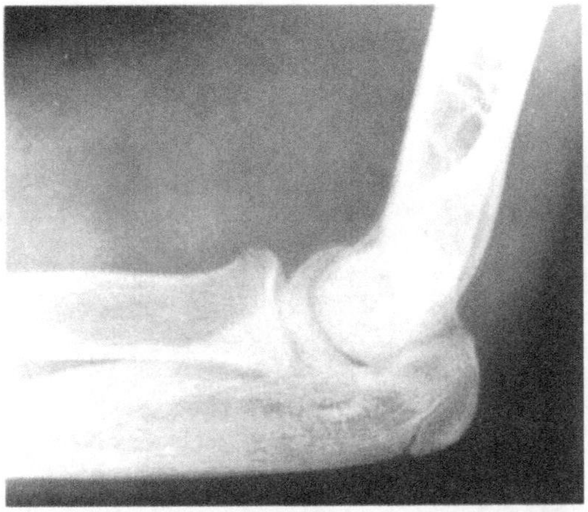

Fig. 11.7. Partial fusion of the epiphysis such as at the olecranon should not be misinterpreted as an incomplete fracture

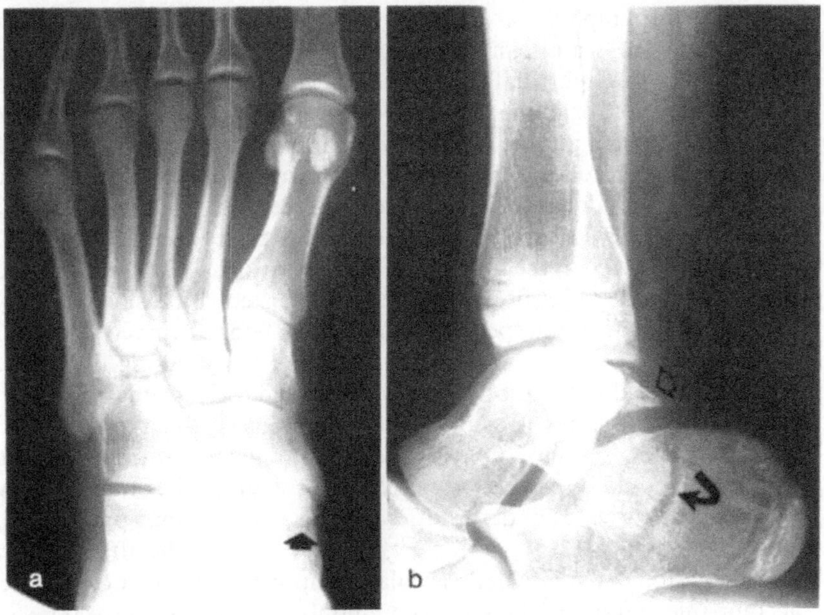

Fig. 11.8 a, b. Accessory ossicles should not be confused for fractures. **a** Os tibiale externum may mimic a fracture of the tarsal navicular. **b** Os trigonum (*open arrow*) may be misinterpreted as a fracture of the talus in this 9-year-old boy who fell out of a tree, landing feet first, and fractured his calcaneus (*closed arrow*)

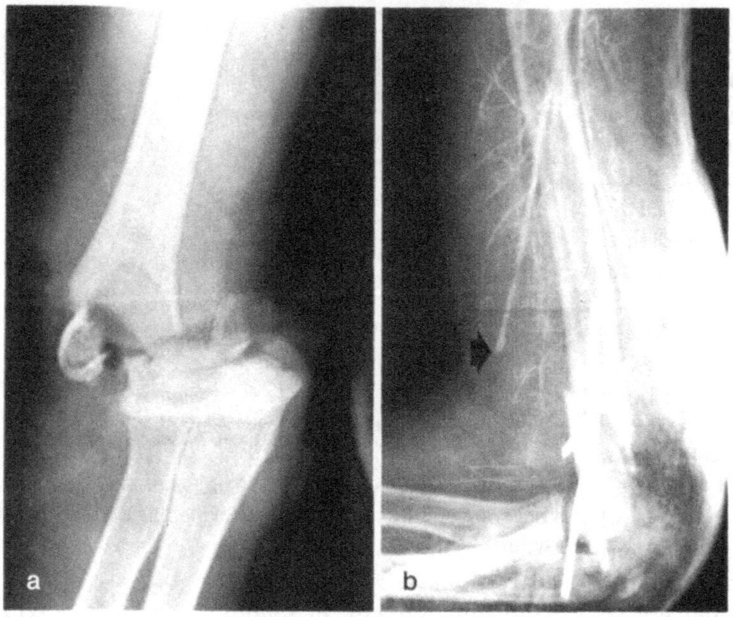

Fig. 11.9. a Thirteen-year-old boy with compound comminuted fracture of elbow. **b** Arterial obstruction is demonstrated on angiography after open reduction and fixation of the fracture

evaluating vertebral fractures and in detecting subtle stress fractures or fracture through an abnormal bone lesion. It is extremely useful in assessing fracture healing if there is concern regarding a new fracture or nonunion.

Arthrography is useful to differentiate dislocation from epiphyseal fracture and separation in neonates when the epiphysis is not yet mineralized. In older children, ligamentous injuries, menisceal tears, enchondral and osteochondral fractures can be evaluated by arthrography.

Radionuclide scans can be useful in detecting occult stress fractures or fractures in bones which may be difficult to examine radiographically [13, 40]. However, the scan may be negative if performed in the first 24–48 h following trauma if vasoconstriction or disruption of osseous circulation is present. Furthermore, as with any diagnostic tests, the result must be interpreted in the light of the clinical setting since a positive scan reflects only increased osteoblastic activity and is not specific for fracture or bone contusion.

Computerized tomography is rarely indicated for fracture diagnosis but if available it may be used instead of linear tomography in certain circumstances. It should be particularly useful in assessing vertebral fractures and deformities of the spinal canal [9, 19].

Angiography is vital when vascular compromise accompanies a fracture. This most commonly occurs with fractures of the distal humerus or distal femur, especially if the fracture segments are sharply pointed and widely displaced [37] (Fig. 11.9). The study localizes the point of vascular obstruction and aids immeasurably in the decision as to whether and where surgical intervention is needed.

11.2 Types of Fracture

Children's bones are not as strong as adult bones but they are more elastic and more plastic. Longitudinal compressive force applied to a long bone in a child will result in a greater degree of gradual bending of a bone before fracture occurs. If the force is released before fracture occurs, the bone will spring back to normal shape. If further longitudinal force which exceeds the maximal strength of the bone is applied but released before fracture occurs, the elasticity of the bone may be exceeded and a bowing deformity of the bone may persist [3]. This *plastic bowing* occurs most commonly in long bones which are slightly curved such as in the forearm [10]. Microfractures along the concave side of the bowed bone may be primarily responsible for the bowed deformity. With healing, some callus has been observed along the concavity of the bowed shaft although no definite fracture line is ever detected (Fig. 11.10). The bowing may prevent reduction of a fracture or dislocation of the affected companion bone in the forearm. Plastic bowing of the femur has also been described [8] and we have observed a bowed fibula accompanying a tibial fracture (Fig. 11.11).

Incomplete fractures such as cortical impactions (torus fractures) and greenstick fractures are more

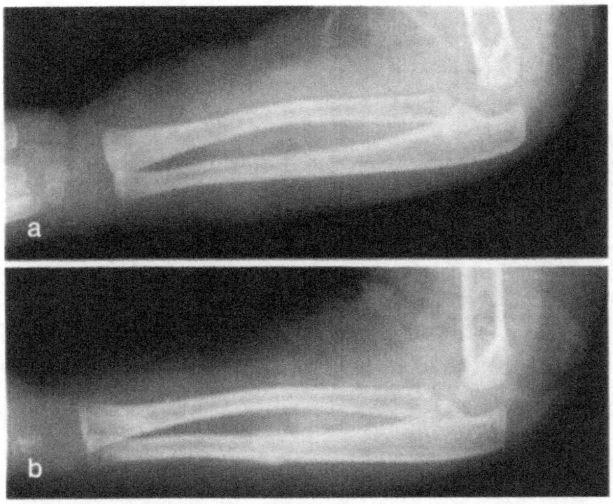

Fig. 11.10. a Mild anterior plastic bowing of the radius with undisplaced fracture of the distal mid ulna in a 4-year-old girl. **b** Three weeks later, film shows ulnar fracture line more clearly and bony callus along ulnar shaft. Faint periosteal reaction is now present in the concavity of the radial bowed deformity

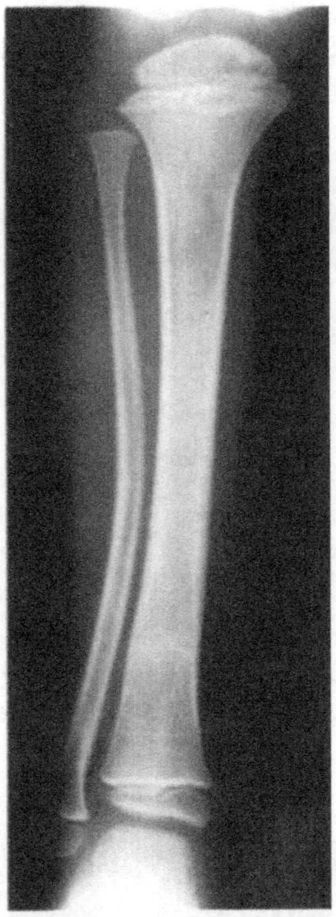

Fig. 11.11. Persistend medial bowing of the fibula with healed fracture of distal tibia in a 3-year-old girl

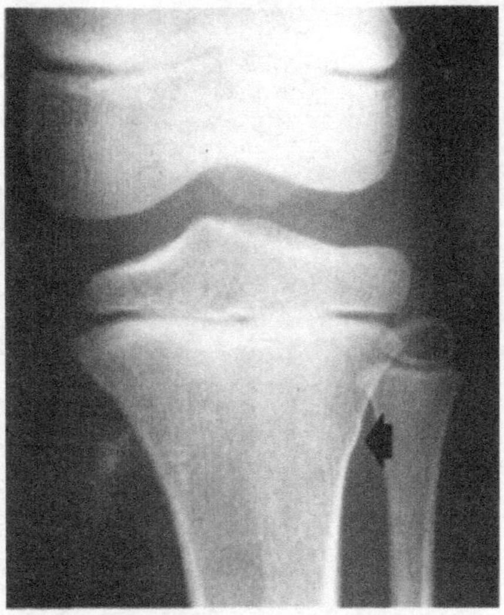

Fig. 11.12. Subtle torus fracture of the proximal tibia seen as a minimal disruption of the normally smooth concave cortical configuration of the metaphysis

common in children than in adults. Cortical impaction fractures may be quite subtle and the normal smooth slightly concave contour of the metaphysis must be carefully inspected to detect any slight disruption (Fig. 11.12). Greenstick fractures occur on the convex side of the bent bone.

Angulated greenstick fractures are common in the distal humerus and radius. In the supracondylar region of the distal humerus, localized soft tissue swelling and bleeding or effusion into the elbow joint with elevation of the posterior fat pad on the lateral view are valuable clues to the location of the injury and should prompt careful inspection of the films for minimal bony changes (Fig. 11.13). The posterior fat pad sign, however, is not pathognomonic of a fracture. Hemarthrosis, pyarthrosis, joint effusion, and synovial thickening from whatever cause will produce swelling of the joint capsule and elevate both the anterior and posterior fat pads [2].

Fat droplets mixed with blood (lipohemarthrosis) can occur in the elbow and other joints following trauma. A fat-fluid interface within the joint space can be demonstrated radiographically if the joint is examined laterally with a horizon beam (Fig. 11.14). The fat comes from the marrow in an intracapsular fracture or from intracapsular extrasynovial tissue through a synovial tear [42]. Fat-fluid levels and post-traumatic fat embolism are relatively uncommon in children, possibly because of the predominance of red marrow compared to yellow marrow in adults.

Subtle anterior or posterior displacement of the distal humeral fragment can be gauged by observing the relationship of the capitellum to the humeral shaft. Normally, the capitellum forms an angle of approximately 140° with the humeral shaft. Rogers et al. [29] proposed the use of the anterior humeral line (AHL) to detect mild dorsal or ventral displacement of the capitellum. In children over 2.5 years of age, a line drawn along the anterior humeral cortex should pass through the middle third of the capitel-

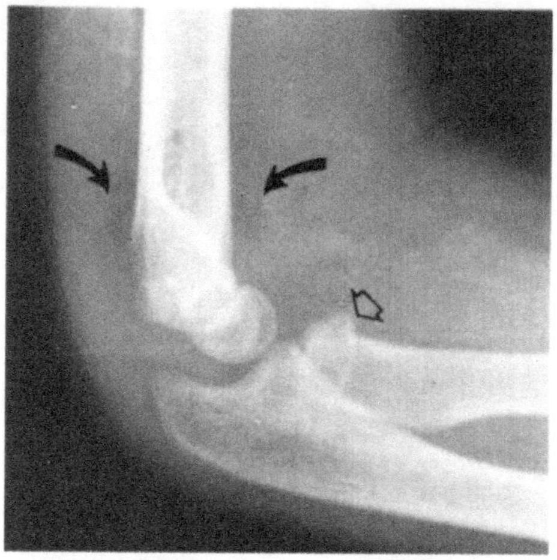

Fig. 11.13. Impacted fracture of the radial neck (*open arrow*) with elbow joint effusion and elevation of the anterior and posterior supracondylar fat pads (*closed curvilinear arrows*)

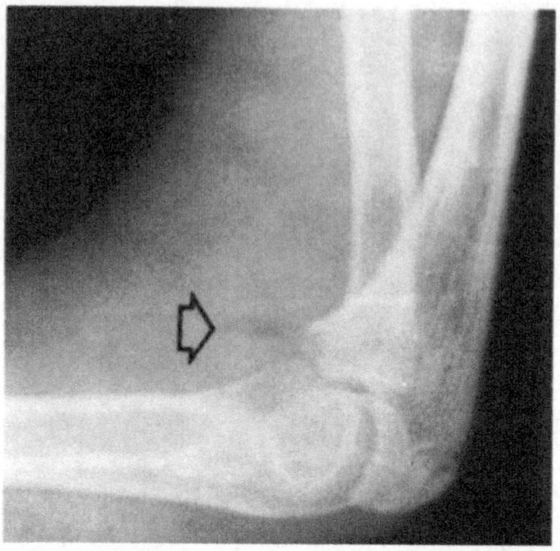

Fig. 11.14. Horizontal beam lateral view of elbow shows fat fluid level (*open arrow*) in the anterior aspect of the elbow joint, indicating traumatic lipohemarthrosis in this 11-year-old girl

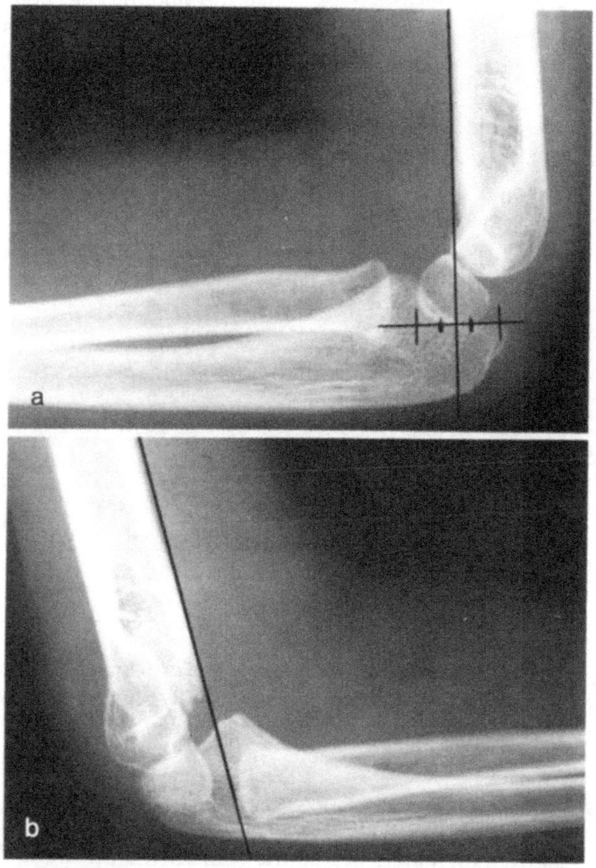

Fig. 11.15 a, b. Seven-year-old boy with elbow injury. **a** Anterior humeral line (AHL) drawn on uninjured side shows line transecting middle third of capitellum. **b** On injured side, AHL lies clearly in front of dorsally displaced capitellum

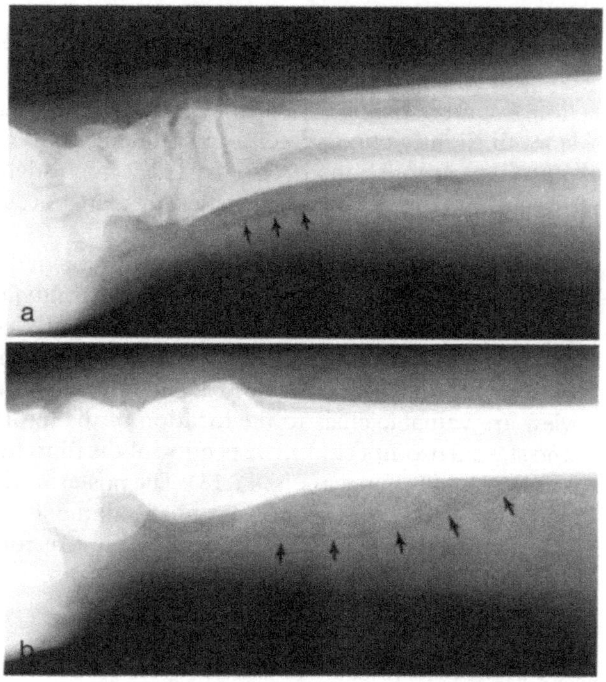

Fig. 11.16. a Normal pronator quadratus fat line in a 14-year-old boy. **b** Displaced pronator quadratus fat line in a boy with obvious impacted radial fracture

lum (Fig. 11.15). Under 2.5 years of age, the AHL may normally pass through the anterior third of the capitellum. Comparison views should be obtained if the findings are equivocal.

Greenstick fractures of the distal radius and ulna are normally easily detected. Displacement of the fat plane overlying the pronator quadratus muscle along the ventral aspect of the distal radius and ulna is a secondary finding resulting from bleeding into or swelling of the muscle (Fig. 11.16). In certain instances, where the incomplete fracture is minor, this soft tissue change may be more obvious and should direct further attention to this region either by close reinspection or additional views [23].

A simple *complete fracture* may be transverse, oblique, spiral, or longitudinal. Complete fractures can, of course, occur in any bone but most frequently, in younger children, the clavicles and upper extremities are involved. Young children cannot verbalize adequately and may suffer from an occult fracture. A child's refusal to bear weight or to move a part should alert the parents to the possibility of a fracture. In young toddlers especially, an unsuspected spiral fracture of the tibia caused by a fall against a coffee table or other low furniture may cause the child to refuse to stand or walk. Since children at this age seem to fall or bump into furniture constantly, a specific episode of injury usually cannot be singled out. This "toddler's fracture" may be quite subtle on the initial examination and needs to be differentiated from the normal nutrient foramen in the upper posterior medial cortex of the tibial shaft (Fig. 11.17). If no fracture is found, a bone scan may be needed to detect an early fracture or to rule out the possibility of diskitis which may similarly present with refusal to bear weight.

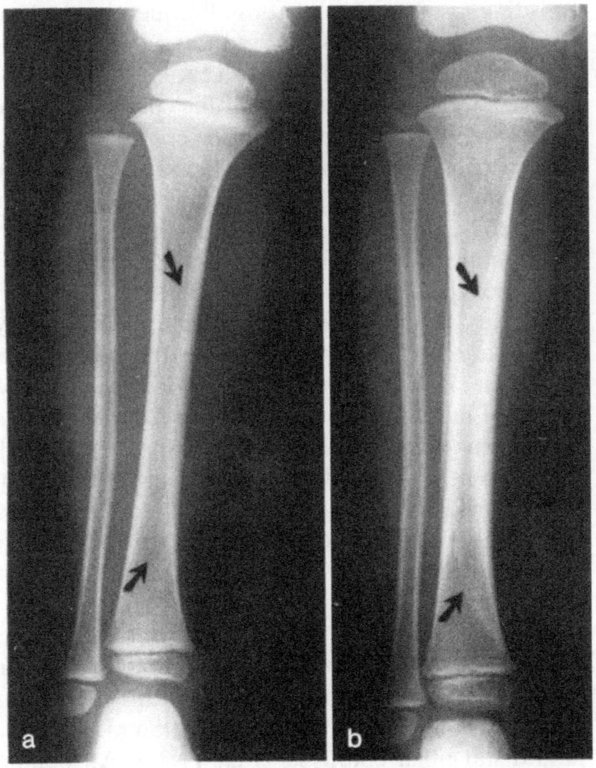

Fig. 11.17. a Faint undisplaced spiral fracture of tibia (toddler's fracture) in 2-year-old boy who suddenly refused to walk. **b** Fracture line is more readily seen as healing occurs

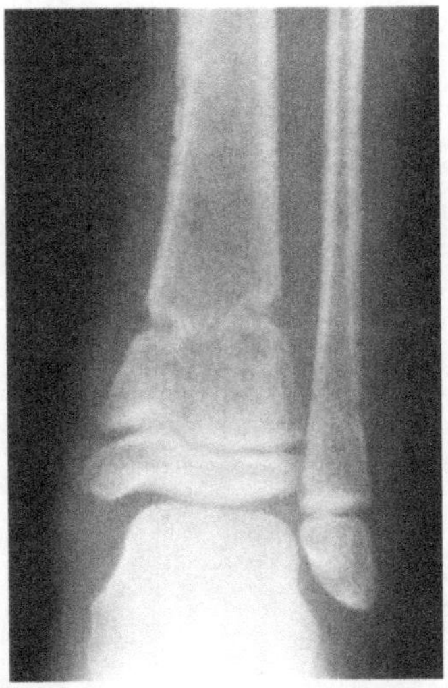

Fig. 11.18. Puncture wounds of distal tibia and fibula in a 6-year-old girl who was severely bitten by a dog. (Courtesy of George R. Barnes, MD, Tacoma, Washington)

A child's bone is less brittle and *comminuted fractures* do not occur as frequently as in adults. Nonetheless, high velocity trauma whether resulting from vehicular accidents or sporting activities such as the current skateboard madness [16, 17] can result in serious comminuted or multiple or open fractures.

A penetrating injury to bone may leave an imprint of the penetrating object or cause a complete simple or comminuted fracture depending on the size and velocity of the penetrating object (Fig. 11.18).

Epiphyseal Fractures

In children, 15% of all fractures involve the epiphyseal growth plate [28]. The weakest part of the growth plate is the zone of hypertrophic cartilage cells just below the zone of provisional calcification, and fractures through the growth plate occur in this plane. Most of the epiphyseal growth plate will thus be displaced with the epiphyseal ossification center.

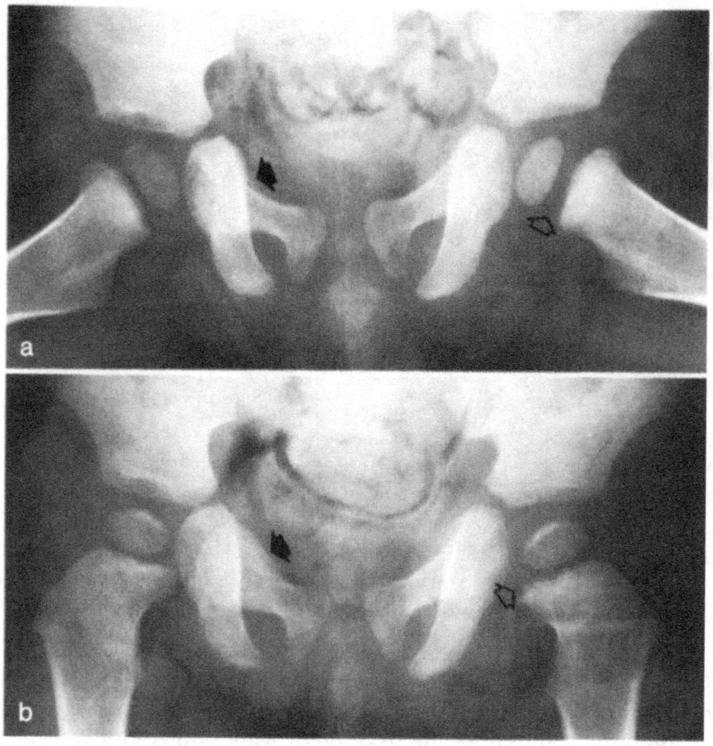

Fig. 11.19. a Salter I fracture of the left proximal femoral epiphysis (*open arrow*) and fracture of right superior pubic ramus (*closed arrow*) in 15-month-old boy. Not widening of left femoral epiphyseal growth plate. **b** Two weeks later, healing is indicated by some calcification along the metaphyseal side of the growth plate (*open arrow*), and by further bony callus in the right suprapubic ramus

The blood supply of the growth plate comes from epiphyseal vessels and if the epiphyseal circulation is not disrupted and the epiphyseal displacement is properly reduced, growth will continue normally. Repeated overzealous attempts to reduce epiphyseal displacement may disturb the blood supply and do more harm than good. Although nearly 85% of epiphyseal injuries will heal without growth disturbance, the risk of complete or partial premature closure of the epiphyseal plate is real and no given case of acute epiphyseal injury can be excluded from this risk [27, 35].

The Salter-Harris classification of epiphyseal plate fractures is the most widely used and should be well known to all radiologists [32]. The classification provides a succinct accurate description of the injury and has prognostic significance.

Type I fracture occurs transversely, completely through the epiphyseal growth plate without a metaphyseal fragment and occurs principally in younger children. It is recognized by widening of the radiolucent growth plate or displacement of the epiphysis (Fig. 11.19). The widening of the epiphyseal plate may be quite subtle and is easily missed unless carefully looked for. Oblique views to prevent overlap by a companion bone and comparison views may be necessary if the findings are equivocal. In neonates, when the epiphysis is not mineralized, complete displacement of the epiphysis may be misdiagnosed as a dislocation. Frequently, the fracture may spontaneously reduce with very little radiographic abnormality at all except for slight soft tissue swelling in the region of the epiphyseal plate. Stress views could reproduce the epiphyseal widening but this is not a universally accepted procedure. With healing, some callus may develop on the metaphyseal side of the plate. Prognosis for this type of fracture is generally favorable.

Type II is most common. The fracture runs obliquely through the metaphysis into the epiphyseal plate and continues through the plate to the opposite side with resultant separation and displacement of the epiphysis and the attached metaphyseal fragment (Fig. 11.20). The periosteum is usually intact on the side of the metaphyseal fragment and aids considerably in accurate closed reduction of the epiphyseal displacement. Subsequent growth disturbance is uncommon unless there is also vascular compromise.

Types III and IV are both intra-articular fractures. A type III fracture is a partial fracture separation of only the epiphysis. This is an uncommon fracture and is found chiefly in the lateral aspect of the distal tibial epiphysis (Fig. 11.21). An oblique view may be needed in order best to demonstrate the fracture if there is minimal displacement of the fragment. Open reduction is frequently required for accurate repositioning and fixing of the fragment. If

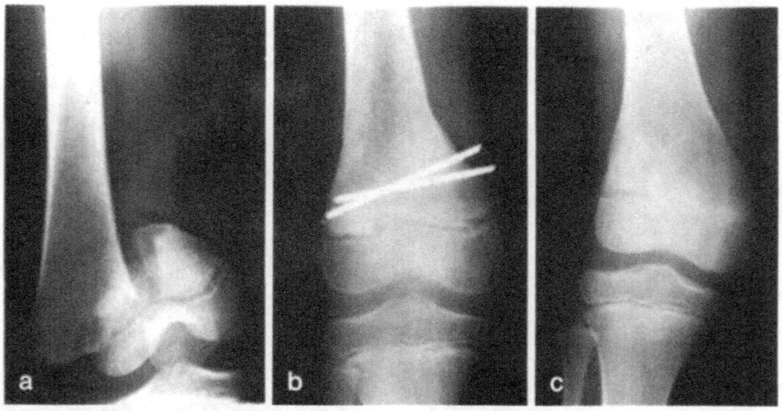

Fig. 11.20 a–c. Salter II fracture of the distal femur in a 10-year-old boy (**a**); postreduction and pin fixation film shows apparently good healing (**b**); one year later, growth retardation in the lateral aspect of femoral metaphysis and epiphyseal plate has resulted in valgus deformity at knee (**c**)

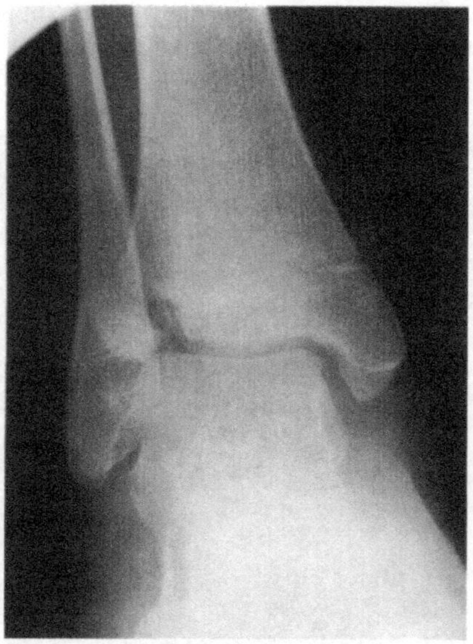

Fig. 11.21. Salter III fracture of distal tibial epiphysis laterally in a 14-year-old girl. This is the most common site for a Salter III fracture

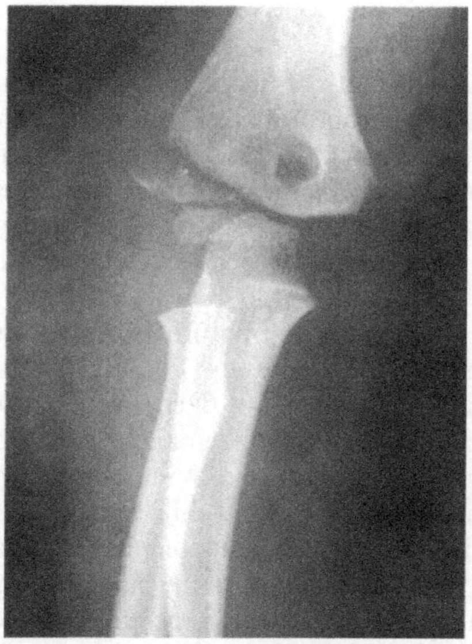

Fig. 11.22. Salter IV fracture of lateral condyle of distal humerus. The fracture line extends through the metaphysis, the epiphyseal growth plate, and the unmineralized distal humeral epiphysis medial to the capitellum. There is slight lateral displacement of the distal fracture segment

the avulsed fragment has maintained its blood supply, prognosis for normal growth is favorable.

Type IV fracture is a complete longitudinal or oblique fracture through the metaphysis, the epiphyseal plate, and the epiphysis to the articular surface. This most commonly occurs through the lateral distal humeral condyle (Fig. 11.22). Open reduction and pin fixation with exact realignment of the epiphyseal growth plate are needed to avert growth disturbance and deformity (Fig. 11.23).

Type V is a localized crush injury to part of the epiphyseal plate. There are no radiographic manifestations and all too often, the injury goes unrecognized. Subsequent premature growth arrest results. Fortunately, this is an uncommon injury which involves primarily the bones at the knees or ankles.

The epiphysis may be injured without involvement of the growth plate [27]. The epiphyseal cartilage is resilient and a comminuted fracture or compression fracture of the articular surface of the epiphysis is uncommon in younger children. The

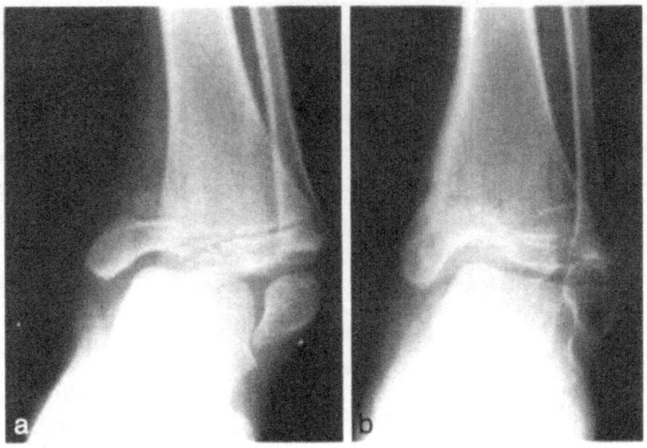

Fig. 11.23. **a** Ten-year-old girl with Salter IV fracture of distal tibia medially and Salter I fracture of distal fibula. The ankle mortise is disrupted. **b** One year later, premature closure of medial aspect of tibial epiphysis is apparent

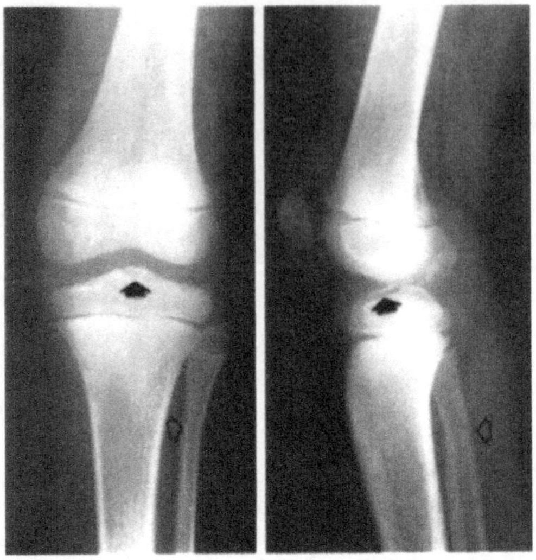

Fig. 11.24. Frontal and lateral views of knee of a 7-year-old boy struck by motorcycle. Avulsion of the tibial eminence and fracture of proximal fibula are noted

relatively greater strength of ligaments and tendons can result in avulsion fractures of the epiphysis at the sites of their attachment (Fig. 11.24). An osteochondral fracture may occur if a shearing force is inflicted on an epiphysis peripherally. A displaced fragment may lie within the joint space and interfere with motion.

Joint dislocation without fracture is much less common in children than in adults (Fig. 11.25). One relatively common type of minor partial dislocation in preschool children is the "nursemaid's elbow" or simply "pulled elbow" syndrome. A sudden jerk or pull on the outstretched arm of a child may cause a tear in the inferior attachment of the annular ligament with entrapment of the radial head through this defect [31]. Characteristically, the child refuses to move the arm and holds the arm in pronation with the elbow flexed. Treatment is simple and easily accomplished by supination of the forearm with the elbow flexed. This treatment is usually unsuspectedly accomplished by the radiologic technologist during positioning of the arm for radiographs. Radiographic studies for this condition are almost always normal.

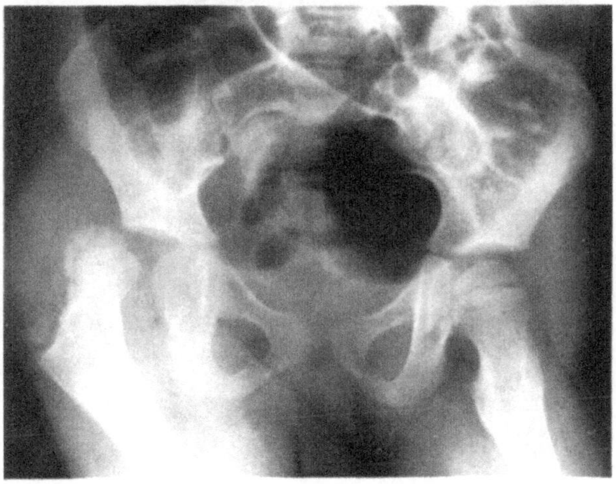

Fig. 11.25. Although dislocation without an associated fracture is uncommon in children, this girl fell on her knee with her hip flexed, resulting in posterior lateral dislocation of the hip

Dislocation accompanying a fracture of the companion bone may be overlooked if attention is distracted by the more obvious fracture. This is a frequent omission in two types of forearm fractures.

Monteggia's fracture dislocation is a fracture of the proximal or mid-ulna association with dislocation of the radial head. The dislocation may be anterior (Fig. 11.26), lateral (Fig. 11.27), or, less frequently, posterior. Radial head dislocation should be easily detected if one remembers that the capitellum-radial head articulation is a ball-and-socket joint and a line drawn through the long axis of the proximal radius should always be in alignment with the capitellum regardless of the projection or obliquity.

Galeazzi's fracture dislocation is less common and consists of fracture of the distal radius with dislocation of the distal ulna (Fig. 11.28).

Dislocation of the shoulder girdle is less common in children than adults. Traumatic dislocation of the humeral head occurs primarily in adolescents after closure of the epiphysis. Neurogenic subluxation of the humeral head may be a complication of Erb's

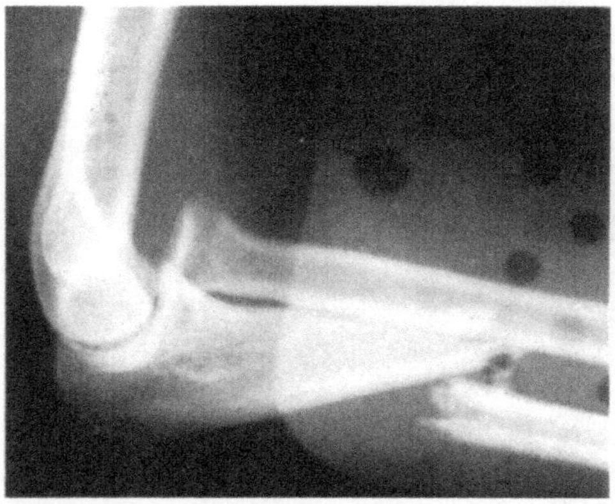

Fig. 11.26. Fifteen-year-old girl with Monteggia's fracture. Anterior angulation of the ulnar fracture has caused anterior dislocation of the radial head

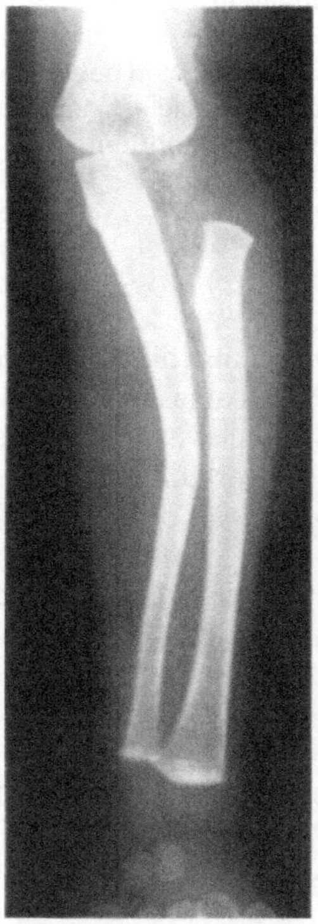

Fig. 11.27. Two-year-old girl with fracture and lateral bowing of the mid ulna, and lateral dislocation of the radial head

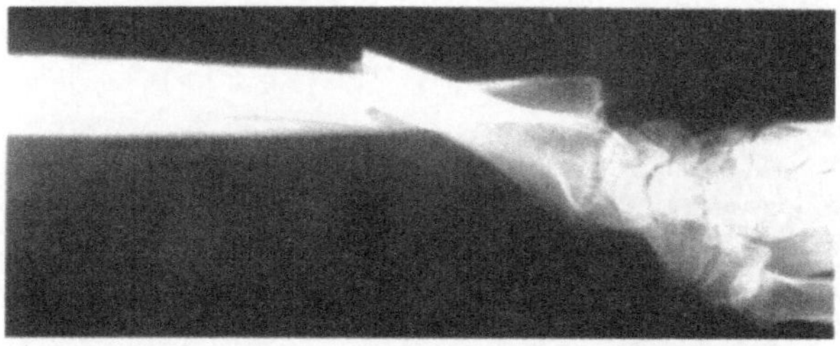

Fig. 11.28. Galeazzi's fracture in a 19-year-old. Fracture of the distal radius with ventral angulation of the distal radial segment and dorsal dislocation of the distal ulna are seen on this lateral view of wrist

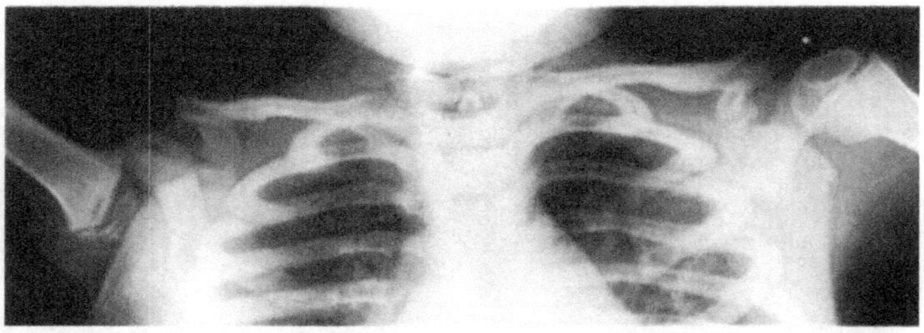

Fig. 11.29. Five-year-old boy with right-sided Erb's palsy. Atrophy of the right shoulder is seen, and neurogenic subluxation of the right shoulder with abduction is demonstrated

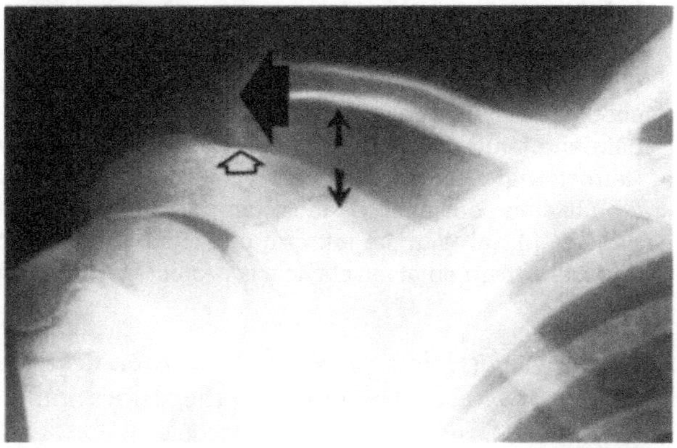

Fig. 11.30. Thirteen-year-old boy with fracture of distal right clavicle (*large black arrow*) and coracoclavicular separation (*smaller black arrows*). The clavicle is displaced upwards but the *open arrow* points to distal clavicular fracture fragment which remains in normal relationship to the acromion, indicating that the acromioclavicular ligaments are intact

palsy (Fig. 11.29). Acromioclavicular separations are uncommon in younger children and may require weight-bearing films to demonstrate it in the older child. Because of the strong ligamentous attachments at the acromioclavicular joints, fracture through the distal clavicle without disruption of the joint but with displacement of the clavicular shaft and separation of the coracoclavicular joint is more common in children than simple acromioclavicular separation [25] (Fig. 11.30). A fall on the shoulder with the line of force directed medially along the axis of the clavicle may occasionally cause dislocation at the sternoclavicular joint. Most of the time, the medial clavicle is dislocated anteriorly but, rarely, retrosternal dislocations can occur with the medial clavicle impinging on retrosternal structures, causing a variety of symptoms. Prompt recognition is required if closed reduction is to be successful. A

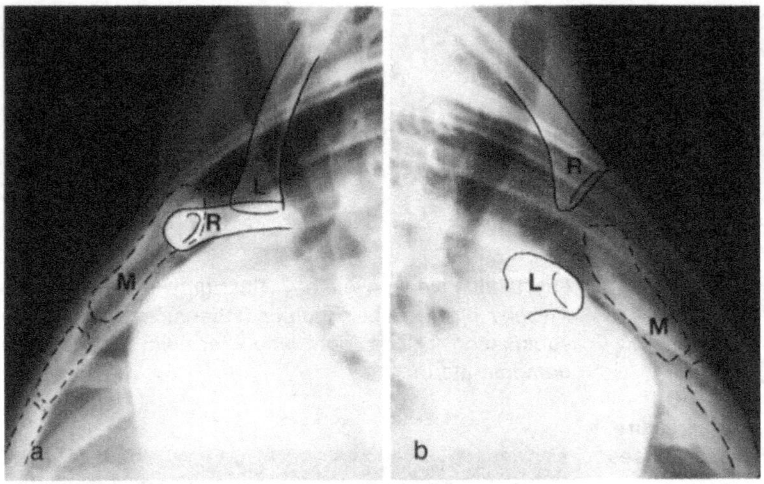

Fig. 11.31 a, b. This 10-year-old boy fell on his left shoulder playing football and immediately experienced pain and tenderness in the left sternoclavicular region. Retrosternal dislocation of the left clavicle is demonstrated utilizing special cross-table lateral view (the Heinig projection). (**a**) With the left arm abducted and the right adducted, the medial left clavicle is projected behind and slightly below the top of the manubrium and the medial right clavicle is projected normally through the manubrium. (**b**) With the left arm adducted and the right abducted, the medial left clavicle is projected behind the manubrium whereas the medial right clavicle is normally projected in line with the top of the manubrium

special view (Heinig projection) has been described which allows easy recognition of the dislocation [21] (Fig. 11.31).

11.3 Types of Trauma

11.3.1 Intrauterine Trauma

The fetal skeleton is usually well protected within the maternal womb. Bowing deformity of long bones and mild calvarial depressions may result from faulty fetal positioning within the uterus [7]. The bowed bone deformities must be differentiated from the various campomelic syndromes [22]. The presence of amniotic bands can cause amputation of fetal extremities, or only mild soft tissue and bony constrictions. Multiple fractures of the fetal skeleton occur only with severe osteogenesis imperfecta.

11.3.2 Birth Trauma

Fractures of normal bones may unavoidably occur during difficult delivery of large babies or babies in abnormal presentation. The clavicle is most commonly fractured during delivery of large babies with wide shoulders. Pseudoparalysis or local swelling and deformity are the usual clinical findings. Healing is usually rapid and uneventful. Congenital pseudarthrosis of the clavicle is uncommon and apart from its lack of symptoms and its occasional bilaterality may be difficult to differentiate from a fracture (Fig. 11.32).

With breech presentation, traction on any part which hangs up in the birth canal can result in fracture or epiphyseal separation. The obstetrician is often aware of the moment of fracture and confirmation of the fracture is usually simple by both physical and radiographic examination. Recognition of epiphyseal separation is more difficult. If the

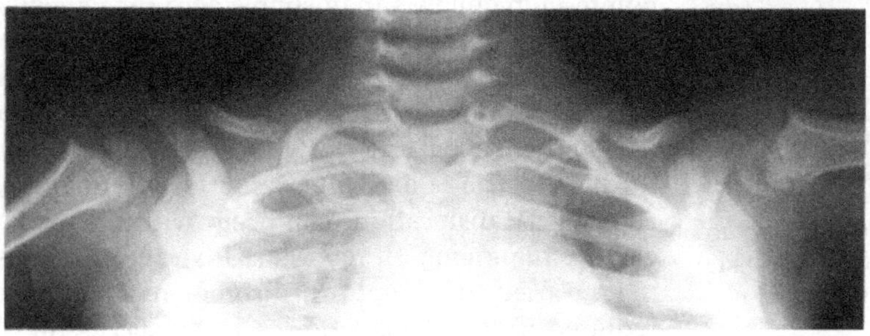

Fig. 11.32. Two-and-a-half-year-old boy with bilateral congenital pseudarthrosis of the clavicles which may be misinterpreted as fractures

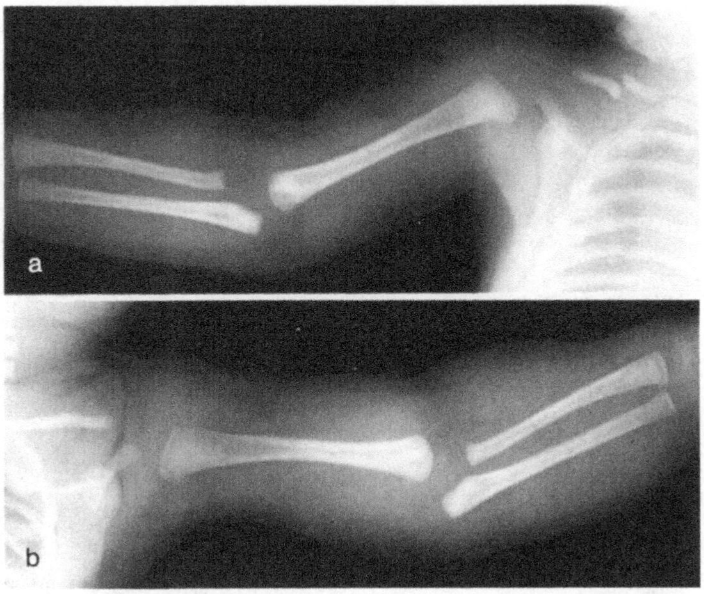

Fig. 11.33 a, b. One-week-old boy delivered after double footling breech presentation refuses to move upper limbs. **a** Film of right upper extremity demonstrates fracture of clavicle. **b** Film of left arm shows marked soft tissue swelling and medial displacement of the radius and ulna at the elbow resulting from medial fracture dislocation of the distal humeral epiphysis rather than dislocation of the elbow. Subsequent films show callus formation in distal humerus. Typically, distal humeral epiphyseal displacement is medial whereas elbow dislocation tends to be lateral [30]

epiphysis is unmineralized, differentiation from a dislocation may not be possible without an arthrogram or until healing begins (Fig. 11.33).

If the head is caught, traction may injure the cervical spine cord either with or without evidence of cervical spine injury. Quadriplegia or death may unfortunately result.

11.3.3 Pathologic Fractures

Pathologic fractures occur through bones which are weakened from any process (Fig. 11.34). Often, the underlying bony abnormality such as a simple bone cyst may be unsuspected until fracture through it occurs. Displacement of a cortical fracture fragment into the fluid-filled lumen ("fallen-fragment sign") is typically diagnostic of a simple bone cyst.

Conversely, a fracture in a bone extensively ravaged by a primary malignancy or metastatic disease or severe osteomyelitis may go unrecognized. Generalized osteopenia, whether from disuse, juvenile rheumatoid arthritis, or steroid therapy subjects the child to a higher risk of fracture. The regenerative anemias cause expansion of the medullar cavities and thinning of the cortices which may become infracted by trivial trauma (Fig. 11.35). Epiphyseal separation occurs frequently with metabolic bone disorders such as scurvy, rickets, and primary or secondary (renal) hyperparathyroidism. Bilateral symmetrical fractures (Looser lines) may also occur in the pelvis, femurs and scapula in rickets (Fig. 11.36).

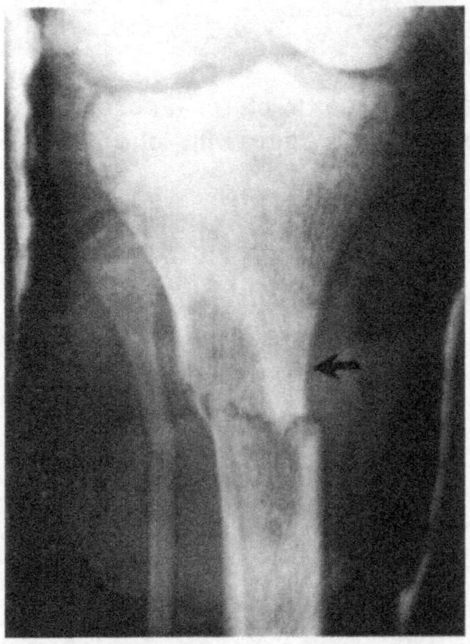

Fig. 11.34. Pathological fracture through a brown tumor in the proximal tibia in a 16-year-old girl with chronic renal disease and renal osteodystrophy. *Arrow* points to local area of subperiosteal bone resorption. Brown tumors occur more commonly with primary hyperparathyroidism

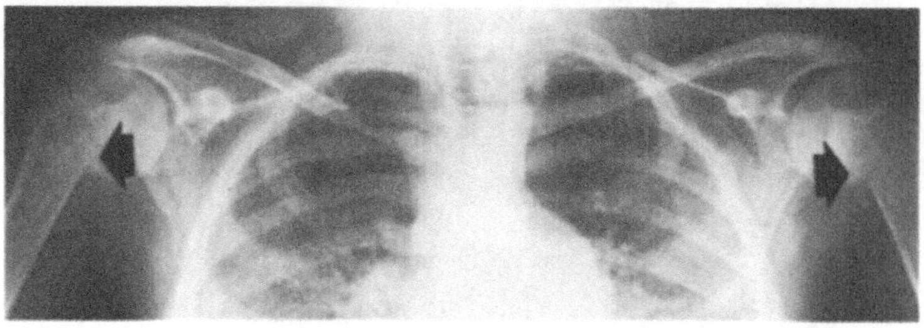

Fig. 11.35. Sixteen-year-old girl with thalassemia major who is confined to a wheelchair because of incipient congestive heart failure. Routine chest film demonstrated cardiomegaly and lung changes of pulmonary hemosiderosis and unsuspected asymptomatic bilateral humeral neck fractures. These presumably developed from the simple stress of propelling the wheelchair

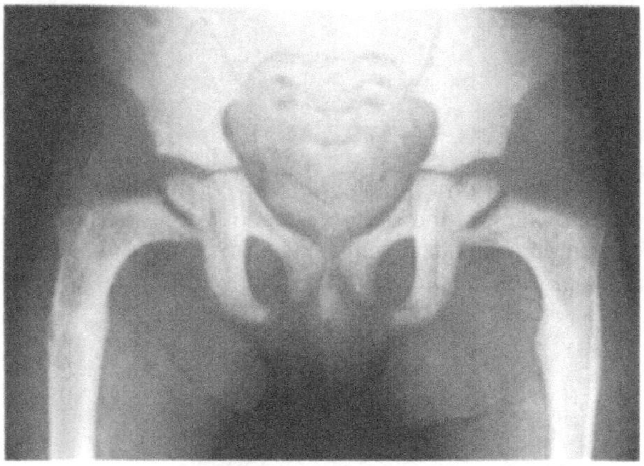

Fig. 11.36. Symmetrical stress fractures (*Looser* lines) in the proximal femurs in a girl with chronic renal osteodystrophy

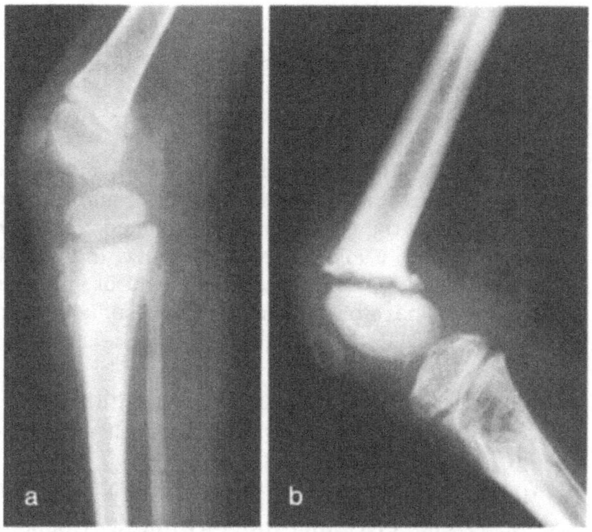

Fig. 11.37 a, b. Neurotrophic fractures in children are typically metaphyseal in location. This girl born with a meningomyelocele shows metaphyseal impaction of the left proximal tibia at 4 years of age (**a**). At 6 years of age, similar fractures developed in the distal left femur (**b**)

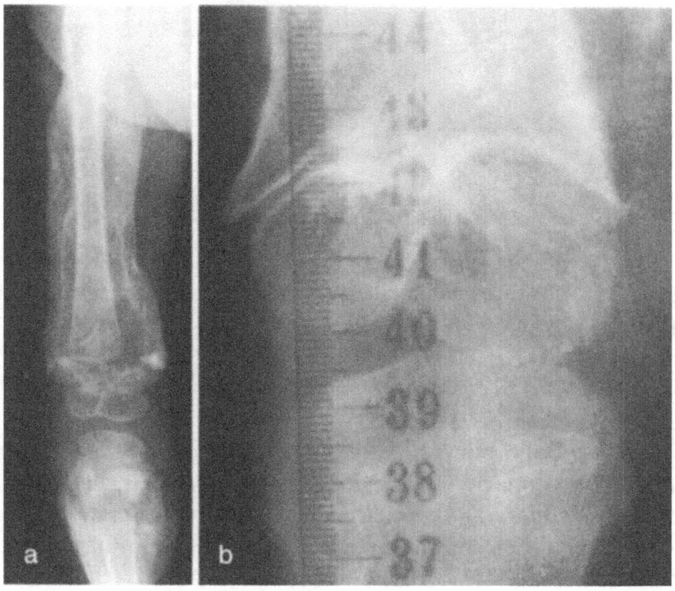

Fig. 11.38 a, b. Four-year-old boy with meningomyelocele shows extensive traumatic involucrum following neuropathic fractures of the distal femur and proximal tibia. **a** The distal femoral epiphysis has been displaced. **b** This resulted in localized central premature closure of the distal femoral epiphysis producing cupped metaphyseal deformity by 7 years of age

Children with neurosensory disturbances may develop extensive comminuted impacted fractures in the region of the metaphysis [14] (Fig. 11.37). By contrast, neurotrophic fractures in adults involve the epiphysis and joint space. Concomitant epiphyseal separation may occur and result in growth disturbance (Fig. 11.38).

Healing of a complete fracture in a child with motor and sensory deficits is usually prompt but remodeling may be markedly delayed owing to absence of the normal muscle tension which plays such an important role in remodeling according to Wolff's law. This neuropathic metaphyseal dysostosis is also exaggerated by the overtubulated appearance of the uninvolved shaft (Fig. 11.39). A bizarre pattern of fractures and soft tissue and bony deformities may be seen in children with congenital indifference to pain [38].

11.3.4 Stress Fractures

Stress fractures result from prolonged repetitive forces exceeding those usually tolerated by a normal bone. This force results from muscular activity on the bone rather than from direct impact. Stress fracture, fatigue fracture, and insufficiency fracture are terms that have been used synonymously and loosely. Daffner [11] divides stress fractures into a fatigue variety where the bone is normal but the force excessive, and an insufficiency type in which normal muscular stress is applied to a bone weakened by various causes. He would reserve the term pathologic fracture only to a bone weakened by a preexisting tumor.

Stress fractures in children occur most frequently in the upper tibia, lower fibula, and the metatarsal bones ("march fracture"). Less commonly, the rib cage, pelvis, and femur are involved. Radionuclide scan is quite sensitive and can detect the site of infraction before radiographic changes develop (Fig. 11.40). Slight periosteal reaction is often the earliest

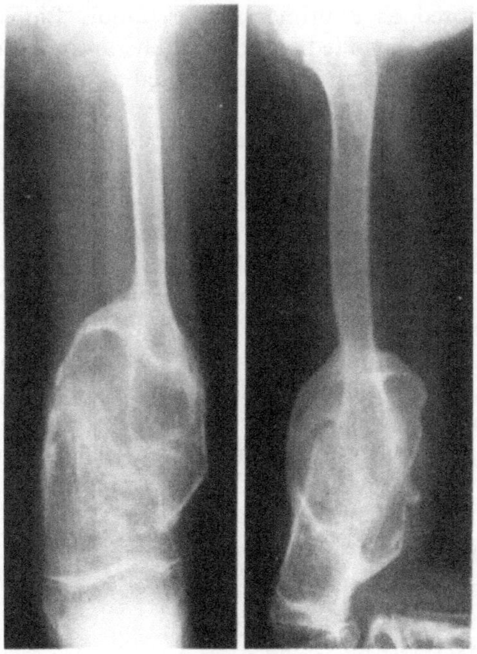

Fig. 11.39. Ten-year-old girl with transverse myelitis. There is rapid healing but frequently delayed remodeling of a fracture in children with neuromuscular abnormalities, resulting in a neuropathic metaphyseal dysostosis. Remodeling will occur eventually

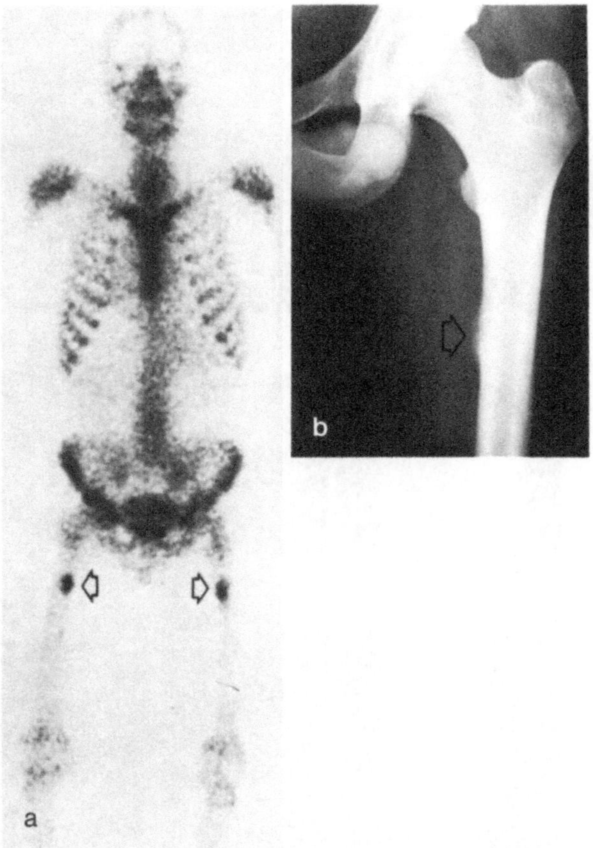

Fig. 11.40 a, b. This 19-year-old usually sedentary college student complained of bilateral medial thigh pains shortly after starting on job as parking lot attendant which required considerable running. Radionuclide skeletal scan demonstrates symmetrical foci of increased uptake in the proximal medial femurs (**a**). Radiograph of the left femur shows localized thickening in the proximal medial cortex indicating cortical stress fracture (**b**). Similar change was noted on the right side. (Courtesy of Sidney Grant, MD, Los Angeles)

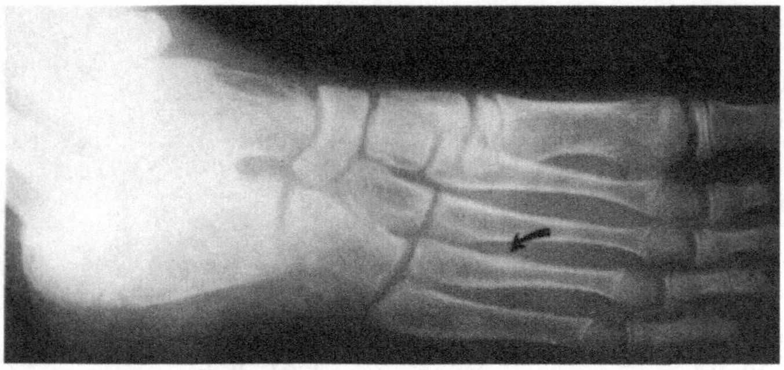

Fig. 11.41. *March* fracture of the fourth metatarsal bone in a 12-year-old boy

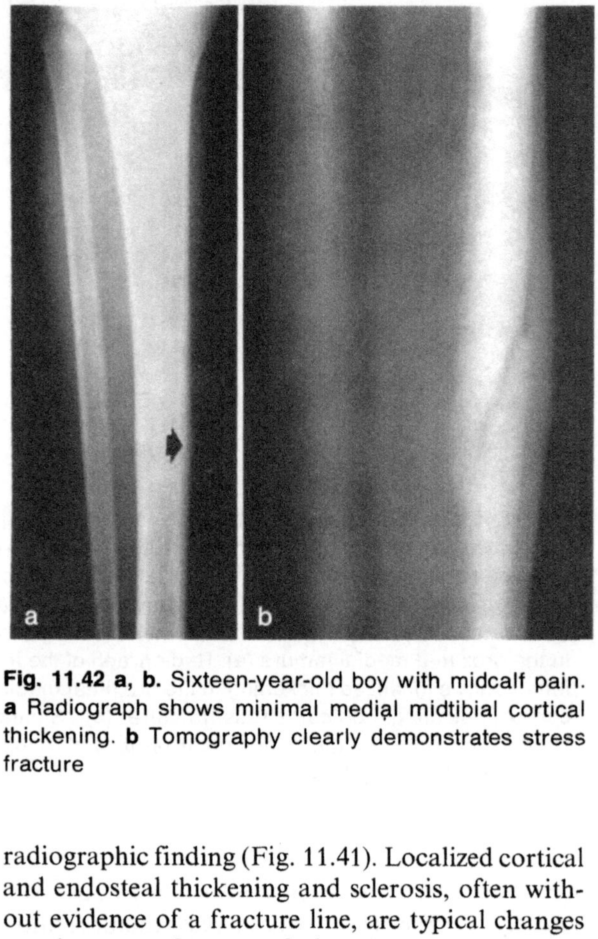

Fig. 11.42 a, b. Sixteen-year-old boy with midcalf pain. **a** Radiograph shows minimal medial midtibial cortical thickening. **b** Tomography clearly demonstrates stress fracture

radiographic finding (Fig. 11.41). Localized cortical and endosteal thickening and sclerosis, often without evidence of a fracture line, are typical changes seen in a stress fracture of a long bone. Tomography through this area may demonstrate the healing fracture line and help differentiate this from an osteoid osteoma or a focus of Garre's sclerosing osteomyelitis (Fig. 11.42).

11.3.5 Athletic Injuries

Athletic injuries, apart from direct blows, are often stress-type injuries. Excessive stress on the sites of muscle origin or insertion secondary to strong muscular contraction can cause avulsion fractures [41]. These most commonly occur among sprinters, hurdlers, jumpers, and football players, and usually affect the pelvic and hip regions. The following sites and their muscle attachments are most frequently involved: (1) the anterior-superior (sartorius) and the anterior-inferior (rectus femoris) iliac spines (Fig. 11.43); (2) the ischial tuberosity apophysis (hamstrings) (Fig. 11.44); and (3) the lesser trochanter apophysis (iliopsoas) (Fig. 11.45). Less commonly involved are the greater trochanter apophysis of the femur (gluteals) and the iliac crest apophysis. An avulsive-type injury causing irregularity and sclerosis of the inferior aspect of the symphysis pubis was recently reported by Schneider et al [33].

With healing, a large bony, sometimes partially cystic, mass may form, particularly if the avulsed fragment was widely displaced. This should not be misdiagnosed as a primary bone tumor. Biopsy should also be avoided since the exuberant reparative bone growth can be misdiagnosed as an osteogenic tumor.

Athletic stress injuries in the upper extremities are uncommon except for the "little leaguer elbow" where avulsion of the medial condylar apophysis occurs during a hard overhand pitch which causes a severe valgus strain at the elbow [4] (Fig. 11.46).

Regional cortical thickening frequently develops in response to a constant abnormal or unusual stress placed on the bone. This is best exemplified by medial cortical thickening of the femurs and tibias with bowed legs, and lateral cortical thickening with knock-knees. Diffuse anterior tibial cortical thickening commonly develops in ballet dancers [34] or from other activity where the anterior tibia is excessively stimulated (Fig. 11.47).

11.3.6 Battered Child Syndrome

The most tragic circumstance for occurrence of skeletal injury results from willfully inflicted trauma to the infant or young child by parents, parent substitutes, or siblings. Unfortunately, these are not

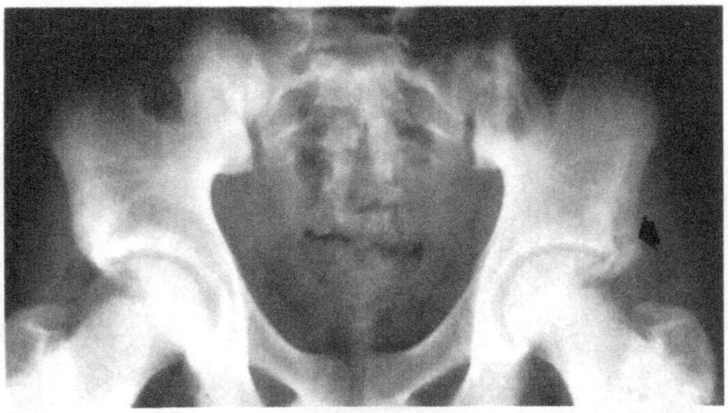

Fig. 11.43. Fourteen-year-old boy with deformity of avulsed anterior inferior iliac spine secondary to abnormal pull of rectus femoris muscle

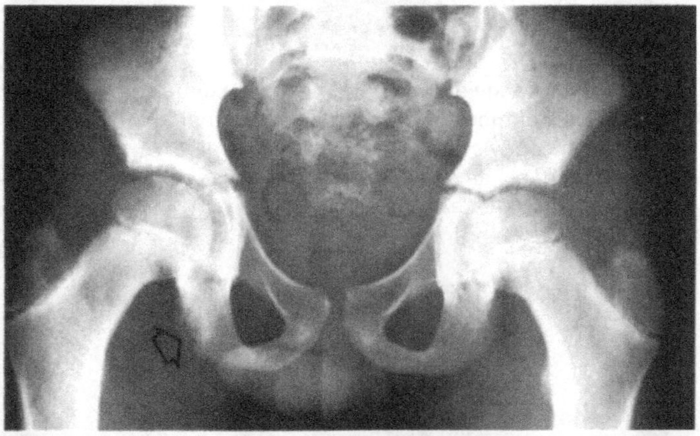

Fig. 11.44. Fifteen-year-old boy who is a hurdler on a track team. Irregularity of right ischium from cortical avulsion by the hamstring muscles may mimic a bone tumor

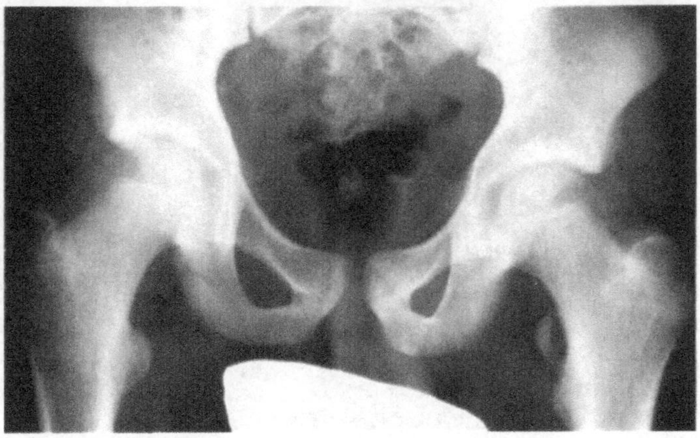

Fig. 11.45. Fifteen-year-old sprinter developed sudden left groin pain while running. Avulsion of left lesser trochanter apophysis at insertion of the iliopsoas muscle is clearly seen

infrequent isolated events. Child battering now appears to be a major pediatric health problem leading to death in 2%–3% of the victims and to severe physical and psychological crippling and brain damage in many others. To place the problem in proper perspective, the mortality rate from battered child syndrome is similar to that of leukemia. Rang [27] suggests that 25% of fractures in children under 3 years of age result from battering. Since child beating tends to be repeated, it is important for the physician to recognize it early to prevent recurrence and, possibly, more serious future injuries.

Infants under 3 years of age are most commonly afflicted. Suspicion of possible battering should be raised whenever injury to a child cannot be adequately explained, or the type and extent of injury are not consistent with the given story. Repeated episodes of injury should also raise suspicion. The physician has a moral and legal obligation to report his suspicion of child abuse to the proper authorities.

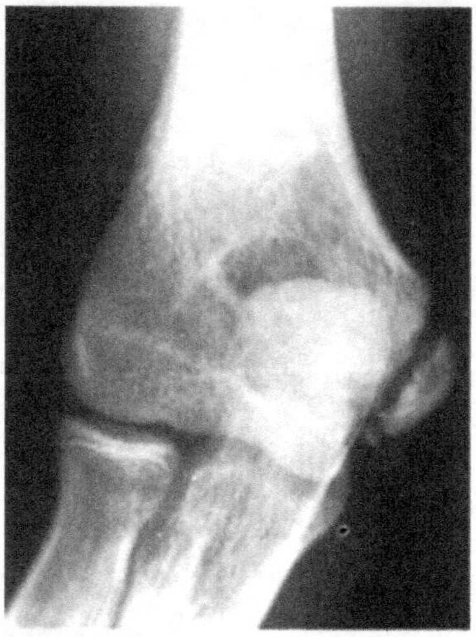

Fig. 11.46. Fifteen-year-old boy developed sudden pain in medial part of elbow while throwing a football. Avulsed medial epicondyle from valgus strain of elbow occurs more commonly among pitchers during baseball season and is called *little leaguer* elbow

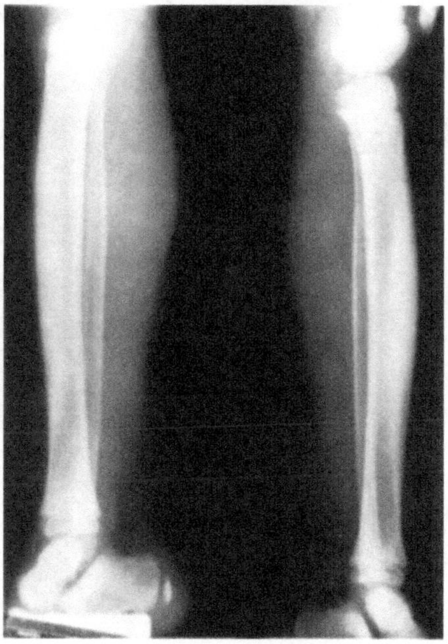

Fig. 11.47. Chronic repetitive subclinical trauma can incite bone reaction. This long-suffering 7-year-old girl was charged with the care of a younger brother who kicks her in the shins almost constantly. There is marked anterior tibial cortical thickening bilaterally which can mimic saber shin deformity of syphilis. Similar changes have been described with ballet dancers

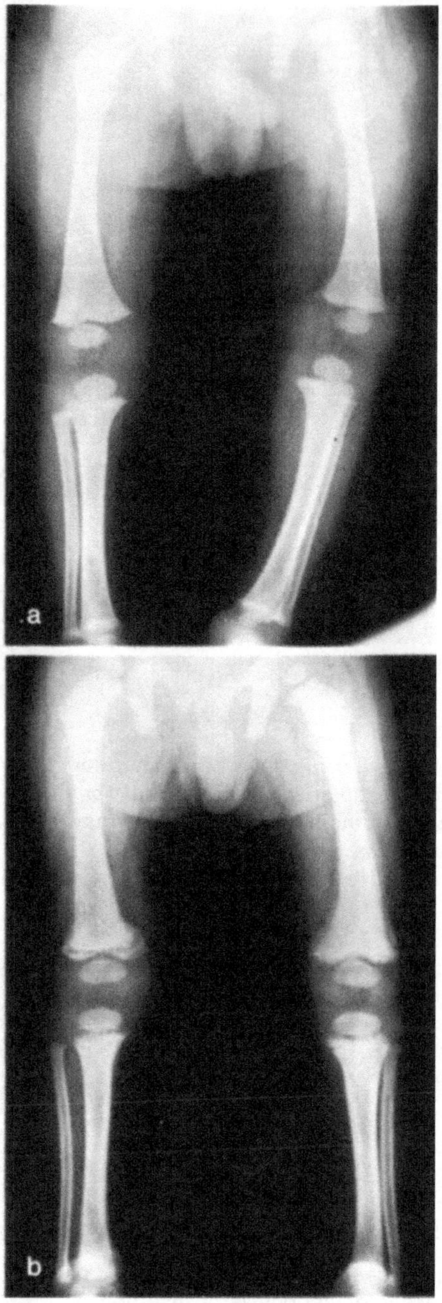

Fig. 11.48 a, b. Frontal view of the lower limbs in a child with multiple bruises shows metaphyseal avulsion off the medial distal left femur (**a**). A follow-up film 6 weeks later (**b**) now shows healing of multiple metaphyseal fractures with typical *bucket handle* tears through distal right femoral and tibial metaphyses. These changes are nearly pathognomonic of inflicted trauma

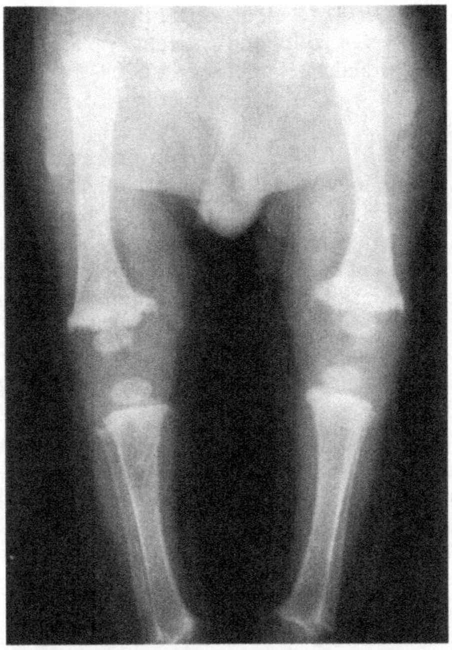

Fig. 11.49. Frontal view of lower limbs in a 4-month-old boy with Menke's kinky hair syndrome shows typical metaphyseal spurs and fragmentation and diaphyseal periosteal reaction. These changes may be confused with the battered child syndrome, but the clinical presentation should permit differentiation

Typically, long bone injuries in infants and young children resulting from battering are from traction forces rather than compression or direct blows [5]. The victim is usually seized by the limbs and the extremities are twisted. This results in avulsion fractures of the metaphyses and often epiphyseal separations. The periosteum is normally loosely attached to the shaft except in the region of the metaphysis and this accounts for the peripheral metaphyseal avulsions and the frequently extensive subperiosteal hemorrhage and bone reaction (traumatic involucrum) along the diaphyses (Fig. 11.48). These widespread metaphyseal and periosteal bone changes may superficially be mimicked by bone changes in Menke's kinky hair syndrome [1, 12, 39] (Fig. 11.49), and other metabolic and inflammatory processes [15]. Spiral fractures of the long bones may also result from twisting of the limbs. Rib fractures result from either direct blows to the chest or from squeezing of the infant's chest. Skull fractures are frequently extensive, but widened cranial sutures resulting from subdural hematomas may be seen without evidence of fractures. The intracranial bleed is thought to occur from tears of vessels crossing the subdural space caused by the violent whip-lashing of the head when the victim is seized and severely shaken by the parent in a fit of rage [6].

If there is any suspicion as to the cause of a skeletal injury, a complete skeletal survey should be obtained to rule out other areas of involvement. Close attention should be paid to the location, number, and age of all the fractures present. In a child with numerous fractures of varying ages, the assumption of inflicted trauma must be accepted until proven otherwise [36].

11.4 Conclusion

The innate differences between the infantile and growing skeleton and a mature skeleton account for the numerous differences in the types of skeletal injuries and the ways in which the bones respond to these injuries. Discussion of many of the more important differences and the potential problems in diagnosis and treatment have been deliberately emphasized in this presentation. A comfortable knowledge of the normal pediatric skeleton is vital to avoid the serious pitfalls of overdiagnosis [37] and of missing potentially serious epiphyseal injuries.

References

1. Adams PC, Strand RE, Bresnan MJ, Lucky AW (1974) Kinky hair syndrome: serial study of radiological findings with emphasis on the similarity to the battered child syndrome. Radiology 112:401–407
2. Bledsoe RE, Izenstark JL (1959) Displacement of fat pads in disease and injury at the elbow. Radiology 73:717–724
3. Borden S IV (1975) Roentgen recognition of acute plastic bowing of the forearm in children. AJR 125:524–530
4. Brogdon BG, Crow NE (1960) "Little leaguers'" elbow. AJR 83:671–675
5. Caffey J (1972) The parent-infant traumatic stress syndrome. AJR 114:217–229
6. Caffey J (1972) On the theory and practice of shaking infants. Its potential residual effects on permanent brain damage and mental retardation. Am J Dis Child 124:161–169
7. Caffey J (1978) Pediatric X-ray diagnosis Year Book Medical Publishers, Chicago
8. Cails WS, Keats TE, Sussman MD (1978) Plastic bowing fracture of the femur in a child. AJR 130:780–782
9. Colley DP, Dunsker SB (1978) Traumatic narrowing of the dorsolumbar spinal canal demonstrated by computed tomography. Radiology 129:95–98

10. Crow JE, Swischuk LE (1977) Acute bowing fractures of the forearm in children: a frequently missed injury. AJR 128:981–984
11. Daffner RH (1978) Stress fractures: current concepts. Skeletal Radiol 2:221–229
12. Danks DM, Campbell PE, Stevens BJ, Mayne V, Cartwright E (1972) Menkes' kinky hair syndrome: an inherited defect in copper absorption with widespread effect. Pediatrics 50:118–201
13. Fordham EW, Ramchandran PC (1974) Radionuclide imaging of osseous trauma. Semin Nucl Med 4:411–429
14. Gyepes MT, Newbern DH, Neuhauser EBD (1965) Metaphyseal and physeal injuries in children with spina bifida and meningomyelocoeles. AJR 95:168–177
15. Haller JO, Kassner EG (1977) The „battered child" syndrome and its imitators. A critical evaluation of specific radiological signs. Applied Radiology 6:88–92, 111
16. Hawkins RW, Lyne ED (1978) Skeletal trauma in skateboard injuries. Am J Dis Child 132:751–752
17. Jacobs RA, Keller EL (1977) Skateboard accidents. Pediatrics 59:939–942
18. Keats TE, Smith TH (1977) An atlas of normal developmental roentgen anatomy. Year Book Medical Publishers, Chicago
19. Kershner MS, Goodman GA, Perlmutter GS (1977) Computed tomography in the diagnosis of an atlas fracture. AJR 128:688–689
20. Kohler A (1968) The borderlands of the normal and the early pathologic in skeletal radiology. Grune & Stratton, New York
21. Lee FA, Gwinn JL (1974) Retrosternal dislocation of the clavicle. Radiology 110:631–634
22. Lee FA, Isaacs H Jr, Strauss J (1972) The campomelic syndrome. Am J Dis Child 124:485–496
23. MacEwan DW (1964) Changes due to trauma in the fat plane overlying the pronator quadratus muscle: a radiologic sign. Radiology 82:866–879
24. McCauley RGK, Schwartz AM, Leonidas JL, Darling DB (1979) An efficacy study for the value of comparison views in extremity injuries in children. AJR 132:307
25. Reed MH (1979) Coracoclavicular fracture separation – the pediatric equivalent of acromioclavicular separation. AJR 132:307
26. Merten DF (1978) Comparison radiographs in extremity injuries of childhood: current application in radiological practice. Radiology 126:209–210
27. Rang M (1974) Children's fractures. Lippincott Philadelphia
28. Rogers LF (1970) The radiography of epiphyseal injuries. Radiology 96:289–299
29. Rogers LF, Malave S, White H, Tachdjian MO (1978) Plastic bowing, torus and greenstick supracondylar fractures of the humerus: radiographic clues to obscure fractures of the elbow in children. Radiology 128:145–150
30. Rogers LF, Rockwood CA Jr (1973) Separation of the entire distal humeral epiphysis. Radiology 106:393–399
31. Salter RB (1970) Injuries of the musculoskeletal system. Williams & Wilkins, Baltimore
32. Salter RB, Harris WR (1963) Injuries involving the epiphyseal plate. J Bone Joint Surg [Am] 45a:587–622
33. Schneider R, Kaye JJ, Ghelman B (1976) Adductor avulsive injuries near the symphysis pubis. Radiology 120:567–569
34. Schneider HJ, King AY, Bronson JL, Miller EH (1974) Stress injuries and developmental changes of lower extremities in ballet dancers. Radiology 113:627–632
35. Siffert RS (1977) The effect of trauma to the epiphysis and growth plate. Skeletal Radiol 2:21–30
36. Silverman FN (1953) Roentgen manifestations of unrecognized skeletal trauma in infants. AJR 69:413–427
37. Silverman FN (1978) Problems in pediatric fractures. Semin Roentgenol 13:167–176
38. Silverman FN, Gilder JJ (1959) Congenital insensitivity to pain: a neurologic syndrome with bizzare skeletal lesions. Radiology 72:176–190
39. Stanley P, Gwinn JL, Sutcliffe J (1976) The osseous abnormalities in Menkes' syndrome. Ann Radiol 19:167–172
40. Wilcox JR Jr, Moniot AL, Green JP (1977) Bone scanning in the evaluation of exercise-related stress injuries. Radiology 123:699–703
41. Wilkinson RH, Kirkpatrick JA (1976) Pediatric skeletal trauma. Curr Probl Diagn Radiol 6:3–38
42. Yousefzadeh DK, Jackson JH Jr (1978) Lipohemarthrosis of the elbow joint. Radiology 128:643–645

Subject Index

GPSR Compliance

The European Union's (EU) General Product Safety Regulation (GPSR) is a set of rules that requires consumer products to be safe and our obligations to ensure this.

If you have any concerns about our products, you can contact us on ProductSafety@springernature.com

In case Publisher is established outside the EU, the EU authorized representative is:

Springer Nature Customer Service Center GmbH
Europaplatz 3
69115 Heidelberg, Germany

Batch number: 10615099

Printed by Printforce, the Netherlands